Treatment of Functional Somatic Symptoms

Treatment of Functional Somatic Symptoms

Edited by

Richard Mayou

*University Department
of Psychiatry
Warneford Hospital,
Oxford*

Christopher Bass

*John Radcliffe Hospital
Oxford*

and

Michael Sharpe

*University Department
of Psychiatry
Warneford Hospital
Oxford*

OXFORD · NEW YORK · TOKYO
OXFORD UNIVERSITY PRESS
1995

Oxford University Press, Walton Street, Oxford OX2 6DP

Oxford   New York
Athens   Auckland   Bangkok   Bombay
Calcutta   Cape Town   Dar es Salaam   Delhi
Florence   Hong Kong   Istanbul   Karachi
Kuala Lumpur   Madras   Madrid   Melbourne
Mexico City   Nairobi   Paris   Singapore
Taipei   Tokyo   Toronto
and associated companies in
Berlin Ibadan

Oxford is a trade mark of Oxford University Press

Published in the United States
by Oxford University Press Inc., New York

A catalogue record for this book is available from the British Library

Library of Congress Cataloging in Publication Data
Treatment of functional somatic symptoms / edited by Richard Mayou,
Christopher Bass, and Michael Sharpe.
1. Somatoform disorders.   I. Mayou, Richard.   II. Bass,
Christopher M. (Christopher Maurice)   III. Sharpe, Michael.
[DNLM: 1. Somatoform Disorders — therapy — congresses. WM 170
T7845 1995]
RC552.S66T74   1995   616',047—dc20   95–873
ISBN 0 19 262499 7

Typeset by Colset Private Limited, Singapore

Printed and Bound by Antony Rowe Ltd., Chippenham, Wiltshire

Preface

This book is based on papers presented to a conference held at Green College, Oxford, in November 1992. This conference was principally concerned with the treatment of patients with functional somatic symptoms, and the development of practical guidelines for both specialist and primary care. Contributors were also asked to review epidemiology and aetiology as a basis of understanding management and the provision of services.

Participants subsequently revised their contributions in the light of discussion. We have further edited the papers to ensure a comprehensive account of the subject and to avoid inconsistencies and overlap. We have written additional chapters to summarize general issues. In this way, we hope to have achieved a book which provides a comprehensive account of the treatment of functional symptoms in general, together with specific information about particular types of treatment.

We are grateful to Dista Pharmaceuticals for generous support of the workshop, to all participants, and to Karine Guest for her considerable help in preparation of the final typescript.

1995   R.M.
C.B.
M.S.

Introduction

Psychiatrists and psychologists have used many terms for symptoms which, in this book, are referred to as functional somatic symptoms. These include hypochondriasis, somatization, and a variety of categories in standard classifications. Such symptoms do not appear to have simple organic explanations. They are very widespread in the general population, and frequently result in consultation with doctors. The extent of this consultation, the limited effectiveness of negative investigations in providing reassurance, and the long-term economic costs are becoming increasingly apparent to both purchasers and providers of healthcare. Even so, the separate clinical and research consideration of individual symptoms and syndromes (such as chronic pain, multiple pains) continues to obscure both the size of the overall problem and the development of general treatment strategies.

There are continuing controversies about the relative contribution of physical, psychological, and social causes and about the role of specialist investigations. Management is frequently difficult, and it is for this reason that this book is principally concerned with treatment.

The book aims to take a comprehensive view of functional symptoms. Contributors show that single and multiple symptoms are prevalent in the general population and in all medical settings. Whilst often transient, a substantial minority persist and are associated with distress, limitations of everyday life, worries about serious physical causes, and considerable use of medical resources.

Aetiology is usually multicausal with an interaction between physical, psychological, and social factors. This approach to causation emphasizes the importance of patients' beliefs, that is to say their attributions or cognitive interpretations. There is also a strong association with psychiatric illness, especially anxiety and depression, but not all patients with chronic disabling symptoms can be given a psychiatric diagnosis. This is partly because of the inadequacies of traditional classifications, but also because the causation of the problem may lie as much in the behaviour of others, especially of doctors and other therapists, as in the patients' own responses.

Our view of aetiology leads to conclusions about management. The authors emphasize the significance of general measures, such as providing appropriate explanations, limiting investigations and offering adequate discussion rather than didactic advice. It also leads to specific drug treatments and psychological interventions. Frequently, treatment involves a variety of elements and it is important that these are closely coordinated.

The scope for improvements in general and specialist care are considered in the concluding chapters which are concerned with delivery of services.

Contents

Contributors

Christopher Bass
Director of the Department of Psychological Medicine, John Radcliffe Hospital, Oxford OX3 9DU, UK

Fiona Blake
Consultant in Liaison Psychiatry (Obstetrics and Gynaecology), Department of Psychological Medicine, John Radcliffe Hospital, Oxford OX3 9DU, UK

Sidney Benjamin
Senior Lecturer in Psychiatry, Manchester Royal Infirmary, Rawnsley Building, Manchester Royal Infirmary, Oxford Road, Manchester M13 9WL, UK

Francis Creed
Professor of Community Psychiatry, Rawnsley Building, Manchester Royal Infirmary, Oxford Road, Manchester M13 9WL, UK

M. Elena Garralda
Professor of Child and Adolescent Psychiatry, St Mary's Hospital Medical School, Horace Joules Building, Central Middlesex Hospital, Acton Lane, Park Royal, London NW10 7NS, UK

Linda Gask
Senior Lecturer in Psychiatry, Avondale Unit, Royal Preston Hospital, PO Box 66, Sharoe Green Lane, Preston PR2 4HT, UK

Dennis Gath
Clinical Reader in Psychiatry, University Department of Psychiatry, Warneford Hospital, Oxford OX3 7JX, UK

Lesley Glover
Clinical Psychologist, Department of Psychology, University College, London WC1E 6AU, UK

Tim E.E. Goodacre
Honorary Clinical Lecturer, University of Oxford, Consultant Plastic Surgeon, Department of Plastic and Reconstructive Surgery, John Radcliffe Hospital, Oxford OX3 9DU, UK

Elspeth Guthrie
Senior Lecturer in Liaison Psychiatry, Rawnsley Building, Manchester Royal Infirmary, Oxford Road, Manchester M13 9WL, UK

Allan House
Consultant and Senior Lecturer in Liaison Psychiatry, Leeds General Infirmary, Great George Street, Leeds LS1 3EX, UK

Wayne Katon
Professor of Psychiatry, Director of the Consultation–Liaison Service, University of Washington, School of Medicine, Department of Psychiatry and Behavioral Sciences, RP-10, 1959 Pacific Street, Seattle, Washington 98195, USA

Chris J. Main
Department of Behavioural Medical Clinical Sciences Building, Hope Hospital, Eccles Old Road, Salford M6 8HD, UK

Richard Mayou
Clinical Reader in Psychiatry, University Department of Psychiatry, Warneford Hospital, Oxford OX3 7JX, UK

Charles Morris
Consultant in Psychiatry of the Elderly, St Andrew's Hospital, Norwich NR7 0SS, UK

Jane Pearce
Consultant in Psychiatry of Old Age, Littlemore Hospital, Littlemore, Oxford OX4 4YN, UK

Shirley Pearce
Professor and Director of Health Policy and Practice Unit, University of East Anglia, Norwich NR4 7TJ, UK

Roy Porter
Professor of the Social History of Medicine, Wellcome Institute for the History of Medicine, 183 Euston Road, London NW1 2BN, UK

Paul Salkovskis
Wellcome Senior Research Fellow, University Department of Psychiatry, Warneford Hospital, Oxford OX3 7JX, UK

Michael Sharpe
Clinical Tutor, University Department of Psychiatry, Warneford Hospital, Oxford OX3 7JX, UK

G. Richard Smith Jr.
Professor of Psychiatry/Vice Chairman, University of Arkansas of Medical Sciences, Department of Psychiatry—Slot 554, 4301 W. Markham Street, Little Rock, Arkansas 72205, USA

Mark Sullivan
Assistant Professor of Psychiatry, University of Washington, Department

of Psychiatry and Behavioral Sciences, RP-10, 1959 Pacific Street, Seattle, Washington 98185, USA

Hilary M.C. Warwick
Senior Lecturer in Behavioural Psychotherapy, Department of Mental Health Service, Jenner Wing, St George's Hospital Medical School, Cranmer Terrace, London SW17 0RE, UK

Simon Wessely
Reader in Liaison Psychiatry, King's College School of Medicine at Psychiatry at the Institute of Psychiatry, Denmark Hill, London SE5 9RS, UK

PART 1 INTRODUCTION

1 Concepts, theories, and terminology

*Michael Sharpe, Richard Mayou,
and Christopher Bass*

In this chapter we review the conceptual issues encountered in a discussion of functional symptoms and briefly review the main theoretical standpoints from which functional somatic symptoms have been viewed. We conclude that there is a need for a comprehensive perspective which goes beyond any particular specialist standpoint and which recognizes the common factors underlying the various theoretical approaches.

Unresolved conceptual issues and conflicting theoretical viewpoints have led to a confusion in terminology. We argue that 'functional somatic symptoms' is currently the least unsatisfactory of the terms available and employ it in the chapters that follow.

Introduction

A person who feels ill and cannot perform their daily tasks is clearly not well. Yet in many such cases the doctor cannot find evidence of organic disease. Such patients constitute a large proportion of those seen in both primary and hospital care (Kroenke and Mangelsdorff 1989). If a person's symptoms are predominantly psychological they may be diagnosed as having a psychiatric illness, but when they are somatic the diagnosis and management is often perceived as problematic by the doctor and unsatisfactory by the patient. This book is devoted to examining better ways of managing these patients.

The literature concerning functional somatic symptoms has been dogged both by unresolved conceptual issues and by lack of agreement about the terminology that should be employed. With the aim of preparing the reader for the chapters that follow, we begin this volume with a review of relevant concepts, followed by a brief discussion of each of the main theoretical approaches. Finally we consider terminology and conclude with the conventions that will be employed in this book.

Basic concepts

Are patients with functional symptoms *really unwell*? Are the symptoms *all in their minds*? Do they *deserve* medical treatment? These issues almost always emerge from a discussion of the treatment of a patient with functional somatic symptoms. Although often expressed in dismissive terms, such statements do reflect important underlying conceptual issues which we will examine further.

Are people with functional symptoms really unwell?

We might seek to define 'unwellness' as the absence of health. Unfortunately there is no generally accepted single definition of health, nor of its absence. It is necessary, therefore, to examine the concept of unwellness from several different viewpoints. These may be broadly divided into the biological, the psychological, and the social, perspectives which correspond approximately to the concepts of disease, illness, and sickness, respectively (Susser 1990). The fact that each of these different aspects or dimensions of unwellness can exist independently of the others often causes serious confusion.

Disease is defined in terms of objective biological abnormalities in the structure and/or function of bodily organs and systems. This apparently objective and scientific biological definition seems at first sight to solve the problem. If we could only define who has disease and who has not, we could determine who was 'really ill'. Doctors often try to avoid the more complex issues associated with illness and sickness by using the presence or absence of conventionally defined disease as an arbiter. This manoeuvre simplifies the question, but also gives rise to a number of important problems.

One problem is that patients present to doctors not with disease, but with illness. *Illness* is the personal subjective perception of unwellness and can be broadly defined as the 'experience of discontinuities in states of being and perceived role performance' (Eisenberg 1977). Therefore, if a person feels ill, they are ill. This subjective experience cannot be abolished by the failure to find objective disease. The individual psychological nature of the illness experience is shaped by the person's previous experience and beliefs, as well as by biological processes.

Another problem is that a person's ability to work, to meet other obligations, and to seek medical help is also influenced by factors other than disease. The socially defined state of unwellness is called the person's sickness. *Sickness* is derived from the concept of the 'sick role' (Parsons 1951), a role that carries certain privileges (for example, to stay away from work), as well as obligations (for example, to seek appropriate medical care and to be seen to be trying to 'get well'). The interpersonal nature of the sick role means that it is shaped by the nature of the person's relationships, by social gains and losses, and by fashion, as well as by disease and by illness.

In conclusion, there is no single measure of health or of its absence. If we are to fully understand what determines 'unwellness', we must consider illness and sickness, as well as disease. These terms are not interchangeable and a person can have one without the other. Thus, one can have a definite disease, such as cancer, yet not feel ill. Conversely one can feel ill, but not have disease. (Most people who adopt the sick role also feel ill whether or not they have a disease. A minority seek the sick role without having either disease or illness and are regarded as having *factitious* symptoms or as *malingering*).

A further complication arises from the arbitrary and changing boundaries of each of these concepts. The illnesses regarded as legitimate tickets to the sick role (and to state benefits) vary with current social norms, fashions, and policies (see Chapter 2 on history and Chapter 16 on chronic fatigue syndrome). Recent examples of such changing fashions include the rise and fall of 'repetitive strain injury' (RSI) in Australia (Brooks 1993; Ferguson 1987) and the controversies surrounding the status of myalgic encephalitis (ME) in the UK (Richmond 1989).

Both these examples also illustrate how social factors can actually influence a person's perception of his or her bodily state. Illness too is subject to fashion (Wessely 1990). What is perhaps less obvious is that even the definition of disease is less objective than it may first appear. Although the diagnosis of disease requires the objective identification of biological disturbance, it is conventionally defined in terms of only a subset of the possible range of measurable bodily changes. For example, although a patient with chest pain and normal coronary arteries may be regarded as having an illness but no disease, they may in fact have abnormal respiration and markedly abnormal blood gas measurements (Sharpe and Bass 1992).

Are functional symptoms 'all in the mind'?

The patient who suffers from an illness for which the doctor can find no demonstrable organic disease is often told that the illness is 'all in his or her mind' (Ware 1992). Thus, if medical investigations are negative, the problem is not 'physical' and if not physical, it is 'mental'. This conclusion is often resented by patients, who see it as implying that their illness is at best psychiatric and at worst imaginary.

This view is, however, flawed by a naïve conceptual separation of mind and body. Because a person's symptoms are not associated with conventionally defined *disease*, they are assumed not to have any biological basis at all and, hence, to reside in the mind. As we have argued above, further physiological assessment may reveal bodily disturbance and even if no bodily disturbance can be identified there are likely to be associated changes in brain function (Eisenberg 1986). We argue that is rarely either accurate or productive to regard a patient's complaints as 'entirely mental' or as 'entirely physical'. Rather it is better to consider biological, psychological, and, indeed, social aspects in every case.

Do patients with functional symptoms deserve medical treatment?

In our experience referrals of patients with functional symptoms often contain an apology. Why is this? Are these patients considered to be a waste of the doctor's time, are they merely 'worried well', or, to paraphrase George Bernard Shaw, the 'undeserving sick'? This view is often associated with the referring doctor's belief, often justified, that the patient would be better managed by a psychiatrist. However, patients with functional somatic symptoms rarely request, and commonly resist a psychiatric diagnosis and psychiatric referral. This is, in part, because the label of psychiatric illness carries a moral connotation. Persons with psychiatric illness, particularly neurotic conditions, are commonly considered to be weak, flawed, and in some way to *blame* for their illness (Goldberg and Bridges 1988). Some doctors may even feel that these patients do not deserve medical treatment and merely take up resources that could be better used on the 'really ill'. There is thus a stark contrast between medical and social attitudes to the person with psychiatric illness, and the person with cancer. In short, the eliciting of both sympathetic medical care and exemption from responsibility is difficult for those in whom organic disease has not been diagnosed. These issues of responsibility for illness are of great importance in the aetiology and management of patients with functional somatic symptoms and will be discussed in other chapters (see Chapter 16 on chronic fatigue syndrome and Chapter 11 on pain).

As we can now see, conflicting definitions of ill health, a persistent aetiological dualism, and pervasive moral attitudes have combined to obscure our understanding and management of the patient with functional somatic symptoms. They are also reflected in the terms used to describe the patients who suffer them.

Theoretical approaches to functional somatic symptoms

Given the conceptual problems described above, it is perhaps not surprising that the extensive literature concerning functional somatic symptoms frequently offers the reader more confusion than clarification. It may be helpful, therefore, to distinguish five distinct (though overlapping) theoretical approaches (Table 1.1). In doing so we take our lead from the comprehensive reviews written by Barsky and Klerman (1983) and by Kellner (1990, 1994).

Table 1.1 Theoretical approaches

---

1. Psychiatric disorder
2. Psychodynamic perspective
   a. Intra-psychic and unconscious emotion
   b. Alexithymia

3. Perceptual and cognitive abnormality
   a. Amplification of normal bodily sensation
   b. Misinterpretation of normal bodily sensation

4. Patho-physiological process

5. Learned social behaviour

Psychiatric disorder

From the standpoint of psychiatric classification, patients with functional somatic symptoms are allocated to categorical diagnoses, each of which is presumed to have a particular aetiology. This approach is used by both the main psychiatric classification systems, DSM-IV and ICD-10 (see Chapter 3). In these classifications patients with functional somatic symptoms may be either categorized as having depressive and anxiety disorders or be placed in diagnostic categories from within the grouping of 'somatoform disorders' (see Chapter 3 for a further discussion of classification). One important advantage of this approach is that patients with functional somatic symptoms are included in a classification. Furthermore, operationally defined categories of 'psychiatric disorder' permit systematic research studies and lead naturally to the use of psychiatric treatment. The disadvantages of the psychiatric approach stem from the questionable implication that all such persons are psychiatrically ill and also from the collapsing of the various aspects of functional somatic symptoms into a categorical psychiatric diagnosis (for example, 'it's really all depression'). This diagnostic simplification risks preventing the consideration of more specific aetiological factors (see also Chapter 3).

The psychodynamic perspective

The term *psychodynamic* refers to the conflict between different psychic processes, both conscious and unconscious. From the psychodynamic standpoint functional somatic symptoms are produced by the unconscious mind to serve a function. The function might be to allow the expression of needs that would be otherwise unacceptable (for example, the expression of dependency needs) or alternatively to defend the person against a threat to his/her psychic equilibrium (for example, protecting self-esteem by avoiding blame for perceived failure). This function has been called *primary gain*. The symptoms may also facilitate a desired change in the patient's external world, for example the avoidance of responsibility at work or even financial advantage. This latter process had been called *secondary gain*.

Furthermore, the actual symptoms reported or exhibited may also have symbolic or representational significance. An example is the 'sexual movements' of pseudo-seizures (Betts and Boden 1992) in persons who were sexually abused as children.

The concept of *Alexithymia* is derived from the psychodynamic approach. This term was introduced to describe patients who have difficulty describing their emotions in words and who focus on the details of external events, at the expense of articulating emotional distress. It is argued that this deficit leads to the expression of psychological distress largely in the form of somatic symptoms (Taylor 1984).

The psychodynamic approach is described more fully in Chapter 8. Its advantages lie in its richness, it's focus on the meaning of the symptoms, and it's linking of childhood and other past experiences with current relationships. It has also led to specific treatments, which although widely practised have undergone little systematic evaluation (but see Chapter 8 for exceptions).

The disadvantages of this approach are that it has the potential to over-complicate the clinical problem and that there are difficulties inherent in conducting research into unconscious processes.

Perceptual and cognitive abnormality

The cognitive behavioural approach conceives of functional symptoms as being the result of interaction between cognition, perception, mood, behaviour, and physiology. The person's beliefs and thoughts (cognitions) are given a particularly prominent role. Symptoms are viewed as selective or *amplified* perceptions of non-pathological bodily changes (Mayou 1976; Barsky 1992) which occur as physiological concomitants of anxiety, depression, and other processes. These symptoms are misinterpreted as evidence of serious disease, which leads in turn to further anxiety and depression, as well as to unhelpful behaviours such as the avoidance of activities that aggravate the symptoms.

The advantage of this perspective is that it identifies explicit processes that can be measured. An example is Barsky's (1992) 'amplifying style'. It also offers a rational approach to treatment. Cognitive behavioural therapy (CBT) has enjoyed considerable success (see Chapter 7) and has been shown to be effective in controlled trials.

The disadvantage of the cognitive behavioural perspective is its tendency to over-simplify often complex clinical problems and to neglect interpersonal and symbolic aspects of functional somatic symptoms.

Pathophysiological approach

Many writers have focused on the role of physiological processes in the aetiology of functional somatic symptoms. These physiological processes commonly involve activity in the autonomic nervous system and skeletal muscle tension (Sharpe and Bass 1992). Examples include increased motility and contractions in the gut of patients with the irritable bowel syndrome (see Chapter 14) and hyperventilation in patients reporting non-cardiac chest pain (see Chapter 18). This approach is useful in complementing other more psychological perspectives and also in encouraging greater exploration of the biology of functional somatic symptoms. It can also lead to rational approaches to treatments, such as biofeedback (Jessup *et al.* 1979).

Taken alone, however, the physiological approach is clearly too narrow to explain the many clinical facets presented by patients with functional somatic symptoms, or to lead to a comprehensive approach to their management.

Learned social behaviour

The social approach focuses on the interpersonal aspects of functional somatic symptoms. Thus, a patient's 'illness behaviour' (Mechanic 1972) is learned from others or from previous experience of disease. The behaviour functions as a social communication by which a person attempts to gain legitimacy for the 'sick role' (Parsons 1951). Validation of the sick role usually requires that it is legitimized by a doctor.

The advantage of the social approach is that it readily encompasses factors that are often clinically apparent, but which are not easily incorporated by other models. It also serves to remind us of the wider social and cultural issues that influence the nature and occurrence of functional somatic symptoms (see Chapter 16 for further discussion of this point). This perspective may also suggest therapeutic approaches including group therapy and the use of in-patient rehabilitation units where interpersonal factors can be manipulated. It also has implications for our understanding of the importance of factors such as State benefits (see Chapter 12).

The disadvantage of the social approach is that it tells us little about the mechanism of symptom production in the individual patient and alone may lead to neglect of biological and psychological processes.

A multifactorial approach

The five approaches outlined clearly overlap and use different terminologies for similar fundamental processes. Rather than competing they are potentially complementary. Along with previous authors (Barsky and

Klerman 1983; Kellner 1990) we consider that effective patient management requires a multifactorial perspective (Engel 1980). The essence of this approach is that the aetiology of functional somatic symptoms is conceived of as involving multiple interacting factors (Mayou 1976, 1991). These factors include physiological (Sharpe and Bass 1992), psychological (Pennebaker 1982), social (Mechanic 1972), and cultural processes (Fabrega 1990; Abbey and Garfinkel 1991). A multidimensional approach to the classification of functional somatic illness is outlined in Chapter 3.

Terminology

The difficulties resulting from unresolved conceptual issues and from conflicting theoretical standpoints are compounded by an unsatisfactory and confusing terminology (see Table 1.2). We therefore briefly review the terms most commonly encountered. One group of terms (hysteria, neurosis, neurasthenia, and hypochondriasis) originally assumed a hypothetical organic disease processes, although all now have connotations of psychogenesis. Another group of terms (psychosomatic, somatization, and illness behaviour) imply a psychosocial aetiology. A third group of terms (somatoform, medically unexplained symptoms, and functional) are less dualist in origin, but have other disadvantages. We will review each in turn.

Table 1.2 Terminology

---

1. Terms originally implying occult disease
    Hysteria
    Hypochondriasis
    Neurosis, nerves, and neurasthenia

2. Terms implying psychogenesis
    Psychosomatic
    Somatization
    Abnormal illness behaviour

3. Other terms
    Somatoform
    Medically unexplained symptoms
    Functional symptoms

Hysteria

This term has a long and varied history (see Shorter, 1992). Its literal meaning refers to the physical migration of the uterus around the body

(Richmond 1989). Because of its misconceived and misogynist origins it is now generally avoided (Lewis 1975). Although rechristened as conversion disorder and dissociative disorder, it continues to pose a problem for taxonomy (see Chapter 3).

Hypochondriasis

Another ancient term which refers literally to the hypochondrium, this term has been used in two ways:

(1) to refer to any person presenting with functional symptoms;

(2) as a primary disorder characterized by an excessive and unjustified fear of or belief in disease (as in the current psychiatric classifications; see Chapter 9).

In this narrowly defined and preferred meaning hypochondriasis focuses on patients' beliefs, rather than on their symptoms (Kenyon 1976; Lloyd 1986). Most patients with functional symptoms are however not hypochondriacal in this sense of the word.

'Nerves', neurosis, and neurasthenia

During the eighteenth and nineteenth centuries, patients with unexplained physical symptoms were often referred to as to being *'nervous'*. Cullen (1772) introduced the related term *neurosis*. Both implied an unknown neurological aetiology and these conditions were initially regarded as the responsibility of the emerging specialty of neurology (Bynum 1985). However, by the beginning of this century they were becoming increasingly viewed as psychological conditions. More recently, the failure of the original organic hypothesis, the rejection of psychodynamic mechanisms of psychogenesis, and the implications of moral weakness have conspired to lead to uncertainty about the utility of the term neurosis. The term was abandoned in the DSM (Editorial 1982), although a plea was subsequently made for its retention, at least in Europe (Gelder 1986). The term neurosis has indeed been retained in the ICD-10 but with little specific meaning.

Neurasthenia, literally weak nerves, is a further variation on the above theme. At the beginning of the century it was seen as an explanation for a wide range of symptoms and was believed to have an (so far undetected) organic substrate (see Chapter 16). It remains prominent in Chinese diagnostic practice and it is of special interest because of its recent renaissance as chronic fatigue syndrome (Wessely 1990).

Psychosomatic

From the dualistic standpoint, the alternative solution to the problem posed by functional somatic symptoms is to imply that the origin of the symptoms is, in fact, mental. The term that implies this most literally is psychosomatic (Bynum 1983). Widely used in the 1930s to describe a number of diseases with definite organic pathology, but for which emotions were thought to play an aetiological role (Lipowski 1986), the term has also been used much more generally to cover all associations between psychological variables and physical symptoms. It is inherently dualistic and may now be both too tainted with psychoanalytic associations and too devalued by overambitious attempts to explain all human illness to be useful for our purpose.

Somatization

This term (Lipowski 1988; Kellner 1990) implies the conversion of psychological distress into somatic symptoms and has become widely if imprecisely used. There are various similar definitions, one of the most widely quoted being 'an idiom of distress in which patients with psychosocial and emotional problems articulate their distress primarily through physical symptomatology' (Katon *et al.* 1984). A more operational definition has also been suggested (Bridges and Goldberg 1985). However, like other terms, somalization remains inherently dualistic (Mumford 1992) and the implication that these illnesses are really 'mental' has, in general, failed to convince physicians and patients alike (Mace and Trimble 1991). Furthermore, concepts of somalization which imply a somatic manifestation of psychological distress are not easily applicable to many non-specific and medically unexplained symptoms for which there is no evidence that psychological distress is in fact the primary cause.

Illness behaviour and abnormal illness behaviour

The term illness behaviour was introduced to describe the ways in which given symptoms may be perceived, evaluated, and acted upon by different types of person (Mechanic 1972). There is no simple relationship between the occurrence of disease and a person's behaviour; some people may become distressed and incapacitated by minor bodily changes whereas others may ignore life-threatening disease. Pilowsky (1969, 1993) suggested the term *abnormal illness behaviour* to describe a category of patients (especially those complaining of chronic pain) whose illness behaviour was thought to be excessive, inappropriate, or maladaptive, irrespective of the presence of disease. There are, however, considerable problems in defining this term, particularly in deciding what is inappropriate and maladaptive and whether patients have received a full medical explanation and reassurance (see Mayou 1989 for a fuller discussion). Although the concept of illness behaviour has been valuable in drawing attention to the behavioural aspects of all illness, it is not specific to patients with functional somatic symptoms.

Somatoform

In their efforts to be atheoretical, the authors of DSM-III introduced the term *somatoform* and used it to embrace a number of symptoms and syndromes in which Somatic symptoms could be found without evidence of organic disease. The term has its merits but retains strong associations with simple psychogenesis. It is also rather ugly. Its use is discussed in more detail in Chapter 3.

Medically unexplained symptoms and medical symptoms unexplained by organic disease

More recently introduced terms have attempted to escape from the dualistic trap, but with only limited success. The terms *unexplained symptoms* (Smith *et al.* 1986) or unexplained physical symptoms (Escobar and Canino 1989) beg the question 'unexplained by what?'. To say they are *medically unexplained* (Mayou 1991) introduces an implicit distinction between physical medicine and psychiatric medicine and assumes that physicians cannot make psychiatric diagnoses. The most explicit term *medical symptoms not explained by organic disease* employed for the purpose of a joint venture between the British Royal Colleges of Physicians and Psychiatrists (Creed *et al.* 1992) is a more precise, almost operational definition, but still begs important theoretical questions about the definition of organic disease. It is also cumbersome to the point of impracticality.

Functional

Another approach to the problem of somatic symptoms without detectable physical pathology is the idea of 'functional illness' (Stearns 1946; Trimble 1982). Functional implies that there is an abnormality in the physical functioning of the body, but this is not of a type or degree that can be detected in terms of gross structural changes. The original meaning of this term has changed so that its current usage by physicians tends to imply psychogenesis (Lipkin 1969). However, a return to its original meaning has been called for (Trimble 1982).

Conclusion

None of the terms in current use is entirely satisfactory. All may be used to dismiss patients' complaints, all are to a greater or lesser extent predicated on a mind–body division, and most are regarded by patients as pejorative. In the remainder of this book we have decided, wherever possible, to employ the term functional somatic symptoms. This has the advantage of not either evoking a hypothetical organic process or indicating that the origin of the patient's symptoms lies entirely 'in the mind'. Rather it implies that there is a real abnormality in the way the organism is functioning and as such sets the stage for a more constructive approach to treatment.

References

Abbey, S.E. and Garfinkel, P.E. (1991). Neurasthenia and chronic fatigue syndrome: the role of culture in the making of a diagnosis. *American Journal of Psychiatry*, **148**, 1638–46.

Barsky, A.J. (1992). Amplification, somatization, and the somatoform disorders. *Psychosomatics*, **33**, 28–34.

Barsky, A.J. and Klerman, G.L. (1983). Overview: hypochondriasis, bodily complaints and somatic styles. *American Journal of Psychiatry*, **140**, 273–83.

Betts, T. and Bodeni, S. (1992). Diagnosis, management and treatment of a group of 128 patients with non-epileptic attack disorder. *Seizure*, **1**, 27–32.

Bridges, K.W. and Goldberg, D.P. (1985). Somatic presentation of DSM-III psychiatric disorders in primary care. *Journal of Psychosomatic Research*, **29**, 563–9.

Brooks, P. (1993). Repetitive strain injury: does it exist as a separate medical condition? *British Medical Journal*, **307**, 1298.

Brown, T. (1989). Cartesian dualism and psychosomatics. *Psychosomatics*, **30**, 322–31.

Bynum, W.F. (1983). Some clinical concepts: "Psychosomatic". In *Handbook of psychiatry 1. General psychopathology*, (ed. M. Shepherd and O.L. Zangwill), pp. 54–5. Cambridge University Press, New York.

Bynum, W.F. (1985). The nervous patient in eighteenth- and nineteenth-century Britain: the psychiatric origins of British neurology. In *The anatomy of madness*. Volume I. *People and ideas*, 89–102. (ed. W.F. Bynum, R. Porter and M. Shepherd). Tavistock Publications, London.

Cullen, X. (1772). *Nosology*. See extracts in I. McAlpine and R. Hunter, *Three hundred years of psychiatry*, pp. 473–9. Oxford University Press, London.

Creed, F., Mayou, R.A., and Hopkins, A. (1992). *Medical symptoms not explained by organic disease*. The Royal College of Psychiatrists and the Royal College of Physicians of London, London.

Editorial (1982). Goodbye neurosis? *Lancet*, **i**, 29.

Eisenberg, L. (1977). Disease and illness. *Culture Medicine and Psychiatry*, 1, 9-23.
Eisenberg, L. (1986). Mindlessness and brainlessness in psychiatry. *British Journal of Psychiatry*, **148**, 497-508.
Engel, G. (1980). The clinical application of the biopsychosocial model. *American Journal of Psychiatry*, **137**, 535-44.
Escobar, J.I. and Canino, G. (1989). Unexplained physical complaints. Psychopathology and epidemiological correlates. *British Journal of Psychiatry*, **154**, Suppl. 24-7.
Fabrega, H.J. (1990). The concept of somatization as a cultural and historical product of Western medicine. *Psychosomatic Medicine*, **52**, 653-72.
Ferguson, D.A. (1987). 'RSI': putting the epidemic to rest. *Medical Journal of Australia*, **147**, 213-14.
Gelder, M.G. (1986). Neurosis: another tough old word. *British Medical Journal*, **292**, 972-3.
Goldberg, D.P. and Bridges, K. (1988). Somatic presentations of psychiatric illness in primary care setting. *Journal of Psychosomatic Research*, **32**, 137-44.
Jessup, B.A., Neufeld, R.W.J., and Mersky, H. (1979). Biofeedback therapy for headache and other pain: an evaluative review. *Pain*, **7**, 225-70.
Katon, W., Ries, R.K., and Kleinman, A. (1984). The prevalence of somatization in primary care. *Comprehensive Psychiatry*, **25**, 208-15.
Kellner, R. (1990). Somatization. Theories and research. *Journal of Nervous and Mental Diseases*, **178**, 150-60.
Kellner, R. (1994). Psychosomatic symptoms, somatization, and somatoform disorders. *Psychotherapy and Psychosomatics*, **61**, 4-24.
Kenyon, F.E. (1976). Hypochondriacal states. *British Journal of Psychiatry*, **129**, 1-14.
Kroenke, K. and Mangelsdorff, D. (1989). Common symptoms in ambulatory care: incidence, evaluation, therapy and outcome. *American Journal of Medicine*, **86**, 262-6.
Lewis, A. (1975). The survival of hysteria. *Psychological Medicine*, **5**, 9-12.
Lipkin, M. (1969). Functional or organic? A pointless question. *Annals of Internal Medicine*, **5**, 1013-17.
Lipowski, Z.J. (1986). Somatization: a borderland between medicine and psychiatry. *Canadian Medical Association Journal*, **135**, 609-14.
Lipowski, Z.J. (1988). Somatization: the concept and its clinical application. *American Journal of Psychiatry*, **145**, 1358-68.
Lloyd, G.G. (1986). Psychiatric syndromes with a somatic presentation. *Journal of Psychosomatic Research*, **30**, 113-20.
Mace, C.J. and Trimble, M.R. (1991). Hysteria, functional or psychogenic? A survey of British neurologists' preferences. *Journal of the Royal Society of Medicine*, **84**, 471-5.
Mayou, R.A. (1976). The nature of bodily symptoms. *British Journal of Psychiatry*, **129**, 55-60.
Mayou, R. (1989). Illness behavior and psychiatry. *General Hospital Psychiatry*, **11**, 307-12.
Mayou, R.A. (1991). Medically unexplained physical symptoms. *British Medical Journal*, **303**, 534-5.

Mechanic, D. (1972). Social psychologic factors affecting the presentation of bodily complaints. *New England Journal of Medicine*, **286**, 1132–9.

Mumford, D. (1992). Does 'somatization' explain anything? *Psychiatry in practice*, pp. 11–14. Spring.

Parsons, T. (1951). *The social system*. Free Press of Glencoe, New York.

Pennebaker, J.W. (1982). *The psychology of physical symptoms*. Springer-Verlag, New York.

Pilowsky, (1969). Abnormal illness behaviour. *Psychological Medicine*, **42**, 347–51.

Pilowsky, I. (1993). Aspects of abnormal illness behaviour. *Psychotherapy and Psychosomatics*, **60**, 62–74.

Richmond, C. (1989). Myalgic encephalomyelitis, Princess Aurora, and the wandering womb. *British Medical Journal*, **298**, 1295–6.

Sharpe, M.C. and Bass, C. (1992). Pathophysiological mechanisms in somatization. *International Reviews in Psychiatry*, **4**, 81–97.

Shorter, E. (1992). *From paralysis to fatigue: a history of psychosomatic illness in the modern era*. Free Press, New York.

Smith, G.R., Monson, R.A., and Ray, D.C. (1986). Patients with multiple unexplained symptoms. *Archives of Internal Medicine*, **146**, 69–72.

Stearns, A.W. (1946). A history of the development of the concept of functional nervous disease during the past twenty-five hundred years. *American Journal of Psychiatry*, **103**, 289–308.

Susser, M. (1990). Disease, illness, sickness: impairment, disability and handicap. *Psychological Medicine*, **20**, 471–73.

Taylor, G.J. (1984). Alexithymia: concepts, measurement, and implications for treatment. *American Journal of Psychiatry*, **141**, 725–32.

Trimble, M.R. (1982). Functional diseases. *British Medical Journal*, **285**, 1768–770.

Ware, N.C. (1992). Suffering and the social construction of illness: the deligitimation of illness experience in chronic fatigue syndrome. *Medical Anthropology Quarterly*, **6**, 347–61.

Wessely, S. (1990). Old wine in new bottles: neurasthenia and 'M.E.'. *Psychological Medicine*, **20**, 35–53.

2 Psychosomatic disorders: historical perspectives

Roy Porter

Heavy thoughts bring on physical maladies: when the soul is oppressed so is the body

Luther

The historian Roy Porter provides a historical background to the major and more recent themes of the remainder of the book. He describes examples from the sixteenth to nineteenth centuries of attempts by physicians, philosophers, and others to explain and categorize in medical and philosophical terms what, in this book, are described as functional somatic symptoms. None of these have satisfactorily resolved fundamental difficulties in understanding the mind–brain relationship.

Porter begins his main argument by discussion of Edward Shorter's recently published account of the influence of cultural factors on symptomatology. Shorter has argued that somatization represents unconscious selection from a wide symptom pool and is determined by individual and cultural factors. Changes in cultural beliefs have been reflected in changes in medical fashion, with doctors usually participating in a tacit acceptance of some underlying physical cause. Freud challenged these views but did so in a way that was offensive and unacceptable to most patients and doctors. Porter emphasizes a second issue — even if cultural background determines the particular mode of presentation of symptoms, we also need to examine the reason why people experience symptoms of any sort.

Porter suggests that hysteria provides a key example. He compares hysteria as a psychiatric disorder as described by Ilza Veith and her views with Szasz's refusal to accept hysteria as a mental illness. Thereafter he reviews the history of hysteria and, in particular, the similarity between medically diagnosed hysteria and possession states and the historical tendency to see hysteria as a problem of women.

Introduction

I wish to sketch in broad terms a historical background for the conceptualization of functional disorders and functional symptoms. Writing not as a psychiatrist but as a historian, I shall look mainly at the period from the sixteenth century to the close of the nineteenth century. The concerns and concepts of those centuries may not map precisely onto those of our own: I may be talking about anxieties and attitudes that may seem only peripherally relevant today. If so, that will be a major marker of historical change. What I shall say will certainly not *solve* our present problems, but it may at least clarify what is specifically contemporary about the pre-occupations of the other chapters in this book.

Modern categorizations of 'psychosomatic conditions' or 'functional disorders' serve, it may be suggested, as extenuating devices masking ignorance of mind–body mediations by grace of a face-saving formula. For such phrases are patently evasions, silent admissions that ideal models of illness (disease regarded as organic lesion or invasion by pathogen) are simplistic. The idea of a functional disorder involves grudging recognition that — at least as of now! — scientific medicine does not know all the answers, since it patently has not cracked the seeming proliferation of non-specific complaints over the last few centuries, be they called the 'vapours', 'nerves', 'stress', or, in recent years, 'chronic fatigue syndrome' and so forth. However problematic the psyche, 'psychogenic illness' has often been viewed as what is left over, once science has done its best to ram sickness into medico-scientific pigeon-holes.

In one of the rich ironies of history, that scholastic or Cartesian 'mind' which reductionist critics in the Enlightenment set out to expose as a 'fiction', fought back and reasserted itself, in surprising and troublesome fashions. For one thing, the mind's pathological face began to reveal itself. Late eighteenth-century medicine began to recognize that lunacy did not simply spring from the blood, nerves, or brain, but might be an authentic *mental* disorder, requiring treatment with 'moral' or, as we would say, psychological means. For another, mind went underground. Inchoate notions of the 'unconscious' budded in the age of sensibility and flowered in the culture of Romanticism. The Age of Reason closed with growing, if grudging, homage to unreason. By a strange paradox, the more medicine has sought to become 'scientific', the more it has had to confront behaviour and complaints that resist its programmes.

The history of what we may call medically unexplained symptoms is therefore especially illuminating. It tells us much about successive attempts, by physicians, philosophers, and the public, to explain phenomena defying authorized medical and philosophical categories — to explain the fact, as Laurence Sterne put it in that great psychological novel, *Tristram Shandy* (1760), that 'a man's body and his mind . . . are exactly like a jerkin and a jerkin's lining, — rumple the one, — you rumple the other'. And its very presence highlights the problematic relations between public presentation (body, mind, malady, and accountability) and the individuals who make use of or trip over this semantic and cultural furniture.

A historical key?

A bold attempt has recently been made to map out the history of functional disorders by the Canadian historian, Edward Shorter in *From paralysis to fatigue. A history of psychosomatic illness in the modern era* (1992). It is cast as a study of 'somatizers', that is, people in Shorter's view suffering from 'pain and fatigue that have no physical cause' — the sort of malady that proves so frustrating to no-nonsense physicians like the early-twentieth century Kentucky doctor who thought a 'good spanking, sometimes even a good "cussing"', was the surest way with hysterical patients. According to Shorter, most of those suffering over the last couple of centuries from conditions variously called 'nervous spine', 'neurasthenia', 'fits', and, nowadays, myalgic encephalomyelitis (ME, 'yuppie flu', or chronic fatigue syndrome) have, in fact, had nothing much organically wrong with them, but have been 'somatizers'. If so, how are we to explain this strange fact? Shorter (1992) claims that, in such cases, the historian should best proceed by assuming that the 'unconscious' selects a convenient suit of somatoform manifestations from a wider 'symptom pool'.

This notion of a historically mutating symptom pool is highly stimulating. Granted that people somatize, what explains the distinct patterns and trends of conversion? Symptoms are not random or unique, but learnt and cultural and it is possible to trace a succession of favoured symptoms. Early in the nineteenth century, motor disorders were most prominent. With some, these showed as immoderate movements — fits, convulsions, spasms, twitches, swoons and seizures — and with others, immobilization — catalepsy, paralysis, and all the stereotyped cases of Victorian ladies collapsing on their bed, literally incapable of standing on their own two feet. In the course of time and in particular by the early twentieth century, such operatic displays quietened into a symptomatological chamber music and 'motor' defects were superseded by more discreet 'sensory' ones: headache, fatigue, pain, and migraine. In its own, successive context, each choice made sense. In the claustrophobic milieu of the Victorian family, nothing less than a melodramatic acting out of abnormalities could command attention and achieve release.

In the twentieth-century individualist environment of the 'lonely crowd', by contrast, the introspective ego finds expression in personal, private pain. In any case, the old florid symptom repertoire was gradually 'found out'. It was exposed as socially vulgar — nowadays only Third World people somatize like Victorian maiden aunts — and, with the refinement of clinical tests for catalepsy, etc., it was also revealed as medically inauthentic, like the notorious 'glove and stocking' hysteria. Modern, 'deeper', sense-oriented symptoms are less vulnerable to medical exposure: the symptom-selecting unconscious, ever adroit at resisting ridicule, silently learns from its mistakes and moves with the times.

Moreover, somatizing modes have their pecking order; stylish symptoms come in and go out of fashion, trickle down the ranks, and finally linger on in the cultural periphery. At the centre, by contrast, Shorter (1992) contends, symptom choice has been propelled by the cream of the medical profession. A melancholy collusion has entangled 'somatizers' and doctors, above all, those elite physicians grasping or cynical enough to spy rich pickings in pandering to the insatiable needs of well-heeled valetudinarians with bank balances to match their imaginations.

As medical theories and illness categories shifted, somatoform symptoms changed with them, thanks to largely unconscious processes of suggestion, legitimation, emulation, and compliance. In the eighteenth century, when the Bath physician, James Adair, noted that medicine 'is become subject to the empire of fashion' (in the sense of directing the beau monde 'in the choice of their diseases'), medicine was preoccupied with the nervous system, hence the rash of nervous complaints. Early in the nineteenth century, spinal irritation and inflammation dominated the scene leading to the infamous paralytic sofa cases. Reflex arc theory then blossomed in the second third of the century, promoting the idea that sickness was triggered by a local lesion. With female patients — easily the majority, some part of the sexual equipment was usually blamed, hence the crop of unnecessary and dangerous gynaecological surgery, including ovariotomies and clitoridectomies. Later the theoretical accent fell on the central nervous system and so neurasthenia became the diagnosis à la mode.

In this succession of medical artefacts negotiated between profession and patient, the constant, the point of rock-solid agreement between patient and practitioner, was a tacit gentleman's agreement or pious fraud, that the body was defective, that the complaint in question was truly physical. Thanks to the success of the medical enterprise or at least its propaganda, sufferers were relieved to hear that their ailments were organic, requiring medical or surgical treatment. This 'medical model' presupposed that a malady with a somatic seat was real; without one it was fictional and fraudulent. It also meant that patients lost no face: there was no hint that they were psychologically shamming and no risk that they be thought to be going quite out of their mind — thus the residual benefits of the Cartesian fall-back. And, of course, this explains the somatizing fad, not just in symptoms but also in treatments. For medical men were unflaggingly inventive in cooking up innovations in minor surgery, spa regimes, and coloured water, all of which could count on the infinite gullibility of patients prepared to believe that each and every organ could spawn dozens of defects. If, over cigars and brandy at the club, doctors derided such patients as hypochondriacs (how else were *physicians* to cope with sufferings for which they had no cure?), in public they manfully upheld the organic doctrine of disease.

In the chronicle of functional symptoms, Shorter suggests that Freudian psychoanalysis forms the great anomaly. For Freud and the Freudians distinctively broke rank and blew the gaffe: fashionable disorders were, in fact, Freud stressed, psychological, all in the mind. Shorter (1992) has an interesting approach to interpreting Freud's bombshell. For, while believing Freud was objectively right, he sees him as tactically naive. A small elite of 'somatizers' — clever patients who could acclimatize to the Freudian gospel or jump on the bandwagon — were genuinely flattered or helped by the notion of sickness being psychogenic. But the gross and offensive tone of Freud's pronouncements (patients, Freud seemed to be saying, were ill because of the sort of people they were, above all because of their infantile and secret sexual selves) put people's backs up; to the popular mind, Freud's message was that neurotics, if not exactly malingerers, were crazy. And the result was that 'any hope of achieving public enlightenment about somatoform illness came to an end'.

But this reading of Freud provokes further reflection. Why in particular were all these people undergoing medically unexplained symptoms in the first place? Why did they express themselves in the idiom of illness, rather than say, of faith, politics, sex, or some other stylistics of the self? Precisely who were the sufferers adopting this particular sick role? Did they constitute groups that were socially coherent and indicative — or were they just a random aggregate of discontented or malcontent atoms? How far should their illnesses be seen as socially induced?

To answer these questions we must go one stage further and integrate the study of medically unexplained symptoms within the wider historical sociology of somatization. We must examine the daily expression of emotions, gestures, body language, and the history of passions with all their local, cultural, and ethnic traditions. Otherwise we will only end up making the psychosomatically ill seem peculiar, albeit they were, in certain ways, perhaps the greatest conformists of all.

The mystery of hysteria

To show how the idea of psychosomatic disorders has been debated, affirmed and resisted over the centuries, it seems worth concentrating attention in the remainder of this chapter upon one particular condition. Hysteria offers the key case. The symptom repertoire associated with hysteria melodramatically mimes the riddle of mind and body in a spectacularly bizarre parody of normal conduct and regular disease.

A skeleton in the cupboard or a ghost in the machine? A phantom like 'the vapours' or a bona fide disease? And if the latter, organic or mental? One essentially extinct or one camouflaging itself in colours ever new? The medical community long remained divided over hysteria (Krohn 1978).

It was ever a tease: elusive, ill-behaved. The hysteria diagnosis, argue sceptics, was hocus-pocus, pinned upon complaints physicians could not fathom. Presented with multiple, bizarre, and unpredictable symptoms — pains in the genitals and abdomen, shooting to the extremities or rising through the thorax to produce the '*globus hystericus*' in the throat; breathing irregularities, twitchings, tics, and spasms; faced with anxiety and emotional lability, tears, and sighs; or worse, confronted by seizures, paralyses, hemiplagia, or catalepsy — all perhaps cascading in dizzying succession and with no manifest root lesion — what was to be done? Such mystery conditions (cynics observed) were wrapped up as 'hysteria'. 'When at any time a sickness happens in a Woman's Body, of an unusual manner, or more occult original, so that its causes lie hid, and a Curatory indication is altogether uncertain', confessed the pioneer seventeenth-century neurologist, Thomas Willis (1684), 'we declare it to be something hysterical ... which oftentimes is only the subterfuge of ignorance'. Nor did things improve. A full century later in 1769, William Buchan was still dubbing hysteria the 'reproach of medicine', since the 'physician ... is at a loss to account for the symptom' (Buchan 1769).

Was hysteria then just a will-o'-the-wisp? Or was it an authentic condition, whose essence lay in its amorphousness, prodigiously protean, a malady in masquerade, mimicking all? (Stallybrass and White 1986). If so, could it truly be a disease at all — and not some monstrous brain-child of medicine's own sick imagination mocking its creator?

Such problems have divided doctors: still they baffle historians. Are we to grant it a historical epidemiology, a rise and fall to be charted, with due semantic sensitivity, down the centuries? Or is hysteria truly the joker in the nosological pack, a flighty diagnostic balloon never moored to a malady — or worse, a spurious issue, a disease name without a disease thing, an alibi for medical ignorance' Indeed, has hysteria been the doctors' Waterloo — a chameleon too clever for clumsy nosologists: the one that got away? (Major 1974; Ey 1982; Roy 1982; Merskey 1983, 1986; Critchley and Cantor 1984; Abse 1987; Micale 1989*a,b*, 1990).

The historian's problems have been exacerbated by the doctors, ever engrossing hysteria's past within their present systems — and why not, for surely science holds Nature's laws to be *universal*, uniform across time as well as space? Thus, as King (1985) has argued, though Hippocratic medicine had no such concept, physicians have commonly fathered their pet notions of hysteria upon the Hippocratics (Palis *et al.* 1985). And Charcot saw his *fin de siècle* hysterics prefigured in the demoniacs of the Counter-Reformation witch trials (Charcot and Richer 1887).

Hysteria as a psychiatric disorder

Historians have taken their cue from the doctors. Down the centuries and across the cultures, the annals of medical history have been rifled to reveal hysterical disorders, permitting the story of the disease to be told as a progression, from ignorance to expertise, from error to enlightenment, from prejudice to psychoanalysis. As its very title proves, the standard English-language history, Veith's *Hysteria. The history of a disease* (1965), is cast within this mould.

Hysteria, Veith (1965) contended, had been known since the Pharoahs and so named by the Greeks. Christian churchmen, to be sure, viewed its symptoms as the stigmata of Satan and, thus, retarded understanding, but great Renaissance physicians like Johannes Weyer brought hysteria back into the medical fold. Even so, misguided medical materialism long misconstrued it as an organic disease — standardly, of the womb or, later, of the nervous system. Veith (1965) particularly deplored the 'increasingly sterile and repetitive neurological basis that had emanated from Great Britain for nearly two hundred years', especially from George Cheyne's early eighteenth-century iatromechanical theory, whose 'affectation and absurdities are such that it scarcely merits elaborate discussion' — even his 'references to his own distress', she complained, 'seem inconsequential'. Not least, somatic hypotheses had been misogynistic. Freud had rightly judged such views had 'long stood in the way of [hysteria] being recognized as a psychical disorder'.

Fortunately, Veith (1965) argued, a counter-theory had arisen. Paracelsus, Edward Jorden, Thomas Sydenham, Franz Mesmer, Philippe Pinel, Ernst von Feuchtersleben, and Robert Carter developed 'anticipations' of Freud's discovery that hysteria was psychogenic, the child of sexual repression. Thanks partly to Freud, modern sexual emancipation has led to the disorder's demise.

The myth of mental illness

This meliorist tale has been challenged over the last generation by fresh scholarship and the anti-psychiatry and feminist movements. Above all, Veith's (1965) reading of the 'history of a disease' — specifically, a 'mental disease' (p. vii) — as a battle between benighted somatists and their enlightened psychological conquerors is now recognized as a Whiggish teleology, culminating in Freud.

Contemporaneously with Veith's, a diametrically opposite account was being developed by Thomas Szasz. Szasz (1961) denied that hysteria was a disease at all, crediting Freud, not with discovering its nature, but with manufacturing its mythology. Drawing upon logical positivism, Parsons's notion of the sick role, ethno-methodology, and a sociology of medical dominance, Szasz (1961) argued in his *The myth of mental illness* that — whether by solecism or false pretences — psychoanalysis had mystified hysteria into a primary psychogenic 'mental illness' marked by somatic conversion. 'I was inclined', reflected Freud, 'to look for a *psychical* origin for all symptoms in cases of hysteria'.

Exposing this psychoanalytic strategy as part of a self-serving 'manufacture of madness', Szasz (1961) counters with a corrosive philosophical critique. By thus privileging the psyche, Freud was in effect revitalizing the hoary Cartesian dualism, resurrecting the old ghost in the machine, or, rather, in the guise of the unconscious, inventing the ghost in a ghost. Yet surely the expectation of finding the aetiology of hysteria in body or mind, worst still in its subterranean chambers, must be a lost cause, a dead-end, and, at bottom, a linguistic error? The 'unconscious' is but a metaphor and Freud was guilty of pictorializing the psyche in terms of hydraulic and electrical models, of reifying the fictive substance behind the substantive.

Properly speaking, contends Szasz (1961), hysteria is not a disease with origins, but a behaviour freighted with meanings. People follow rules and play games; the hysterical role threads in and out of norm-governed activities, no less communicative for being largely non-verbal. Not illness but idiom, it pertains not to a Cartesian ontology but to a semiotics, being communication by *complaints*. Since the hysteric is engaged in social performances following, while challenging, expectations, we must ask not about the aetiology of hysteria, but its uses.

Side-stepping mind–body dualisms, Szasz (1961) thus recasts hysteria as social performance, a problem of conduct, communication, and context. Freud believed mind–body problems were real, though mystified and attempted to resolve them. Szasz (1961) dismisses them as *questions mal posées*, deriving from linguistic confusion or bad faith and aims to dissolve them.

However idiosyncratic, Szasz's (1961) analysis is manifestly a child of its time. Modern linguistic philosophy, behaviourism, and structuralist antihistoricism all query the aetiological quest. Origins, individuals, intentions are discounted; systems, conventions, meanings brought to the fore. Such a paradigm switch does not, of course, magically switch off uncontrollable sobbing, fits, tantrums, and paralyses. But it offers new readings of what such actions signify, while undermining expectations that we shall get at root causes, that hysteria will afford the key to the riddle of mind and body.

Szasz's (1961) solution is bracing, but it reduces hysteria's past to pantomime: sufferers become the puppets of their parts and medics knaves or fools. Why is this? Because, for Szasz, the bottom line is medical materialism (disease is disease if and only if it is organic). Were hysteria — were *any* so-called mental illness — somatically based, it would have a real history. Lacking organic credentials, its past, rather like those of trans-substantiation or perpetual motion machines, is a blot, a disgrace, a chronicle of enthusiasm, superstition, and fraud worthy of some philosopher's pen.

Hysteria and the economy of medical knowledge

Thus, for equal but opposite reasons, Veith and Szasz both short circuit the history of functional disorders. Believing *hysteria* psychogenic, Veith (1965) recounts her 'history of a disease' as the road to the Freudian triumph. Believing *disease* must be somatic, Szasz (1961) paints the history of hysteria as the pageant of a dream. Both approaches trivialize the complex texture of hysteria down the ages, whose true understanding must respect its mystery nature, the enigmas of multiform pain in a culture within which mind–body relations have been supercharged and devilish problematic.

It is not for historians to shower bouquets and brickbats upon neurologists or gynaecologists. History does not show whether the condition was psychogenic or somatogenic, but, rather, it does demonstrate that hysteria's conditions of existence lay in discourses in which the scope, meanings, and boundaries of 'psyche' and 'soma' were ever contested, ever reconstituted. *Pace* Veith and Szasz, the psychic and the somatic are not self-evident, timeless Platonic ideas. Constructs of the wider culture, they demand analysis laying bare their implications for health, gender differentiation, moral autonomy, legal responsibility, and human dignity. The story of hysteria is no technical series of internal, medical skirmishes over nerves and neurones, passions and pathogens. Far more has been at stake.

Biological explanation

For one thing, medicine's own authority resides in its sovereignty over the body. The organism explains its own behaviour: in this, as Entralgo (1955) has emphasized, lay the message of Greek medicine to its inheritors. Diseases are in and of the organism, caused by some physical lesion, displacement, or imbalance; material therapies – drugs, surgery – will relieve or cure. 'In the beginning, was the body': abandon this article of faith and the kingdom of medicine vanishes with it. Unless sickness speaks exclusively in the idiom of organic laws and lesions, why should it not be open to all – priests, philosophers, charlatans?

Hence, the investment of post-Renaissance 'scientific' medicine in anatomy and physiology, even though the therapeutic fruits long remained nugatory. Hence also nineteenth-century medicine's favourite metahistory, a positivist schema of evolutionary stages, rising from theological and metaphysical up to biological explanations. What first had been misattributed to spirit possession, witchcraft, etc., only to be later mystified into formulaic verbiage (humours, animal spirits), had finally been rendered, argued Charcot, into the patho-anatomical laws of hysteria.

Mind over matter   Medicine's theoretical practice laid claim to the body. Yet obvious dangers lay herein. For the wider culture traditionally enthroned spirit over what preachers denigrated as the 'flesh', forever too, too solid (Bottomley 1979; Brown 1988). Idealism was hegemonic, philosophically buttressed by Platonism and the Cartesian *cogito*, underwritten by Christian theology, and, in secular garb, still the metaphysical foundations of right-thinking men.

Idealism's postulates are familiar. Its hierarchical, dualistic models set mind over matter, thinking over being, head over hand, the mental over the corporeal. Macrocosmically, the Divine Mind, commanding immaterial powers, governs brute matter; in a microcosmic analogy, the achievement of *mens sana in corpore sano* requires self-control by mind as captain of the soul. As many historians have argued, from their various standpoints, the 'civilizing process' or the 'march of mind' entailed ever stricter physical discipline, stringent subjection of the body (Adorno and Horkheimer 1972; Foucault 1979; Elias 1983).

Thus, medicine occupies an ambiguous niche within the larger ontology. For it risks establishing its comprehensive organic expertise at the price of a nobler dignity — witness Coleridge's damnation of the doctors for their debasing reductionist somaticism: 'They are *shallow* animals; having always employed their minds about Body and Gut, they imagine that in the whole system of things there is nothing but Gut and Body' (Griggs 1956, p. 256; Porter 1990).

Complementary models   Of course, medicine has its ways of bridging these incommensurable cultures. Doctors live in the world and medicine is not without status. Accommodations are reached, ensuring that cultural idealism and medical materialism collude rather than collide. Thus, medicine itself stipulated that mind should be in the saddle, physicians prescribing will-power (healthy mindedness, positive thinking, self-control) as the recipe for 'whole person' well-being. Victorian doctors, as Clark (1981, 1988) has brilliantly shown, characterized the sound individual as one exercising body restraint, cultivating obliviousness to their body, and channelling their energies, in true Aristotelian fashion, into public activity — in stark contrast to hysterics morbidly meditating upon themselves and their metabolisms (Bynum 1985). Sickness is seen as the loss of rational control — either because the organism is highjacked (for example, in epidemics) or because civil war erupts within, precipitating insanity.

Cultural idealism and medical materialism may thus be worlds apart, but they have rarely been daggers drawn, for each finds roles for the other within its symbolic system. They should be seen less as incompatible paradigms than as complementary packages of values, ideological imperatives, rhetorical resources, and prescriptions for action, symbiotically shaping images of the constitution of man, soma and psyche, sanity, salubrity and sickness, and, not least, determining the politics of the moral–physical interface.

For, at bottom, doctors operate in the public domain, jostling with rivals, judged by their clients. Medicine cannot hide its head in sprains and pains, but must engage with broader values — religious, ethical, social, and cultural. The sick — society too — demand explications no less than medications and medicine accommodates with its just-so stories about the nature of man and the order of things.

Accommodations, but tensions too, are ever prominent in formulations of hysteria. Take Freud. Encultured within mid-century aggressive medical materialism, Freud was steeped, as Sulloway (1979) has emphasized, in the German neurophysiology of Helmholtz and Meynart, in Charcot's positivism, and in English Darwinism. Life's laws had to be grounded in the body or science ceased. Nevertheless, despite the materialist cast of his 1895 'Project', Freud's theorizings of neuroses and hysteria steadily became more psychodynamic; his battery of mentalist neologisms — the unconscious, the *ego*, *id*, and *super ego*, the death wish, etc. — have ever been derided by logical positivists, notably Karl Popper, as throwbacks to the Comtean metaphysical stage. His therapeutics moved from pharmaceuticals (for example, cocaine), through hands-on, pressure-point hypnosis, to the purely psychical (free speech associations) (Sulloway 1979; Rubinstein 1983; Knight 1984; McGrath 1986).

In increasingly privileging the psyche as *primum mobile*, Freud offended the biomedicalism of his day, being forced, as he saw it, into the position of persecuted heretic. Yet while alienating medical science, he gained the plaudits of modern high culture, disposed to believe that psychological explanations of behaviour — however dark and devious — must be more profound, humane, sensitive, more titillating even, and true than mere mechanical causation. Psychoanalysis' 'discovery of the unconscious' (Whyte 1962; Ellenberger 1970), unlocking the sphinxian secrets of human nature, retains its allure in the mythologies of modernity.

Yet Freud — as Gay (1988) has stressed, a child of the Enlightenment — dismissed theology, distrusted philosophy, but embraced 'science'. With his views of the libido and the unconscious, of course he could not countenance the Christian–Platonic divine right monarchy of the mind or accept face-value idealizations of love and altruism: psychoanalysis must expose such 'illusions' (Gay 1988). Nevertheless', the cutting edge of Freudian psychodynamics — his point of departure from Breuer and Fliess, no less than from Charcot — lay in denying the sufficiency of biochemical or hereditarian inputs to explain behavioural complexities. The hysterical

Hence, hysteria is not a thing with a single, uniform, chronological 'history'. It was not recognized by the Hippocratics: the noun rarely surfaced before the seventeenth century, nor did the person dubbed 'the hysteric' appear till the mid eighteenth century. Ironically, today's diagnostic manuals boast the full-blown disease concept, but there are few takers: *ou sont les grandes hystériques d'hier*? Even accepting the real presence theory, hysteria has had, it appears, an unusually chequered career, whose rise and fall cry out for interpretation within the larger histories of patients and practitioners. If 'mind' and 'body' are not cast-iron categories, but rather triangulations between culture, medicine, and society, our task must be to explore the different meanings successively assumed by 'hysteria' where and when the politics of mind–body relations were in contention and medicine was battling to extend its sway.

I emphasize this last point, not to imply that hysteria was 'made up' by a mendacious medical mafia, but because it was, beyond doubt, a condition crystallized by the medical gaze, from the expert witnesses at witch trials, through Enlightenment specialists in 'nervous' patients, to the heads of institutions such as the Salpetriere. Cynical about patients — they were 'actresses' — Victorian doctors reflected that nature knew no such creature as a solitary hysteric: it was a complaint presupposing an audience and ultimately a medical audience. Was hysteria, then, purely iatrogenic? I do not suggest this, though would anyone deny that the nineteenth century was hysteria's golden age, precisely because it was then that the doctor became guardian as never before of intimate lives?

'*L'Hystérie a toujours existé*', declared Charcot, '*en tous lieux et en tous temps*' (Trillat 1986, p. 272). By contrast, proposing no single history of hysteria, but many, I wish to explore, in the remainder of this chapter, the situations and the pressures, which gave rise to special, distinctive formulations of the mind–body duo in hysteria.

Hysteria and possession   In their *Les Démoniques dans l'art*, Charcot and Richer (1887) contended that religious mystics, witches, etc., had typically been hysterics. Their view, supported by Freud, by Zilboorg, and by modern psychohistorians (Carroy-Thirard 1980, 1981; Maire 1981, Goldstein 1982, 1987; Brais 1990), is not one I would endorse. Nevertheless, it was in the context of witchcraft and demonology that hysteria was first formulated as a somatic affliction. In early modern possession accusations, much hinged upon interpretation of the *stimata diaboli*, the bodily and behavioural symptoms of the victim. In reading these, meticulous courtroom procedures aimed to sift demoniacs from frauds, the suggestible, and the sick.

Doctors did not disbelieve in demons. But familiarity with the mysteries of the organism and professional rivalry with the clergy sometimes led them to insist that supposed signs of possession — convulsions, anaesthesias, trances — were due not to Satan but to sickness, Ambroise Paré and Johannes Weyer, for instance, pointing to disorders such as melancholia (Veith 1965, p. 114; Anglo 1977). A medical aetiology was particularly urged by the English physician, Edward Jorden (1578–1632).

With three other practitioners, Jorden testified in the case of Elizabeth Jackson, accused of bewitching a teenage girl, Mary Glover, who had begun to suffer from 'fittes ... so fearfull, that all that were about her, supposed that she would dye'; rendered speechless and temporarily blind, her left side was anaesthetized and paralysed. Classic symptoms, but was it the Devil or disease? Initially treated by college physicians, Glover failed to respond, whereupon they predictably pronounced that there was something 'beyond naturall' in it. Jorden demurred, finding for disease (Jorden 1603).

When Justice Anderson — a notorious hammer of witches — overrode his testimony, Jorden (1607) defended himself in a book whose title highlighted his contentions: *A briefe discourse of a disease called the suffocation of the mother. Written uppon occasion which hath beene of late taken thereby, to suspect possession of an evill spirit, or some such like supernaturall power. Wherein is declared that divers strange actions and passions of the body of man, which in the common opinion are imputed to the Divill, have their true naturall causes, and do accompany this disease.*

Jorden (1603) diagnosed Glover's condition as the 'suffocation of the mother' (that is, matrix or womb) or simply 'the mother', tags interchangeable with 'hysteria': all pointed, etymologically and clinically, to the womb. In contending that such conditions as the esophagian ball, respiratory and digestive blockages, panic, suffocation, and constrictions, indicated a uterine pathology, Jorden (1603) drew heavily upon ancient authority.

He did not subscribe to Aretaeus's notion of the womb as an 'animal within the animal' (the somatic analogue, perhaps, of Freud's free-floating unconscious, the 'mind within the mind'). He gave some airing to the Hippocratic and Platonic idea of the wandering womb. But Jorden chiefly argued, following Galen, that uterine irregularities — menstrual blockage, amenorrhoea, the retention of putrescent 'seed', and other 'obstructions' — bred 'vapours' rising through the cavities, paining the extremities, abdomen, and even the brain — an effect facilitated by 'sympathies' linking the womb to the head, the seat of the imagination, to the senses, which determined feelings, and, finally, to the 'animal soul', which governed motion — thereby producing the twitchings, paroxysms, palsies, convulsive dancing, stretchings, yawnings, etc., so often misattributed to possession, yet properly explained by 'the mother'.

Noting his belief that 'the perturbations of the minde are oftentimes to blame for this and many other diseases' and his advocacy of therapeutic comfort and counsel, Veith (1965) praises Jorden's precocious psychological understanding. But this is misleading. Jorden's recognition of the complicity of the consciousness was neither new — it was standard humouralist holism — nor properly 'psychogenic'. Jorden's aim, rather, was to establish a *natural* theory, to convince the vulgar, 'who are apt to make every thing a supernaturall work which they do not understand', that Glover's '*passio hysterica*' was a mundane disorder. 'I doe not deny but that God doth in these days worke extraordinarily, for the deliverance of his children, and for other endes best knowne unto himself', he piously insisted,

and that among other, there may be both possessions by the Divell, and obsessions and witchcraft, etc. and dispossession also through the Prayers and supplications of his servants, which is the onely meanes left unto us for our reliefs in that case. But such examples being verie rare now adayes, I would in the feare of God advise men to be very circumspect in pronouncing of a possession: both because the impostures be many, and the effects of naturall diseases be strange to such as have not looked throughly into them.

'Consider a little', he invited readers, 'the signes which some doe shew of a supernaturall power in these examples':

One of their signes is Insensibilitie, when they doe not feele, being pricked with a pin, or burnt with fire, &c. Is this so strange a spectacle, when in the Palsie, the failing sickenesse, Apoplexis, and diverse other diseases, it is dayly observed?

In thus touting constitutional causes, Jorden was a man of his times, as is made clear by the case-books of his contemporary, Richard Napier (MacDonald 1981) and Robert Burton's *Anatomy of melancholy* (1621) (Burton 1948; Babb 1959; Evans 1972). Williams's (1990) recent study of Stuart case histories confirms that medicine simultaneously implicated body, passions, and mind in hysteria diagnoses. After all, upon the Chain of Being man was the great amphibian, a unique, ineffable amalgam of matter and spirit.

The Glover case was not a fist fight between medicine and theology. Jorden's physician rivals found for possession, whereas Jorden himself endorsed the stance adopted by the Anglican hierarchy, who were embarrassed by demoniacal possession, since it provided ready ammunition for Papists and Puritans. In the later climates of Restoration conservatism and Enlightenment rationalism, medics felt powerful professional, as well as political, pressures to promote naturalistic interpretations of marvels and monsters — forwarding Weber's 'demystification of the world', by enlarging the empire of 'disease' and treating it as essentially physical.

Thereby, doctors themselves assumed a certain 'witch-hunting' function.

If Jorden may be seen as a humane defender of Elizabeth Jackson, the profession increasingly saw in hysteria tell-tale signals of moral corruption and erotic danger. It was an outlet for female lasciviousness, frustrated, for example, by widowhood; worse it could turn into the *furor uterinus*, 'metromania', or nymphomania (Rousseau 1982). Thus, the somatization of hysteria proved ambivalent. While exculpating them from diabolism, it incriminated women of possession by a lewdness within.

Hysteria and the woman question   This difficulty applies particularly to the somatic views of hysteria in nineteenth-century psychiatry and gynaecology. As needs no restating, medicine played a prominent part in rationalizing the subordinate position of women within Victorian patriarchy. In such contexts, the concept 'hysterical' could almost become a synonym for 'female', by intimate association with the female reproductive system, especially once greater understanding of ovulation and the menstrual cycle heightened the enigmas of female sexuality. Hysteria became the archetypal disease of female difference (Showalter 1987).

Ever regarded as a charade of disease, hysteria came to be viewed as Eros in disguise. Its swoonings, jerks, and convulsions obscenely simulated arousal, affording surrogate outlets under the cover of sickness. In the throes of a fit, the hysteric was bound to be touched, pampered, and subjected to medical examination and treatment, all recognized as erotically gratifying.

Nineteenth-century gynaecology and psychophysiology blamed the sexual organs for producing a hysteria commonly believed to lead to moral insanity. In 'females who become insane', argued Haslam (1817), apothecary to Bethlem, 'the disease is often connected with the peculiarities of their sex' (pp. 4–5) and Burrows (1828) in particular drew attention to 'various sanguiferous discharges, whether periodical, occasional, or accidental', which 'greatly influence the functions of the mind' (pp. 146–8) Herein lay the key, for 'every body of the least experience must be sensible of the influence of menstruation on the operations of the mind' — 'the uterine action and periodical discharge' affected 'the due equilibrium of the vascular and nervous systems', thereby disrupting 'the cerebral functions'. It was thus no less than the 'moral and physical barometer of the female constitution' (Burrows 1828, p. 146).

Ripeness for childbearing marked the healthy woman. By contrast, Burrows (1828) emphasized, once menstruation were interrupted, for example in amenorrhoea, 'the seeds of various disorders are sown'. Menopause was equally hazardous, where, once again, it was the physiological change that was primary (Burrows 1828, p. 146):

The whole economy of the constitution at that epoch again undergoes a revolution. The moral character, at the age when the menses naturally cease, is much changed to what it was on their first access; and every care or anxiety produces a more depressing and permanent impression on the mind. There is neither so much vital nor mental energy to resist the effects of the various adverse circumstances which it is the lot of most to meet with in the interval between puberty and the critical period.

Nevertheless, here, as elsewhere, physiological changes were exacerbated by typically female character weaknesses, for, suggested Burrows (1828, p. 148), at menopause:

the age of pleasing in all females is then past, though in many the desire to please is not the less lively. The exterior alone loses its attractions, but vanity preserves its pretensions. It is now especially that jealousy exerts its empire, and becomes very often a cause of delirium. Many, too, at this epoch imbibe very enthusiastic religious notions; but more have recourse to the stimulus of strong cordials to allay the uneasy and nervous sensations peculiar to this time of life, and thus produce a degree of excitation equally dangerous to the equanimity of the moral feelings and mental faculties.

The menopause meant double jeopardy.

Hysteria was thus the stigma of the peculiar tribulations of female sexuality: 'Nervous susceptible women between puberty and thirty years of age, and clearly the single more so than the married' judged Burrows (1828), 'are most frequently visited by hysteria'. It often led, he believed, to 'mental derangement, or perhaps epilepsy', for if hysterical fits repeated themselves, 'the brain at length retains the morbid action, and insanity is developed'. In short, 'habitual hysteria clearly approximates to insanity' (Burrows 1828, p. 191).

This 'Hysteric's Progress' from womb to tomb, was imaged most fearfully by that gloomy giant', Henry Maudsley. What were the signs? 'Great restless, rapid and disconnected but not entirely incoherent conversation, sometimes tending to the erotic or obscene . . . laughing, singing, or rhyming, and perverseness of conduct, which is still more or less coherent and seemingly wilful' (Maudsley 1886). What was the cause? It was due to 'the effect of some condition of the reproductive organs on the brain' (Maudsley 1886). Not surprisingly, Maudsley linked hysterical insanity to nymphomania, both of them proceeding from 'the irritation of the ovaries or uterus' (Maudsley 1886, p. 464).

Such misogyny — singling out women and blaming the uterus — was far from confined to these shores. In Germany, Griesinger (1987) regarded hysteria as a disease of the reproductive apparatus, especially local disorders of the uterus, ovaries, and vagina. Certain women shammed hysteria; *authentic* hysteria, however, was somatic, involving the 'morbid action of . . . the brain' (Griesinger 1867; Schiller 1982), generally provoked by vaginal erotic stimulus, itself in turn sparked by menstrual pain, irregularities in the courses, strictures, and stoppages, and exacerbated by masturbation.

Thus, gynaecology and psychological medicine supported that rehabilitation of uterine theories so prominent throughout the nineteenth century, leading to increased surgical interventions: hysterectomy and ovariectomy and, notoriously if exceptionally, clitoridectomy, touted as radical solutions — and even prophylactics — to *mental* disorders no less than to local infections. Faced by the 'woman problem', aggressive medicalization blamed the problem woman.

But if, in certain specialisms, organic theories of hysteria served to pathologize women, it would be a mistake to assume that somatic theories were automatically scapegoating. Consider medicine in Enlightenment Edinburgh. Veith (1965) has deprecated the somatic slant there prominent. Because William Cullen 'clung . . . firmly to the somatic etiology', implicating the uterus once more, his work, she suggests, 'had a retarding effect' (Cullen 1779–1784; Veith 1965, pp. 170, 179; Pinero 1983). Yet this judgment is surely undermined by Guenter Risse's account of the use of the hysteria diagnosis in the Edinburgh Infirmary. Hysteria cases were routinely admitted: women presenting with multiple physical symptoms — breathing and swallowing difficulties, nervous coughs, bronchial problems, menstrual troubles, chest constriction, etc. — exacerbated by emotional irregularities. They were evidently perceived as exhausted, undernourished labouring women, suffering from weakened systems, amenorrhoea, and stress. The hysteria diagnosis secured them recuperative bed-rest, supplemented by a nourishing diet. The organic substrate implied in constituting their hysteria as 'nervous' safeguarded these patients from insinuations of shamming. The supportive treatment accorded them shows that Veith's disappointment at not finding psychogenic theories in Edinburgh teaching is misplaced (Risse 1985, 1988).

In any case, is it clear, as Veith (1965) contends, that psychogenic and psychodynamic theories were less gender stigmatizing? Psychological theories of hysteria largely developed in the context of bourgeois private practice. No surprise. Such practices necessitated protracted, intimate contact with patients, women above all, doubtless veterans of family and medical politics. Drenched in sensibility, affluent sufferers were often introspective, articulate, and vocal in their complaints, rationalizations, and demands. Were not the affinities between the emotional intensities of the bourgeois dolls house and the appearance of hysterical symptoms staring physicians in the face? Maybe, but in their daily practice most doctors refused this association. By professional reflex equating sickness with the somatic, many tacitly chose, presumably for their patients' peace of mind, to render complaints as somatic ailments ('nervous stomach'). A few however, broke with this convention. The consequences were radical.

For, decoding hysteria into a malady of the mind changed the rules of the game at a stroke. Hysteria was reduced from disease to deceit, exculpation became indictment, and a dark psychopathology loomed of the fake hysteric, habitually female. Hysteria as the disease-mimicking disease made way the hysterical woman who pretends to be ill.

Hysteria and theories of psychogenesis   This transformation appears most starkly in the writings of Robert Carter, praised by Veith (1965) for his 'clear insight into the psychopathology of hysteria', a man who, by his 'advanced' discovery of sexual aetiology, helped effect 'a greater stride forward' than 'all the advances made since the beginning of its history'.

Robert Carter   A young Leytonstone general practitioner, Carter published his *Hysteria* in 1853 (Carter 1853; Kane and Carlson 1982). Analysis of all previous theories proved 'the disease itself is too shifting and variable to depend upon any definite change in any individual organ'. Above all, attempts to ground it in 'irritation of the uterus and ovaria [were] ... utterly untenable'. Hysteria, in short, was not somatic at all, but psychological: 'the emotional doctrine affords an easy and complete solution of the difficulty'.

What was it? Drawing upon W.B. Carpenter and other psychophysiologists, Carter (1853) explained that strong emotions find healthy outlet in physical release: tears, laughter, flight, etc. Sexual passions should find natural fulfilment in orgasm. This rarely posed problems for males. In civilized society, however, the double standard commonly denied women such relief. Without such a 'safety valve', women bottled up their longings, suffering what Carter called 'repression'. Crises (for example, a broken engagement) could burst the emotional dam, leading to uncontrollable sobbing, shaking, fits, and temper, providing the relief of what Carter called 'primary hysteria'.

Hysteria did not stop there, however. For 'the suggested or spontaneous remembrance of the emotions' attending the primary fit easily provoked further attacks: 'secondary hysteria'. In this case, medical attendance was prudent, to prevent patients from habituating themselves to its compensatory pleasures, above all, narcissistic attention seeking.

For the danger was that 'tertiary hysteria' would follow, a condition 'designedly excited by the patient herself through ... voluntary recollection, and with perfect knowledge of her own power to produce them' (Carter 1853). It meant the despotism of the ego over others. The tertiary hysteric, in the depths of moral depravity, manipulated all around her, gratifying her whims and basking in the 'fuss and parade of illness' (Carter 1853). Somatically camouflaged, this exercise of will compelled sympathy, free of suspicions of shamming. The greater the sympathy, the greater the tyranny. Hysterics grew expert: 'hair will often be so fastened as to fall at the slightest touch', a testament to the 'ingenuity of the performer' (Carter 1853).

Such a minx, manipulating a 'self-produced disease' wherein the patient herself had full 'power over the paroxysm' and showing a 'mendacity that verges on the sublime', was not, however, easily vanquished. Medical means were futile; psychological warfare needed. The hysteric had to be incarcerated in the physician's home. Once there, under no circumstances should the doctor 'minister to the hysterical desire'. Tantrums, convulsions, fasts, acts of self-mutilation, and, above all, the hysteric's cravings for surrogate sexual gratification, through endless demands for vaginal examinations with a speculum — all had to be ignored.

No holds were barred. The hysteric was mistress of duplicity, hence, the physician would reciprocally be obliged to 'completely deceive her'. And at bottom he had to find tactful ways of communicating that she had been rumbled and her game was up. If done diplomatically, this would allow her to surrender with honour, thereby putting herself 'completely in the power of her interlocutor', after which she might, as the prodigal daughter, be received back into the bosom of the bourgeoisie — whose constraints and double standards, by Carter's own admission, were responsible for hysteria in the first place.

Several aspects of this taming of the shrew deserve attention. Carter (1853) conceived a triangle of elective affinities, pregnant for the future, linking (1) psychological explanation with (2) female nature and (3) a sexual aetiology ('sexual emotions are those most concerned in the production of the disease'). In other words, tertiary hysteria was a matter of *mental* acts (frauds), perpetrated by *women*, to achieve surrogate *sexual* gratification. Was it an accident that the first psychogenic theory of hysteria was misogynistic and victim blaming?

Carter (1853) developed a psychogenic theory of hysteria, viewing the sufferer as manipulating others through body manipulation mimicking true illness, enjoying all the 'secondary gains' of the 'sick role'. Carter, of course, was not Freud and it would be a travesty to liken his image of the wanton malice of the hysterical mind to Freud's grasp of the almost unfathomable cross-purposed dynamics of a multilayered psyche, struggling from birth with desire and denial. Carter might possibly have said with Freud, 'hysterical patients suffer from reminiscences', but he would have meant something radically different. Carter's vixens knew only too well what they are doing, they just wouldn't own up; Freud's hysterics didn't even know what they ought to confess. Nevertheless, the parallels have some resonances.

We have seen hysteria reduced to a somatic complaint and to a psychiatric disorder. In both cases, such a resolution, I suggest, mastered the condition, penalized the patient, and empowered the physician. This was not the inevitable scenario of hysteria. There were other circumstances, other resolutions, depending on other configurations, intellectual, clinical, and social. What were these? Much hinged, of course, upon the socio-economic nexus governing patient and doctor. The wealthier, the more independent, the patient, the more individual moods and needs were respected by the physician; 'hysteria' could there prove a medium for negotiating special sickness entitlements. Such moves are evident in the context of emergent fashionable private practice, as can be gauged from the writings, for instance, of Thomas Sydenham.

Thomas Sydenham and the English disease   By pioneering of the 'natural history' of 'diseases', Sydenham in turn highlighted residues of bizarre and unpredictable symptoms resistant to taxonomic pigeon-holing. These he labelled 'hysteria', thereby delineating disorders without fixed careers, ones whose 'regularity', as it were, lay in their irregularity. 'This disease', he stressed', 'is not more remarkable for its frequency, than for the numerous forms under which it appears, resembling most of the distempers wherewith mankind are afflicted'. Thus. hysteria became anomalous, *sui generis* amongst the ranks of diseases, the diagnostic correlate for *sui generis* patients, authenticating their individuality (Dewhurst 1966; Boss 1979).

Veith (1965) praised Sydenham for psychologizing hysteria: 'the definite inclusion of hysteria itself amongst afflictions of the mind was the contribution of Thomas Sydenham'. His view was, however, more complex. Neither mind nor body had priority; it was an affliction of interaction — neither diabolical nor fanciful, fashionable though not fictional, an ailment with allure, exuding a certain *je ne sais quoi* which, because its essence was held in suspension, could exercise fascination over both patient and physician. It remained tactful, however, as George Cheyne was to emphasize, for the physician to give a certain somatic anchorage to his diagnosis — 'hysterick colic' or 'hysterick gout' — to reassure patients that it was not hinted their conditions were imaginary (Cheyne 1722, 1733, 1740, 1742).

This suspension of aetiologizing pervades Enlightenment discussions. As imputations of diabolism were dispelled, pressures upon medics to anchor 'hysteria' in the womb likewise receded. Rather physicians explored sympathetic symbioses and what Whytt (1767) called the 'laws of union between the soul and the body', emphasizing how the 'shapes of *proteus*, or the colours of the *chameleon*, are not more numerous and inconstant, than the varieties of the hypochondriac and hysteric disease'. If Enlightenment thinkers professed bafflement at the Sphinxian riddles of psyche-soma affinities — 'the action of the mind on the body, and of the body on the mind', noted an authority on madness, 'after all that has been written, is as little understood, as it is universally felt' — such ontological equivocations, such suspended judgments, were what the doctor ordered in the context of a private practice in which, as Jewson (1974, 1976) has stressed, some parity governed patient–practitioner relationships. In other words, the historial sociology of Enlightenment hysteria is epitomized by the clinical encounter between sensitive patient and sympathetic physician. It was elitist and, not least, it was, in essence, unisex.

The industrial age This clinical rapport between fashionable doctors and wealthy patients did not lapse in 1800: far from it. The private practices of a Sydenham or a Heberden found their successors — capitalized, organized, and bureaucratized as befitted the industrial age — in the rest-cure 'clinics', 'spas', and 'sanatoria' devoted to neurasthenia mushrooming in the late nineteenth century. From Baglivi to Beard, from Mandeville to Weir Mitchell, the astute clinician knew that the hysteric's prime needs were escape and attention, rest and recuperation, strengthening — physical, moral, and mental alike. Hysteria was their first protection; the sympathetic physician their second. No wonder Weir Mitchell spoke of 'mysteria' (Mitchell 1877, 1881, 1888; Walter 1970; Levin 1971).

This parity, this tension or suspension, between patient and practitioner, medicalized in the nervous theory of hysteria, was mirrored, odd as it may seem, by Charcot's practice at the Salpêtrière. Surely a preposterous idea! After all, was not Charcot the Napoleon of the neuroses, his patients working-class waifs? Surely Charcot had the power to reduce his hysterical patients to silly shammers or inflamed wombs?

But he didn't. For Charcot needed his Blanche Wittmans no less than they needed him. His claim to fame, his career, lay not in demystifying hysteria but in displaying it, showing off its every twist and turn (like a good magician, he never explained his tricks). Hence, Charcot had to preserve its mystery in the only way a positivist knew, by approaching it from the viewpoint of patho-anatomy, insisting that it was grounded in the organization of the nervous constitution and tracking its laws. If Sydenham had seen hysteria as the *exception* to the natural history of diseases, the positivist Charcot, by contrast, believed he could incorporate it within such a taxonomy.

Conclusion

In this chapter, I have not addressed the question of why people 'somatize'. This may itself be a highly dubious notion, freighted with questionable psychodynamic and psychosomatic prejudices — though I certainly agree that suffering and sufferers' symptom repertoires demand more attention than I have afforded them. My concern, rather, has been to argue that hysteria and other medically unexplained symptoms could be fashioned as disorders, precisely because the general culture created images of tense and ambiguous relations between representations of mind and body, which were reproduced in the hierarchical yet interactive ontologies of morality and medicine and in their turn reflected by the social realities of doctor-patient clinical encounters. In hysteria, as with other disorders, different fields of force break in distinctive ways. Sometimes medicine's mission has been reductionist, resolving hysteria now into the womb, now into mere wilfulness. In other circumstances, medicine seeks to render hysteria real, protecting its mysteries. In hysteria, mind and body may be seen as sublimations of doctors and patients.

From this one major conclusion suggests itself. History shows the rise and fall of various medically unexplained symptoms. These may, perhaps, appear and disappear for authentic biomedical reasons. They may also come and go because of profound general social changes (for example, the domestication and then the emancipation of women). But they also arise and then repeat themselves, because of psychosocial aspects of the culture of medical and of clinical set-ups. Medically unexplained symptoms can thus also be artefacts of clinical encounters. In that respect, the medicine of each era gets the functional symptoms it deserves.

References

Abse, D.W. (1987). *Hysteria and related mental disorders*. Wright, Bristol.

Adorno, T.T. and Horkheimer, M. (1972). *Dialectic of enlightenment*. Herder and Herder, New York.

Anglo, S. (ed.) (1977). *The damned art. Essays in the literature of witchcraft*. Routledge and Kegan Paul, London.

Babb, L. (1959). *Sanity in bedlam: a study of Robert Burton's anatomy of melancholy*. Michigan State University Press, East Lansing.

Boss, J.M.N. (1979). The seventeenth-century transformation of the hysteria affection, and Sydenham's Baconian medicine. *Psychological Medicine*, 9, 221–34.

Bottomley, F. (1979). *Attitudes to the body in Western Christendom*. Lepus Books, London.

Brais, B. (1990). The making of a famous nineteenth century neurologist: Jean-Martin Charcot (1825–1893). M Phil thesis, University College, London.

Brown, P. (1988). *The body and society: men, women and sexual renunciation in early Christianity*. Columbia University Press, New York.

Buchan, W. (1769). *Domestic medicine, or a treatise on the prevention and cure of diseases by regimen and simple medicines*, p. 561. Balyou, Auld, & Smellie, Edinburgh.

Burrows, G.M. (1828). *Commentaries on insanity*. Underwood, London.

Burton, R. (1948). *The anatomy of melancholy*, (ed. F. Dell and P. Jordan-Smith). Tudor Publishing Co., New York.

Bynum, W.F. (1985). The nervous patient in eighteenth and nineteenth century

Britain. The psychiatric origins of British neurology. In *Anatomy of madness*, i, (ed. W.F. Bynum, R. Porter, and M. Shepherd), pp. 89–102. Tavistock, London.

Carroy-Thirard, J. (1980). Possession, Extase, Hystérie au XIX siècle. *Psychanalyse a l'Université*, 499–515.

Carroy-Thirard, J. (1981). *Le Mal de Morzine. De la Possession a l'hystérie*. Soin, Paris.

Carter, R.B. (1853). *On the pathology and treatment of hysteria*. John Churchill, London.

Charcot, J.-M. and Richer, P. (1887). *Les Démoniques dans l'art*. Delahaye and Lecrosnier, Paris.

Cheyne, G. (1722). *An essay of the true nature and due method of treating the gout*. G. Strahan, London.

Cheyne, G. (1733). *The English malady; or, a treatise of nervous diseases*. G. Strahan, London. Reprinted (1990), (ed. R. Porter). Routledge, London.

Cheyne, G. (1740). *An essay on regimen*. C. Rivington, London.

Cheyne, G. (1742). *The natural method of cureing diseases of the body and the disorders of the mind*. G. Strahan, London.

Clark, M. (1981). The rejection of psychological approaches to mental disorder in late nineteenth century British psychiatry. In *Madhouses, mad-doctors and madmen*, (ed. A. Scull), pp. 271–312. Athlone Press, London.

Clark, M. (1988). 'Morbid introspection', unsoundness of mind, and British psychological medicine, c. 1830–1900. In *Anatomy of madness*, iii, (ed. W.F. Bynum, R. Porter, and M. Shepherd), pp. 71–101. Routledge, London.

Critchley, E.M.R. and Cantor, H.E. (1984). Charcot's hysteria renaissant. *British Medical Journal*, **289**, 1785–8.

Cullen, W. (1779–1784). *First lines in the practice of physic*, 2 vols. Creech, Edinburgh.

Dewhurst, K. (1966). *Dr Sydenham 1624–1689*. University of California Press, Berkeley.

Elias, N. (1983). *The civilizing process*. Basil Blackwell, Oxford.

Ellenberger, H.T. (1970). *The discovery of the unconscious*. Allen Lane, London.

Entralgo, P.L. (1955). *Mind and body*. Harvill, London.

Evans, B. (1972). *The psychiatry of Robert Burton*. Octagon Books, New York.

Ey, H. (1982). Hysteria: history and analysis of the concept. In *Hysteria*, (ed. A Roy), pp. 3–19. John Lesley and Sons, Chichester.

Foucault, M. (1979). *Discipline and punish*. Penguin, Harmondsworth.

Gay, P. (1988). *Freud. A life for our time*. Dent, London.

Goldstein, J. (1982). The hysteria diagnosis and the politics of anticlericalism in late nineteenth century France. *Journal of Modern History*, **54**, 209–39.

Goldstein, J. (1987). *Console and classify. The French psychiatric profession in the nineteenth century*. Cambridge University Press, Cambridge.

Griesinger, W. (1867). *Mental pathology and therapeutics*, (trans. C.L. Robertson and J. Rutherford). New Sydenham Society, London.

Griggs, E.L. (ed.) (1956). *Collected letters of Samuel Taylor Coleridge*, i. Clarendon Press, Oxford.

Haslam, J. (1817). *Considerations on the moral management of insane persons*. R. Hunter, London.

Hunter, R. and Macalpine, I. (1963). *Three hundred years of psychiatry, 1535–1860*, p. 473. Oxford University Press, London.

Jewson, N. (1974). Medical knowledge and the patronage system in eighteenth century England. *Sociology*, **8**, 369–85.

Jewson, N. (1976). The disappearance of the sick man from medical cosmology 1770–1870. *Sociology*, **10**, 225–44.

Jorden, E. (1603). *A briefe discourse of a disease called the suffocation of the mother. Written uppon occasion which hath beene of late taken thereby, to suspect possession of an evill spirit, or some such like supernaturall power. Wherein is declare that divers strange actions and passions of the body of man, which in the common opinion are imputed to the Divill, have their true naturall causes, and do accompany this disease.* John Windet, London. Reprinted (1990) with an introduction by Michael MacDonald. Routledge, London.

Kane, A. and Carlson, E. (1982). A different drummer: Robert B. Carter on nineteenth century hysteria. *Bulletin of the New York Academy of Medicine*, **58**, 519–34.

King, H. (1985). From Parthenos to Gyne. The dynamics of category. PhD thesis, University of London.

Knight, I.F. (1984). Freud's *Project*: a theory for *Studies on Hysteria. Journal of the History of the Behavioral Sciences*, **20**, 340–58.

Krohn, A. (1978). Hysteria: the elusive neurosis. *Psychological Issues*, **45/46**. International Universities Press, New York.

Levin, K. (1971). S. Weir Mitchell: investigations and insights into neurasthenia and hysteria. *Transactions and Studies of the College of Physicians of Philadelphia*, **38**, 168–73.

MacDonald, M. (1981). *Mystical Bedlam: madness, anxiety and healing in seventeenth century England*. Cambridge University Press, Cambridge.

McGrath, W.J. (1986). *Freud's discovery of psychoanalysis. The politics of hysteria*. Cornell University Press, Ithaca.

Maire, C.-L. (1981). *Les Posedées de Morzine 1857–1873*. Presses Universitaires de Lyons, Lyons.

Major, R. (1974). The revolution of hysteria. *International Journal of Psycho-Analysis*, **55**, 385–92.

Maudsley, H. (1886). *The pathology of mind*. Appleton, New York.

Merskey, H. (1983). Hysteria: the history of an idea. *Canadian Journal of Psychiatry*, **28**, 428–33.

Merskey, H. (1986). The importance of hysteria. *British Journal of Psychiatry*, **149**, 23–8.

Micale, M. (1989a). Hysteria and its historiography: a review of past and present writings (part 1). *History of Science*, **27**, 223–61.

Micale, M. (1989b). Hysteria and its historiography: a review of past and present writings (part 2). *History of Science*, **27**, 319–50.

Micale, M. (1990). Hysteria and its historiography: the future perspective. *History of Psychiatry*, **1**, 33–124.

Mitchell, S. Weir (1877). *Fat and blood. An essay on the treatment of certain forms of neurasthenia and hysteria*. Lippincott, Philadelphia.

Mitchell, S. Weir (1881). *Lectures on the diseases of the nervous system, especially in women.* Lea, Philadelphia.

Mitchell, S. Weir (1888). *Doctor and patient.* Lippincott. Philadelphia.

Palis, J., Rossopoulos, E., and Triarkou, L.-C. (1985). The Hippocratic concept of hysteria: a translation of the original texts. *Integrative Psychiatry,* **3**, 226-8.

Piñero, J.M.L. (1983). *Historical origins of the concept of neurosis,* (trans. D. Berrios). Cambridge University Press, Cambridge.

Porter, R. (1990). Barely touching: a social perspective on mind and body. In *The languages of psyche. Mind and body in enlightenment thought,* (ed G.S. Rousseau), pp. 45-80. University of California Press, Berkeley.

Risse, G. (1985). *Hospital life in enlightenment Scotland.* Cambridge University Press, Cambridge.

Risse, G. (1988). Hysteria at the Edinburgh infirmary: the construction and treatment of a disease, 1770-1800. *Medical History,* **32**, 1-22.

Rousseau, G.S. (1982). Nymphomania, Bienville and the rise of erotic sensibility. In *Sexuality in eighteenth-century Britain,* (ed. P.-G. Boucé), pp. 95-120. Manchester University Press, Manchester.

Roy. A. (ed.) (1982). *Hysteria.* John Wiley and Sons, Chichester.

Rubinstein, B.B. (1983). Freud's early theories of hysteria. In *Physics, philosophy and psychoanalysis: essays in honor of Adolf Grünbaum,* (ed. R.S. Cohen and L. Laudan), pp. 169-90. D. Reidel, Dordrecht.

Schiller, F. (1982). *A Moebius strip. Fin de siècle neuropsychiatry and Paul Moebius.* University of California Press, Berkeley.

Shorter, E. (1992). *From paralysis to fatigue. A history of psychosomatic illness in the modern era.* Free Press, New York.

Showalter, E. (1987). *The female malady. Women, madness and English culture, 1830-1980.* Virago, London.

Stallybrass, P. and White, A. (1986). Bourgeois hysteria and the carnivalesque. In *The politics and poetics of transgression,* pp. 171-90. Methuen, London.

Sulloway, F. (1979). *Freud. Biologist of the mind.* Basic Books, New York.

Szasz, T. (1961). *The myth of mental illness.* Paladin, New York.

Trillat, E. (1986). *Histoire de l'hystérie.* Seghers, Paris.

Veith, I. (1965). *Hysteria. The history of a disease.* University of Chicago Press, Chicago.

Walter, R.D. (1970). *S. Weir Mitchell, MD, neurologist. A medical biography.* Thomas, Springfield, II.

Whyte, L.L. (1962). *The unconscious before Freud.* Doubleday, New York.

Whytt, R. (1767). *Observations on the nature, causes and cure of those disorders which have been commonly called nervous, hypochondriac, or hysteric.* Balfour, Edinburgh.

Williams, K.E. (1990). Hysteria in seventeenth century primary sources. *History of Psychiatry,* **1**, 383-401.

Willis, T. (1684). *Essay of the pathology of the Brain,* p. 69.

3 Overview of epidemiology, classification, and aetiology

Richard Mayou, Christopher Bass, and Michael Sharpe

The editors emphasize the need to take a comprehensive view of the many types of acute and chronic functional symptoms which occur both in the general population and in all medical settings. They suggest that existing psychiatric and other classifications are inadequate and restrict and distort discussion. Instead it is proposed that functional symptoms can be more satisfactorily classified in terms of five separate dimensions. The aetiology of functional somatic symptoms is reviewed and a multicausal and an interactive model, which includes both physical and psychological factors, is proposed. This approach avoids arbitrary distinctions between organic and psychological causations. Variants of this model are implicit in most of the other chapters in this book.

Introduction

The experience of changes in bodily perceptions and functions is part of daily life. Usually these sensations are transient and cause little concern or disability, but a small proportion are regarded as symptoms of illness. Symptoms are 'perceptible changes in the body or its functions indicating disease' (Oxford English Dictionary). This definition encompasses two elements: first, a perception of change in the body or its function and, second, an interpretation of that symptom as indicating disease. Only a small proportion of such changes are regarded by the person experiencing them as evidence of disease, that is, as a *symptom*. Mechanic (1980) has pointed out that the process of coming to regard a bodily change as a symptom is not a simple mechanical one, but a complex process that is influenced by upbringing, psychosocial stress, and physiological state.

Once a person regards him/herself as symptomatic he or she may respond in a number of ways. These responses include ignoring the symptom or making minor life-style adjustments such as an increase in exercise or a change in diet. Alternatively, the person may perceive himself or herself as ill and seek exemption from daily duties, a diagnosis, and treatment. Most people who experience symptoms take no action unless the symptom affects their functioning, or provokes fear of serious disease. Sometimes, friends and relatives are consulted, frequently self-medication

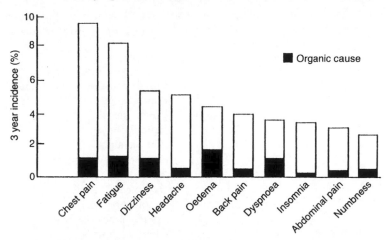

Fig. 3.1 Three year incidence of ten common symptoms and proportion of symptoms with suspected organic disease (Kroenke and Mangelsdorff 1989)

is used, and occasionally treatment is sought from practitioners of complementary medicine. Only a minority will seek a medical consultation.

To summarize, whilst the perception of bodily changes is a universal and almost daily experience, only a small proportion of such changes come to be regarded as symptoms of illness and an even smaller proportion result in a medical consultation. Of those symptoms presented to doctors only a minority can be explained by organic disease (Kroenke and Mangelsdorff 1989) (Fig. 3.1).

In this chapter we review the prevalence of functional complaints, the difficulties encountered in attempts to classify them, and their aetiology.

Epidemiology of functional symptoms

Epidemiological studies have been concerned with a wide range of complaints (not all of them accepted as functional) (Table 3.1), with multiple symptoms, and also with numerous alleged syndromes such as compensation neurosis, post-concussional neurosis, multiple allergy (see Chapter 16), and repetitive strain injury. Other chapters consider specific aspects of epidemiology; this chapter is concerned with the overall picture.

General population

Everyone experiences changes in their bodies that do not result from organic disease (Crook *et al.* 1984; Von Korff *et al.* 1988). Between 80 and

Table 3.1 Range of specific symptoms (and syndromes) studied in epidemiological surveys of patients with functional somatic syndromes

Pain	Tinnitus
Low back	Repetitive strain injury
Neck	Post-concussional syndrome
Chest	Fibromyalgia
Abdomen	Premenstrual tension
Headache	Irritable bowel syndrome
Mastalgia	Fibromyalgia
Pelvic	Conversion, dissociative symptoms
Facial	Breathlessness
Palpitations	Dysphagia
Dizziness	Dysmenorrhoea
Fatigue	Epidemic health anxiety
Non-ulcer dyspepsia	Factitious injuries

90 per cent of the general population experience at least one symptom per week (Anderson *et al.* 1968; Hannay 1978). However, research studies have typically not clearly differentiated between bodily changes accepted as having no special significance and those of sufficient concern to be regarded as symptoms.

Von Korff *et al.* (1988) found that 41 per cent of enrollees in a large health maintenance organization in the USA reported suffering back pain in the previous 6 months, 26 per cent headaches, 17 per cent abdominal pain, 12 per cent chest pain, and 12 per cent facial pain. Although the complaints were mainly of no more than mild to moderate intensity and did not usually limit activities, up to 40 per cent of subjects reported days during the the six month period when they had been unable to carry out their usual activities, because of the pain. Analysis of data gathered in the American Epidemiologic Catchment Area (ECA) study revealed that approximately one-quarter of the general population had suffered at least one of each of a number of somatic symptoms at some time in their lives. In each case the symptom was of sufficient concern for the patient to do something, such as taking medicine, changing diet or life-style, or con-sulting a doctor (Kroenke and Price 1993) (Table 3.2). Furthermore, these figures are undoubtedly an underestimate of the extent of functional symptoms both because of the difficulties that lay interviewers and patients have in defining 'functional' and because the Diagnostic Interview Schedule does not distinguish between acute episodes and chronic illness.

It was common for individuals in the ECA study to report multiple somatic symptoms. The prevalence of the DSM-IIIR (Diagnostic and Sta-tistical Manual, 3rd edition, revised) category of multiple chronic symp-toms (somatization disorder), was 0.38 and 4.4 per cent (depending on the number of symptoms required) (Swartz *et al.* 1986; Escobar *et al.* 1989).

Table 3.2 Lifetime prevalence of functional somatic symptoms from ECA study (Kroenke and Price 1993)

Symptom	Per cent
Joint pains	37
Back pain	32
Headache	25
Fatigue	25
Chest pain	25
Arm and leg pain	24
Abdominal pain	24
Dizziness	23

Only a minority of symptoms result in consultation. Banks *et al.* (1975) found that in a health diary study of women aged 20–44 years, on average, women reported symptoms as occurring on 10 out of 28 days, but they only consulted a doctor once for every 37 symptom episodes. Another surprising finding was that there was no clear association between the *frequency* of a symptom and medical consultation. For example, of 184 episodes of headache only one resulted in medical consultation, compared with one in 14 episodes of chest pain. The implication is that many symptoms are perceived as mild and relatively unobtrusive, and factors other than the frequency of the symptoms determine whether people interpret bodily sensations as a sign of illness (see Craig and Boardman 1990). The processes which result in consultation with doctors have also been studied in relation to specific symptoms and syndromes such as the irritable bowel syndrome (Drossman and Thompson 1992) (see also Chapter 14).

Primary care

As many as one in five new consultations in primary care are for somatic symptoms for which no specific cause can be found (Bridges and Goldberg 1985). Whilst many complaints are transient, a sizeable proportion are persistent and associated with both distress and considerable use of medical resources (Craig *et al.* 1993).

In a series of reports from a primary care internal medicine clinic at a US Army Medical Centre, Kroenke and his colleagues (Kroenke and Mangelsdorff 1989; Kroenke *et al.* 1990; Kroenke 1992) described the frequency of 14 common non-specific symptoms. The most striking findings were that less than one in five patients with such complaints were given an organic diagnosis and that many patients were dissatisfied at not receiving 'helpful' therapy. The cost of investigating these symptoms was considerable.

Emergency departments

Patients frequently present to hospital emergency departments with acute symptoms for which no physical cause is found. A small proportion are admitted for further investigation of certain symptoms, particularly chest (Lee *et al.* 1992) and abdominal pain (Gray and Collin 1987).

Hospital out-patient clinics

Non-specific physical complaints are among the commonest reasons for out-patient referral from primary care in the United Kingdom (Bradlow *et al.* 1992).

Most of these patients do not receive a specific psychological diagnosis however (Mayou and Hawton 1986). Van Hemert *et al.* (1993) assessed 191 newly referred medical out-patients and diagnosed psychiatric disorder in 38 per cent of those who presented with 'unexplained' physical complaints, as compared with 15 per cent of those with clear evidence of organic disease. Functional complaints are especially frequent in certain specialist clinics, in particular abdominal and bowel symptoms in gastroenterology clinics and chest pain and palpitations in cardiac out-patients. They are notably common among patients referred to pain clinics (Benjamin and Eminson 1992; Keefe *et al.* 1992).

Contrary to what many physicians believe, follow-up studies suggest that many patients who present to out-patient clinics with worry about physical problems are *not* reassured by negative physical investigations. In particular, the subgroup with multiple somatic complaints are difficult to reassure and use very considerable amounts of general hospital care over long periods of time (de Gruy *et al.* 1987; Katon *et al.* 1990).

Hospital in-patient units

The proportion of hospital in-patients with predominantly functional complaints would appear to be low. Non-specific symptom diagnoses are made for a small minority of discharges of in-patients, (between 1 and 2 per cent of all discharges in Oxford). However, such patients frequently report persistent symptoms and have a greater than expected use of subsequent psychiatric care. In a linked case register study Mayou *et al.* (1991) found that patients discharged from general hospitals with several types of non-specific physical diagnoses used psychiatric services at rates considerably greater than that expected for the population in the year before, and in the year following the index general hospital admission. The nature and extent of this morbidity has been particularly well demonstrated following normal coronary angiograms (Chambers and Bass 1990; Potts and Bass 1993).

Although the number of patients is small, they consume a considerable amount of medical resources. Fink (1992*a*,*b*) used Danish case registers to document the use of medical and surgical treatment resources used by the relatively small number of patients who, during an 8-year period, were admitted at least ten times to general hospitals for physical symptoms for which no organic case was found. They had consumed 3 per cent of the budget for admissions to non-psychiatric departments. Interestingly, one-fifth of these patients were admitted at least once for a factitious disorder. From these findings, the estimated frequency of persistent multiple functional complaints (somatization disorder) in the general population was 0.6 per 1000 in men and 3.2 per 1000 in women. These figures are remarkably similar to the prevalence reported in the American ECA study (Escobar *et al.* 1989).

Consultation–liaison services

All accounts of consecutive consultations by consultation–liaison (CL) services (Katon *et al.* 1984; Slavney and Teitelbaum 1985) have noted that the assessment of unexplained physical symptoms is among the most common reasons for referral. These symptoms are much more often associated with anxiety and depression than with somatoform disorders (Katon *et al.* 1984; de Leon *et al.* 1987; Snyder and Strain 1989). However, it is worth recalling that most CL units concentrate on in-patients, whereas medically unexplained symptoms are more common in medical out-patients. There have been few accounts of CL out-patient services (Fava *et al.* 1987).

Classification

Patients with medically unexplained symptoms have never been satisfactorily accommodated in either medical or psychiatric classifications. As a result physicians and psychiatrists have used different terms and diagnoses (see Chapter 1).

Physicians' 'syndrome descriptions' have reflected their specialist interests, for example irritable bowel syndrome (Manning *et al.* 1978), hyperventilation syndrome (Lum 1976), fibromyalgia syndrome (Yunus 1989); chronic pelvic pain (Beard and Reginald 1990), and non-specific abdominal pain (Gray and Collin 1987). These syndromal diagnoses overlap however, especially if studied in community settings (Kirmayer and Robbins 1991*b*).

Psychiatrists, on the other hand, have focused on associated psychological symptoms and used standard psychiatric diagnostic categories.

Table 3.3 Psychiatric disorder and functional somatic symptoms

No psychiatric disorder	Major depression
General anxiety	Somatoform disorder
Panic disorder	Factitious disorder

The psychiatric classifications

The International Classification of Disease (ICD-IO) and DSM-IV psychiatric classifications are not well suited to the classification of functional symptoms (Table 3.3). There are two general difficulties.

1. The clinical descriptions of specific psychiatric disorders are derived from hospital-based experience and are not applicable to the large number of people with functional complaints in community and primary care settings. Most of these have subthreshold emotional problems or adjustment disorders of less than 6 months duration. This means the glossaries do not satisfactorily accommodate the vast majority of patients.

2. Medically unexplained symptoms can occur in the *absence* of psychiatric diagnosis (especially in primary care), even though abnormal illness beliefs and pathophysiological processes may be apparent.

Somatoform disorder   In patients with functional somatic symptoms, the traditional psychiatric syndromes of anxiety, panic disorder, and depression can frequently be diagnosed, but some patients with apparent psychiatric disorder are more difficult to categorize. One approach has been to suggest that somatization is an atypical presentation of a traditional psychiatric syndrome, especially depression. This device is unproven and unsatisfactory. Another approach is to regard them as suffering from somatoform disorders. The American Psychiatric Association introduced this new class of psychiatric disorder in DSM-III with the essential feature of 'physical symptoms suggesting physical disorder for which there are no demonstrable organic findings or known physiological mechanisms and for which there is positive evidence, or a strong presumption, that the symptoms are linked to psychological factors or conflicts'. The ICD-10 has followed the American lead. Unfortunately, despite the recent close collaboration in the preparation of ICD-10 and DSM-IV, differences have arisen between the two classifications of somatoform disorders (Table 3.4).

Furthermore, there are serious difficulties with the *concept* of somatoform disorder.

Table 3.4 Somatoform disorders in DSM-IV and ICD-10

DSM-IV	ICD-10
Somatoform disorder	Multiple somatization disorder
Conversion disorder	–
Hypochondriasis	Hypochondriasis
Body dysmorphic disorder	–
Pain disorder	Pain syndromes without specific organic
Undifferentiated somatoform disorder	cause
	Undifferentiated somatoform disorder
Somatoform disorder. Not otherwise specified	Other psychogenic disorders of sensation, function, and behaviour
	Psychogenic autonomic dysfunction

1. The lack of any clear operational definition of the whole category and the haphazard division of subcategories. Many of the defining concepts, including medical help-seeking behaviour, number of somatic symptoms, and hypochondrial attitudes are better described in *dimensional* rather than categorical terms.

2. Some of the types of somatoform disorders are so chronic and enduring (especially body dysmorphic disorder, hypochondriasis, and somatization disorder) that it would make more sense to classify them as personality disorders (axis 2), than as mental state disorders (axis 1). Hypochondrial attitudes and behaviours are chronic maladaptive patterns which begin early and continue throughout life (Tyrer *et al.* 1990.)

3. Most patients have clinical features which fit criteria for several diagnostic categories simultaneously (somatoform and other disorders).

Specific subcategories of somatoform disorder

1. Conversion disorder. The diagnostic criteria for conversion disorder (CD) include the presence of psychological conflicts and primary and secondary gain. However, emotional stress before onset, secondary gain, improvement with suggestion or sedation, histrionic personality, and *la belle indifference* all fail to predict the absence of physical disease in patients suspected of having conversion disorder (Cloninger 1986).

2. Hypochondriasis. In contrast to non-specialist usage, hypochondriasis is defined by both DSM-IV and ICD-10 in very narrow terms. It is frequently uncertain that the criterion of 'appropriate medical evalua-

tion and reassurance' has been satisfied. Individual hypochondriacal symptoms occur in many psychiatric syndromes, most commonly anxiety and depression. A number of workers have reported variants of DSM hypochondriasis. Barsky *et al.* (1992) have described more transient forms, and Kellner (1991) refers to recurrent hypochondriasis. Barsky and colleagues (1992) also noted considerable co-morbidity and also provided empirical support for primary and secondary types of this disorder. Continuing uncertainty about the status of this category means that it is rarely used in general medical practice (Noyes *et al.* 1993).

3. Body dysmorphic disorder. DSM-IIIR introduced a category of patients who present with 'excessive concern' about a trivial or non-existent physical abnormality, which they believe renders them misshapen or ugly. But neither DSM-IIIR nor DSM-IV criteria guide the clinician in judging what is excessive concern. Such judgements are not medical but aesthetic and are likely to vary between doctors.

4. Somatization disorder. There is no doubt that the diagnostic criteria for the subcategory of somatization disorder (SD) are too restrictive for clinical use, particularly outside the USA (Deighton and Nichol 1985; Escobar *et al.* 1989). As a consequence many patients with chronic functional complaints end up in a residual category (undifferentiated somatoform disorder), which clinicians and researchers are understandably reluctant to use to classify a common clinical problem. Modifications in DSM-IV fail to solve this problem.

5. Pain disorder. In many ways this is the most unsatisfactory somatoform category since it is limited to symptoms of pain. DSM-IIIR required the presence of 'preoccupation with pain', but offered no guidance about the meaning of this term, leaving it open to individual interpretation. Furthermore, clinicians and researchers encounter problems in attempting to determine whether the patient's pain exceeds what would be expected. DSM-IV requires that: 'Psychological factors are judged to have an important role in the onset, severity, exacerbation, or maintenance of the pain.' The diagnosis also excludes the large number of patients with acute pain for which there is also substantial evidence of the role of psychological factors (Phillips and Grant 1992). King and Strain (1992) have proposed a new diagnostic grouping for pain, which takes account of the contribution of psychological and organic factors, as well as the duration of pain.

6. Factitious disorder. This uncommon, but certainly under-recognized,

disorder results in considerable morbidity and substantial use of health resources. It is most often diagnosed in hospital settings following prolonged investigation, but less severe forms are probably not uncommon in primary care. It is an important differential diagnosis of functional somatic symptoms, but it is not considered further in this book (see Sutherland and Rodin 1990).

A proposed new multidimensional classification

We conclude that existing classifications are unsatisfactory. They are based either on psychiatric systems (such as DSM and ICD) which are not comprehensive and result in multiple, inconsistent, poorly defined diagnoses, or on medical syndromes (such as irritable bowel syndrome and chronic fatigue syndrome) of doubtful specificity and homogeneity. These problems are well illustrated in a study by Kirmayer and Robbins (1991*b*) who found three types of somatization associated with different sociodemographic and illness behaviour characteristics

1. *Functional somatization*, that is, high levels of functional somatic distress, measured by the Somatic Symptom Index (SSI) of the Diagnostic Interview Schedule (DIS).

2. *Hypochondriasis*, that is, elevated scores on an 'illness worry' scale in the absence of serious ilness.

3. *Exclusive somatic presentations* in patients with current major depression or anxiety.

We advocate a multidimensional classification based in part on the three-systems model of Lang (1978) for anxiety disorders, and on the work of Kirmayer and Robbins (1991*a*) in primary care. Although many dimensions might be considered, we suggest that five deserve special attention (Table 3.5). Disorders are classified as acute (less than 6 months duration) or chronic (greater than 6 months) and then coded on each of five dimensions. This system may be used to assess individual patients and guide treatment. It may also provide the basis for a revised classificatory system.

Aetiology

The pursuit of single specific cause for hypothetical functional syndromes has resulted in many futile controversies. For example, the explanations of non-cardiac chest pain have included panic disorder (Beitman *et al*. 1988), oesophageal spasm (Swift *et al*. 1991), and microvascular angina

Table 3.5 Proposed multidimensional classification of patients with functional somatic symptoms

---

1. Somatic symptoms
   Number of symptoms (single system, multiple systems)
   Type (for example, sensory, motor)

2. Mental state
   Depression
   Anxiety and panic
   Other psychiatric disorder

3. Cognitions
   Fear of disease
   Conviction of disease

4. Behaviour and functional impairment
   Avoidance
   Illness behaviour
   Use of health services

5. Pathophysiological disturbance
   Identifiable mechanisms (for example, hyperventilation, vasospasm)
   Organic disease

Disorders are classified as acute (less than 6 months' duration) or chronic (greater than 6 months) and then coded on each of the five dimensions.

(Cannon 1988). In fact it is more likely that multiple factors interact and that all the factors mentioned above may make a contribution. We (and the contributors to this book) therefore prefer a multicausal, interactive aetiological model, which includes biological and psychological and social factors. The use of the model in clinical formulation is discussed in Chapter 10.

In many cases there will be an interaction between

(1) normal and/or abnormal physiological processes, for example, extrasystoles or tremulousness induced by caffeine;

(2) psychological factors; that is, the way in which the somatic sensations are perceived, interpreted and acted upon;

(3) the behaviour and reactions of doctors and others.

Table 3.6 lists aetological factors under the groupings of predisposing, precipitating, and perpetuating.

Table 3.6 Aetiological factors

Predisposing factors
  Genetic
  Personality traits, for example excessive health consciousness
  Illness beliefs
    Childhood experience and family attitudes to illness
    Knowledge and beliefs about illness
  Major physical illness

Precipitating factors
  Physiological and pathological factors
    Minor physical pathology
    Benign tissue lumps and inconsistencies
    Arousal: benign and hormonal
    Muscle tension
    Hyperventilation
    Inactivity
    Poor sleep
    Physiological consequences of diet, alcohol
    Side-effects of medication
  Epidemic health anxiety
  Psychiatric disorder
  Stressful events
  Chronic difficulties
  Social support
  Problems in coping

Perpetuating factors
  Psychiatric disorder (primary or secondary)
  Continuing physical and psychological factors

  Reactions of others:
    Lack of confidants
    Relatives and friends
    Iatrogenic medicine
    Other therapists, for example complementary medicine
    Litigation and financial gain

Genetic factors

It has been claimed that certain somatoform syndromes are associated with psychopathology in a biological parent (Cloninger 1986). Although familial associations between somatization, alcohol abuse, and antisocial personality have been noted in a number of studies, genetic transmission is not proven (Bohman *et al.* 1984).

Personality

Personality may also predispose to the development of functional somatic symptoms. Excessive health concern is a common personality trait which is frequently associated with repeated seeking of reassurance from doctors. For example, patients with a tendency to introspection and anxiousness, characterized by Watson and Pennebaker (1991) as 'negative affectivity', have higher rates of somatic symptoms reporting during their lifetimes (Costa and McCrae 1985). Tyrer *et al.* (1990) have argued the need for a category of hypochondriacal personality disorder for which there is some empirical support.

Illness beliefs

Childhood experience   There are several retrospective studies that suggest that adults who report functional somatic symptoms have witnessed more physical illness in family members. This includes an excess of

(1)   somatic complaints by parents;

(2)   illness or complaints of illness in the family generally;

(3)   family complaints of pain;

(4)   a history of family members with physical handicap and deformity (Blumer and Heilbron 1981; Hartwig and Sterner 1985).

Particularly striking is the similarity between children's symptoms and those of their parents — especially for abdominal pain, headache, and backache (see Benjamin and Eminson (1992) for a more detailed review of this field). There is also evidence to suggest that adults with chronic intractable pain are more likely to have been hospitalized as children (Pilowsky *et al.* 1982).

Childhood experience of illness is a more powerful risk factor for adult somatization when it is associated with lack of parental care. In a recent study Craig *et al.* (1993) found that the best predictors of adult somatization were parental lack of care and childhood illness. Craig and colleagues (1993) have speculated that each of these risk factors contribute to adult somatization in different ways. In this hypothetical model, lack of care is a risk factor for the development of emotional disorder in the face of adversity, while their early childhood exposure to illness predisposes them to interpretations of the symptoms of emotional disorder as indicative of physical illness. These factors would combine at onset of depression, the mood disorder both producing novel symptomatic sensations and lowering

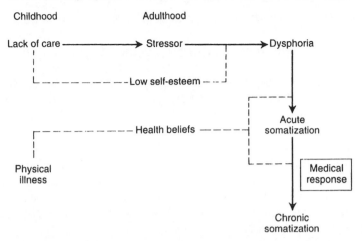

Fig. 3.2 Hypothetical model of the aetiology of chronic somatization (see text for further details) (Reproduced with permission from Craig *et al.* 1993)

the threshold for the tolerance of somatic discomfort. Whilst this model may help to explain the evolution of some of the more chronic somatoform disorders, simpler explanations are needed for the more common acute and subacute functional symptoms (Fig. 3.2).

Certain kinds of early trauma appear to be particularly damaging (see Barsky *et al.* 1994. Kirmayer *et al.* 1994 have reviewed the significance of personality variables.) For example, pelvic pain and abdominal functional symptoms are more common in women who have been sexually abused in childhood (Drossman and Thompson 1992; Walker *et al.* 1992). Childhood abuse is especially important in 'Munchausen's syndrome by proxy', in which a parent knowingly presents a child to doctors with claimed symptoms or signs which are in fact induced by the parent (Taylor 1991). Often the symptoms claimed by the parent to afflict the child induce doctors to investigate and thereby interfere physically with the child. Anecdotal evidence (Meadow 1983) suggests that such children develop chronic somatoform syndromes.

Knowledge and illness experience   An individual's beliefs are influenced by their culture and by press and television, as well as by childhood and later personal experience (Hunt *et al.* 1989). Doctors need to be aware of the range of illness beliefs in the population (Hadlow and Pitts 1991). Previous experience of physical illness, either direct or vicarious, has repeatedly been noted as an important aetiological factor. For example, a patient with non-cardiac chest pain may not respond to reassurance because

(1)   a friend at work of the same age has just died of a heart attack;

(2)   there is a strong family history of premature heart disease;

(3)   a close relative died 1 year previously of a non-cardiac cause (cancer) after having been reassured that the symptoms were not related to serious disease.

All these personal experiences of illness and disease will influence perceptions, causal attributions, and expectations. However, it may be not only experience of illness, but also a greater awareness and preoccupation with it, that predisposes to functional somatic symptoms, as people without functional symptoms can recall similar experiences but have taken much less notice of them.

Major physical illness

Those who have suffered major physical illnesses are particularly alert to bodily sensations and understandably liable to misinterpret benign perceptions as evidence of serious illness. For example, non-cardiac chest pain is a common cause of concern and disability in those who have suffered myocardial infarction or undergone cardiac surgery (Mayou 1989).

Epidemic health anxiety

Functional symptoms may occur in acute epidemics in small communities (such as schools) and in less dramatic form in the wider population following episodes of pollution, disasters, and other major events (Cooper 1993; David and Wessely 1995). Public fears and assumptions about physical causes and threats of litigation often hinder rational discussion (see Chapter 10).

Pathophysiological mechanisms

Although psychological factors are of undoubted importance in the production of somatic symptoms, parallel physiological processes that give rise to increased bodily sensations can be identified, These processes include autonomic arousal, increased smooth muscle and striated muscle contraction, hyperventilation, vascular changes, sleep disorders, the effects of inactivity, and the cerebral processing of information. Many terms have been used to refer to individual variation in the perception of pain and other bodily perceptions: pain threshold, appraisal, bodily awareness, etc. Psychological experiments have consistently supported the clinical observation that anxious and hypochondriacal patients are more aware of bodily sensations than others, and more likely to perceive these as severe and threatening (Tyrer *et al.* 1980). These processes and their relationship to psychosocial mechanisms are described in more detail elsewhere (Sharpe and Bass 1992).

Psychiatric disorder

Medically unexplained symptoms may be associated with almost any form of psychiatric disorder, but most commonly with anxiety, depression, and phobic disorders (Simon and Von Korff 1991).

The associations with psychiatric disorder have already been considered in relation to classification and are discussed in greater detail in other chapters. Psychiatric disorder is especially common in patients with chronic multiple symptoms (Chapter 10) and in those seen in specialist medical settings.

Stressful life events

Psychological factors may be either primary or secondary causes of functional somatic symptoms. For example, a distressing life event may lead to anxiety or low mood which may make an individual more aware of a benign subcutaneous lump of long-standing or abdominal bloating and flatulence. This heightened awareness leads in turn to increasing concern about the bodily sensation and consultation with doctors. Creed (1990) has suggested such a model for irritable bowel syndrome (Chapter 14).

Coping

Research on chronic pain has emphasized the role of coping (Jensen *et al.* 1991) (Chapter 11) as an important explanation of the differences in functioning between individuals attending pain clinics. It has been shown that the patient who believes that they can control their pain, avoids a catastrophic view of the condition, and also believes that they are not severely disabled, tends to function much better than the patient with more pessimistic views.

Lack of confiding

In a series of recent studies Pennebaker and colleagues (1988) have shown that inhibition of emotion and lack of confiding may cause physiological arousal, somatic symptoms, and physical disease. For example, among individuals whose spouses died unexpectedly by suicide or car accident, the more the survivors had talked to others about the spouse's death, the healthier they reported being (Pennebaker and O'Heeron, 1984).

Family

The patient's own family can have an important bearing on the course of functional somatic symptoms. Their own knowledge and experience of illness and concern about the patient's well-being may reinforce the patient's worries and disability. Therapeutic efforts can be subverted by family members, who may act as an important impediment to successful rehabilitation in patients with chronic pain (Benjamin and Eminson 1992).

Iatrogenic factors

The importance of iatrogenic factors in the initiation and maintenance of medically unexplained symptoms should not be underestimated. Doctors' uncertainty about aetiology, concern about not missing major physical illness, and feelings of therapeutic impotence make it difficult to respond to patients' demands authoritatively and constructively. In many instances the underlying misinterpretation of bodily sensations arise not only from the patient's own misconceptions but also from the doctor's failure to provide a satisfactory alternative explanation for the patient's somatic symptoms. Indeed, the doctor may have contributed to the misunderstanding by inconsistent or ambiguous advice or behaviour, for example continuing to prescribe anti-anginal medication in patients with non-cardiac chest pain.

Litigation and financial gain

Patients who receive sickness benefits, pensions or other disability payments remain disabled longer than those who have no such insurance, even with diseases of similar severity (Better *et al*. 1979; Chapter 12). These findings suggest that disability payments reduce the incentive to return to full-time employment.

There is inconsistent evidence that litigation increases the reports of severity of pain. However, there is no evidence that it induces or aggravates symptoms or prolongs the duration or that a legal settlement leads to amelioration of symptoms in patients involved in compensation claims (Mendelson 1984).

Lishman (1988) has pointed out the relative contribution of physical and psychogenic factors in the genesis of post-concussional syndrome as follows: 'organic factors are chiefly relevant in the early stages, whereas long-continued symptoms are perpetuated by secondary neurotic developments, often of a complex nature'. Compensation, which is often seen as a major aetiological factor in low back pain and 'accident neurosis', should be interpreted in this manner and seen as one of a variety of psychological and social determinants (Mills and Horne 1986).

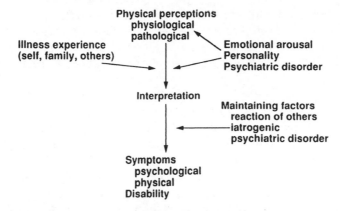

Fig. 3.3 An aetiological model of functional somatic symptoms

A multicausal interactive aetiological model

The factors outlined above may be combined in an overall model of the aetiology of functional somatic symptoms. The central tenet of this model (see Fig. 3.3) is that subjective symptoms, physical and psychological, are the results of patients' interpretation (or attribution) of somatic perceptions (Benedict 1989; Rowland *et al.* 1992). These underlying perceptions may be due to minor physical pathology or excessive awareness of normal physical and bodily processes. They may also be due to the somatic consequences of anxiety or other primary psychiatric disorder.

There are many psychosocial variables which make it more likely that individuals will misinterpret their bodily perceptions as more threatening than is in fact the case. These can be grouped into long-standing predisposing, and acute precipitating factors. Once established, these or other factors may then maintain the misinterpretation. Two important groups of predisposing and precipitating factors have been identified: these are illness knowledge and experience, and emotional arousal.

1. *Illness knowledge and experience.* This includes knowledge of illness and experience of previous disease and illness, family history of disease, models of disease in friends and neighbours, general experience of doctors, and satisfaction with medical care.

2. *Emotional arousal.* This group of predisposing and precipitating factors are those resulting from interaction between personality and stress, grouped in Fig. 3.3 under the heading of emotional arousal. This category covers illness worry and autonomic arousal as well as diagnosable psychiatric syndromes. However, the latter are common

and include adjustment disorders, anxiety disorders, with or without panic attacks, major depressive illnesses, and the various somatoform disorders, in which the most prominent feature is persistent concern about physical symptoms, despite the absence of relevant organic disease.

Once symptoms are established, they may be maintained or reinforced by the patients' persistent awareness of the minor physical perceptions or by factors such as secondary anxiety, the reactions of friends and relatives, and the reactions and behaviour of doctors. Each of these factors may lead a patient who has suffered temporary physical discomfort in their back, abdomen, or chest to experience prolonged overconcern.

This multicausal interactive model (shown diagrammatically in Fig. 3.3) includes both the biological basis of symptoms and also individual illness beliefs, personality, and life circumstances. It also points to ways in which medical intervention could reduce distress and disability by modifying the patient's interpretations of their symptoms. It is not satisfactory to simply reassure the patient that there is no serious physical cause — this is often ineffective. What is important is to provide the patient with a satisfactory alternative explanation and appropriate advice. Sometimes the misinterpretations are so persistent that there is a need for specialist psychiatric treatment (see, for example, Chapter 9).

Conclusion

In this chapter the prevalence of functional somatic symptoms in patients attending in a variety of different medical settings has been discussed. Particularly high rates have been described in hospital out-patient clinics.

Diagnostic classification and glossaries have never adequately accommodated patients with functional somatic symptoms and some of the reasons for this are discussed. We describe the limitations of current classification systems (which are essentially categorical) and propose a new multidimensionnal classification which considers not only somatic symptoms but also psychological states, attitudes and beliefs, functional impairment, and possible pathophysiological mechanisms. The latter have been neglected by both ICD-10 and DSM-IV.

Finally, we argue against unitary causal theories. Instead, we propose a multicausal, interactive aetiological model which takes account of a number of relevant physical, psychological, and social factors.

References

Anderson, R., Anderson, O.W., and Smedby, B. (1968). Perception of an response to symptoms of illness in Sweden and the United State. *Medical Care*, **6**, 18-30.

Banks, M.H., Beresford, S.A., Morrell, D.C., Waller, J.J., and Watkins, C.J. (1975). Factors influencing demand for primary medical care in women aged 20-44 years: a preliminary report. *International Journal of Epidemiology*, **4**, 189-95.

Barsky, A.J., Wool, C., Barnett, H.C., and Cleary, P.D. (1994). Histories of childhood trauma in adult hypochondriasis patients. *American Journal of Psychiatry*, **151**, 397-401.

Barsky, A.J., Wyshak, G., and Kleman, G.L. (1992). Psychiatric comorbidity in DSM-III-R hypochondriasis. *Archives of Senses Psychiatry*, **4**, 101-08.

Beard, R.W., and Reginald, P.W. (1990). Chronic pelvic pain. In *Gynaecology*, (ed. R. Shaw). Churchill Livingstone.

Beitman, B.D., Basha, I.M., Trombka, L.H., Jayaratna, M.A., Russell, B.D., and Tarr, S.K. (1988). Alprazolam in the treatment of cardiology patients with atypical chest pain and panic disorder. *Journal of Clinical Psychopharmacology*, **8**, 127-30.

Benedict, R.H.B. (1989). The effectiveness of cognitive remediation strategies for victims of traumatic head-injury: a review of the literature. *Clinical Psychology Review*, **9**, 605-26.

Benjamin, S., and Eminson, D.M. (1992). Abnormal illness behaviour: childhood experiences and long-term consequences. *International Review of Psychiatry*, **4**, 55-70.

Better, S.R., Fine, P.R., Simison, D. (1979). Disability benefits as disincentives to rehabilitation. *Health and Society*, **57**, 412-27.

Blumer, D., and Heilbron, M. (1981). The pain prone disorder. A clinical and psychological profile. *Psychosomatics*, **22**, 395-98.

Bohman, M., Cloninger, C.R., and von Knorring, A.L. (1984). An adoption study of somatoform disorders: II Cross-fostering analysis and genetic relationship to alcoholism and criminality. *Archives of General Psychiatry*, **41**, 872-78.

Bools, C.N., Neale, B.A., and Meadow, R. (1993). Follow up of victims of fabricated illness (Munchhausen Syndrome by Proxy). *Archives of Diseases of Childhood*, **69**, 625-30.

Bradlow, J., Coulter, A., and Brookes, P. (1992). *Patterns of referral. A study of referrals to out-patient clinics from general practices in the Oxford Region*, Health Services Research Unit, Oxford.

Bridges, K.W., and Goldberg, D.P. (1985). Somatic presentation of DSM-III psychiatric disorders in primary care. *Journal of Psychosomatic Research*, **29**, 563-9.

Cannon, R.O., and Epstein, S.E. (1988). Microvascular angina as a course of chest pain and angiographically normal coronary arteries. *American Journal of Cardiology*, **61**, 1338-43.

Chambers, J.B., and Bass, C. (1990). Chest pain and normal coronary anatomy: review of natural history and possible aetiologic factors. *Progress in Cardiovascular Disease*, **33**, 161-84.

Cloninger, C.R. (1986). Classification of the somatoform disorders: a critique of DSM-III. In *Diagnosis and classification in psychiatry*, (ed. G. Tischler). pp. 243–59. Cambridge University Press, New York.

Cooper, B. (1993). Single spies and battalions: the clinical epidemiology of mental disorders. *Psychological Medicine*, **23**, 891–907.

Costa, P.T., and McCrae, R.R. (1985). Hypochondriasis, neuroticism and ageing. When are somatic complaints unfounded? *American Psychologist*, **40**, 19–28.

Craig, T.K.J., Boardman, A.P. (1990). *Somatization in primary care settings*. In *Somatization: Physical symptoms and psychological illness*, (ed. C. Bass), pp. 73–103. Blackwells, Oxford.

Craig, T.K.J., Boardman, A.P., Mills, K., Daly-Jones, O., and Drake, H. (1993). The South London somatization study: I longitudinal course and the influence of early life experiences. *British Journal of Psychiatry*, **163**, 570–88.

Creed, F. (1990). *Functional abdominal pain*. In *somatization: physical symptoms and psychological illness*, (ed. C. Bass), pp. 141–70. Blackwells, Oxford.

Crook, J., Rideout, E., and Browne, G. (1984). The prevalence of pain complaints in general population. *Pain*, **18**, 299–314.

David, A.S., and Wessely, S.C. (1995). The legend of Camelford. *Journal of Psychosomatic Research*, **39**, 1–10.

de Gruy, F., Crider, J., and Hashimi, D.K. (1987). Somatization disorder in a university hospital. *Journal of Family Practice*, **25**, 579–84.

Deighton, C.M., and Nicol, A.R. (1985). Abnormal illness behaviour in young women in a primary care setting: is Briquet's syndrome a useful category? *Psychological Medicine*, **15**, 515–20.

de Leon, J., Saiz-Ruiz, J., and Chinchilla, A. (1987). Why do some psychiatric patients somatize? *Acta Psychiatrica Scandinavica*, **76**, 203–9.

Drossman, D.A., and Thompson, W.G. (1992). The irritable bowel syndrome: Review and a graduated multicomponent treatment approach. *American College of Physicians*, **116**, 1009–16.

Escobar, J.I., Rubiio-Stipec, M., Canino G., and Karno, M. (1989). Somatic symptom index (SSI): a new and abridges somatization construct. Prevalence and epidemiological correlates in two large conununity samples. *Journal of Nervous and Mental Diseases*, **177**, 140–6.

Fava, G.A., Trombini, G., Grandi, S., Bernardi, M., and Canestrari, R. (1987). A psychosomatic outpatient clinic. *International Journal of Psychiatry in Medicine*, **17**, 261–7.

Fink, P. (1992a). Surgery and medical treatment in persistent somatizing patients. *Journal of Psychosomatic Research*, **36**, 439–47.

Fink, P. (1992b). Physical complaints and symptoms of somatizing patients. *Journal of Psychosomatic Research*, **36**, 125–36.

Gray, D.W., and Collier, J. (1987). Non-specific abdominal pain as a cause of acute admission to hospital. *British Journal of Surgery*, **74**, 239–42.

Hadlow, J., and Pitts, M. (1991). The understanding of common health terms by doctors, nurses and patients. *Social Science and Medicine*, **32**, 193–6.

Hannay, D.R. (1978). Symptom prevalence in the community. *Journal of the Royal College of General Practitioners*, **28**, 492–9.

Hartwig, P., and Sterner, G. (1985). Childhood psychologic environmental exposure in women with diagnosed somatoform disorders. A case control study. *Scandinavian Journal of Social Medicine*, **13**, 153-7.

Hunt, L.M., Jordan, B., and Irwin, S. (1989). Views of what's wrong: diagnosis and patients' concepts of illness. *Social Science and Medicine*, **28**, 945-56.

Jensen, M.P., Turner, J.A., Romano, J.M., and Karoly, P. (1991). Coping with chronic pain: a critical review of our literature. *Pain*, **47**, 249-83.

Katon, W., Ries, R.K., and Kleinman, A. (1984). Part II: a prospective DSM-III study of 100 consecutive somatization patients. *Comprehensive Psychiatry*, **25**, 305-14.

Katon, W., Von Korff, M., Lin, E., Lipscomb, P., Wagner, E., and Polk, E. (1990). Distressed high utilizers of medical care DSMIII-R diagnoses and treatment needs. *General Hospital Psychiatry*, **12**, 355-62.

Keefe, F.J., Dunsmore, J., and Burnett, R. (1992). Behavioral and cognitive-behavioural approaches to chronic pain: recent advances and future directions. *Journal of Consulting and Clinical Psychology*, **60**, 528-36.

Kellner, R. (1991). *Psychosomatic syndromes and somatic symptoms*. American Psychiatric Press, Washington DC.

King, S.A., and Strain, J. (1992). Revising the category of somatoform pain disorder. *Hospital and Community Psychiatry*, **43**, 21-19.

Kirmayer, L., and Robbins, J.M. (1991a). *Current concepts of somatization. Research and clinical perspectives*. American Psychiatric Press, Washington DC.

Kirmayer, L.J., and Robbins, J.M. (1991b). Three forms of somatization in primary care: prevalence, co-occurence, and sociodemographic characteristics. *Journal of Nervous Mental Disorder*, **179**, 647-55.

Kirmayer, L.J., Robbins, J.M., and Pain, J. (1994). Somatization disorders. Personal and social matrix of sample districts. *Journal of Abnormal Pschology*, **103**, 125-36.

Kroenke, K. (1992). Symptoms in medical patients: an untended field. *American Journal of Medicine*, **92**(1A), 3-6.

Kroenke, K., and Mangelsdorff, D. (1989). Common symptoms in ambulatory care: incidence, evaluation, therapy and outcome. *American Journal of Medicine*, **86**, 262-6.

Kroenke, K., and Price, R.K. (1993). Symptoms in the community. Prevalence, classification, and psychiatric comorbidity. *Archives of Internal Medicine*, **153**, 1474-80.

Kroenke, K., Arrington, M.E., and Mangelsdorff, D. (1990). The prevalence of symptoms in medical out-patients and the adequacy of therapy. *Archives of Internal Medicine*, **150**, 1685-9.

Lang, P.J. (1978). Anxiety: Toward a psychophysiological definition. In *Psychiatric diagnosis: Exploration of biological predictions*, (ed. H.S. Akiskal and W.L. Webb), Spectrum, New York.

Lee, T.H., Ting, H.H., Shammash, J.B., Soukup, H.R., and Goldman, L. (1992). Long-terms survival of emergency department patients with acute chest pain. *American Journal of Cardiology*, **69**, 145-51.

Lishman, W.A. (1988). Physiogenesis and psychogenesis in the post-concussional syndrome. *British Journal of Pschiatry*, **153**, 460-9.

Lum, L.C. (1976). The syndrome of chronic hyperventiliation. In *Modern trends in psychosomatic medicine*, (ed. O. Hill). Butterworths, London.

Manning, A.P., Thompson, W.G., Heaton, K.W., and Morris, A.F. (1978). Towards positive diagnosis of the irritable bowel. *British Medical Journal*, **ii**, 653–4.

Mayou, R.A. (1989). Invited review: atypical chest pain. *Journal of Psychosomatic Research*, **33**, 373–406.

Mayou, R.A., and Hawton, K.E. (1986). Psychiatric disorder in the general hospital. *British Journal of Psychiatry*, **149**, 172–90.

Mayou, R.A., Seagroatt, V., and Goldacre, H. (1991). Use of psychiatric services of patients in a general hospital. *British Medical Journal*, **303**, 1029–32.

Mechanic, D. (1962). The concept of illness behaviour. *Journal of Chronic Disease*, **15**, 189–94.

Mechanic, D. (1980). The experience and reporting of common physical complaints. *Journal of Health and Social Behaviour*, **21**, 146–55.

Mendleson, G. (1984). Follow-up studies of personal injury litigants. *International Journal of Law and Psychiatry*, **7**, 179–88.

Mills, H., and Horne, G. (1986). Whiplash-manmade disease? *New Zealand Medical Journal*, **99**, 373–4.

Mumford, D.B. (1993). Somatization: a transcultural perspective. *Internal Review of Psychiatry*, **5**, 231–42.

Noyes, R. Jr., Kathol, R.G., Fisher, M.M., and Thomas, P.G. (1982). The validity of DSM-III-R hypochondriasis. *Archives of General Psychiatry*, **50**, 961–70.

Phillips, H.C., and Grant, L. (1991). Acute back pain: A psychological analysis. *Behaviour Research and Therapy*, **29**, 429–34.

Pilowsky, I., Bassett, D.L., Begg, M.W., and Thomas, P.G. (1982). Childhood hospitalisation and chronic intractable pain in adults. A controlled retrospective study. *International Journal of Psychiatry in Medicine*, **12**, 75–84.

Potts, S.G., and Bass, C.M. (1993). Psychosocial outcome and use of medical resources in patients with chest pain and normal or near-normal cononary arteries: a long-term follow-up study. *Quarterly Journal of Medicine*, **86**, 583–93.

Pennebaker, J.W., and O'Heeron, R.C. (1984). Confiding in others and illness rate among spouses of sucide and accidental-death victims. *Journal of Abnormal Psychology*, **93**, 473–76.

Pennebaker, J.W., and Susman, J.R. (1988). Disclosure of traumas and psychosomatic processes. *Social Science and Medicine*, **26**, 327–32.

Rowland, N., Beveridge, A., and Maynard, A. (1992). Screening for patients at risk of alcohol related problems: the results of the York District Hospital Alcohol Study. *Health Trends*, **24**, 99–102.

Sharpe, M., and Bass, C. (1992). Pathophysiological mechanisms in somatization. *International Review of Psychiatry*, **4**, 81–97.

Simon, G.E., and Von Korff, M. (1991). Somatization and psychiatric disorder in the NTMH epidemiologic catchment area study. *American Journal of Psychiatry*, **148**, 1494–5.

Slaveney, P.R., and Teitbaum, M.L. (1984). Patients with medically unexplained symptoms: DSM-III Diagnoses and demographic characteristics. *General Hospital Psychiatry*, **7**, 21–5.

Snyder, S., and Strain, J.J. (1989). Somatoform disorders in the general hospital impatient setting. *General Hospital Psychiatry*, **11**, 288–93.

Sutherland, A.J., and Rodin, G.M. (1990). Factitious disorders in a general hospital setting: clinical features and a review of the literature. *Psychosomatics*, **31**, 392–414.

Swartz, M.S., Blazer, D.G., George, L.K., and Landerman, R. (1986). Somatization disorder in a community population. *American Journal of Psychiatry*, **143**, 1403–8.

Swift, G.L., Alban-Davies, H., Mckirdy, H., Lowndes, R., Lewis, D., and Rhodes, J. (1991). A long-term clinical review of patients with oesphageal pain. *Quarterly Journal of Medicine*, **295**, 937–44.

Taylor, D. (1991). Outlandish factitious illness. In *Recent advances in paediatrics*, (ed. T. David), pp. 63–77. Churchill Livingstone, London.

Tyrer, P., Fowler-Dixon, R., Ferguson, B., and Kelemen, A. (1990). A plea for the diagnosis of hypochrondrial patients. *Psychological Medicine*, **10**, 171–4.

Van Hemert, A.M., Henegeveld, M.W., Bolk, J.H., Rooijmans, H.G., and Vandenbrouche, J.P. (1993). Psychiatric disorders in relation to medical illness among patients of a general medical out-patient clinic. *Psychological Medicine*, **23**, 167–73.

Von Korff, M., Dworkin, S.F., Le Resche, L.L., and Kruger, A. (1988). An epidemiologic comparison of pain complaints. *Pain*, **32**, 173–83.

Walker, E.A., Katon, W., Jemelka, R.P., and Roy-Byrne, P.P. (1992). Comorbidity of gastrointestinal complaints, depression, and anxiety in the epidemiological catchment area (ECA) study. *American Journal of Medicine*, **92**, 26S–9S.

Watson, D., and Pennebaker, J.W. (1989). Health complaints, stress, and distress: exploring the central role of negative affectivity. *Psychological Review*, **96**, 234–54.

Yunus, M.B. (1989). Fibromyalgia syndrome: new research on an old malady. *British Medical Journal*, **298**, 474–5.

4 An overview of the treatment of functional somatic symptoms

Michael Sharpe, Christopher Bass,
and Richard Mayou

In this chapter we offer an overview of the treatment of patients with functional somatic symptoms with the aim of providing an introduction and context for the chapters that follow. We discuss where patients should be treated, who should treat them, and how they should be treated. A review of the different forms of therapy available is preceeded by a consideration of non-specific aspects of treatment. The chapter concludes with an outline of practical management.

Introduction

The intention of this chapter is to provide the reader with an overview of the treatment of functional somatic symptoms. In contrast to other chapters which are devoted to specific syndromes and to specific forms of treatment, this chapter aims to provide a description of, and practical guide to, the general principles of the management of functional somatic symptoms in general.

We consider treatment as encompassing all aspects of patient management. It begins, therefore, with the patient's first contact with the medical services, includes the process of history taking, examination and investigation, the giving of an explanation and advice to the patient and, if appropriate, the prescription of medication or psychotherapy. Throughout this process the doctor–patient relationship is of crucial importance.

Where should patients be treated?

Functional symptoms and functional illnesses are extremely common in the population (Escobar and Canino 1989). They are usually transient and most persons experiencing them do not seek any treatment. Others follow folklore remedies offered by families and friends, purchase 'over the counter' remedies, or seek help from alternative practitioners (see Chapter 23). Only a minority of patients with functional somatic symptoms make contact with the conventional medical services (Anderson *et al.* 1968; Eisenberg *et al.* 1993). Indeed it has been suggested, not unreasonably, that

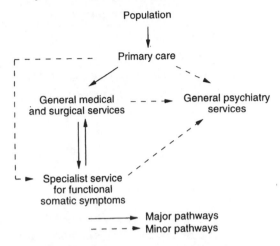

Fig. 4.1 Services used by patients with functional somatic symptoms and pathways to care

if everybody who suffered from a functional somatic symptom were to attend a doctor, the health services would rapidly collapse under the demand (Kleinman *et al.* 1978). The pathways the patients may follow within the health service are shown in Fig. 4.1.

Primary care

Most patients initially present to a primary care physician. This person plays a critical role in the patient's subsequent management (see Chapter 21). He or she has the opportunity to provide effective care and occasionally to make a referral to hospital. By acting as gatekeeper to hospital services the primary care physician can prevent the patient from being subjected to unproductive and expensive investigations and treatments (Smith *et al.* 1986) and can also guide those patients with emotional disorders towards more appropriate services. For patients with established chronic functional syndromes long-term follow-up by the primary care physician rather than repeated referral to hospital may be the best management (Smith 1991).

The primary care doctor can also make the problem worse and increase the risk of the patient developing chronic illness by dismissing the patient's concerns, making an inaccurate disease diagnosis, instigating excessive investigation, or making inappropriate hospital referrals (Todd 1984*a*,*b*). The role of the primary care physician is summarized in Table 4.1.

Table 4.1 The role of the primary care physician

1.	To give appropriate advice for acute functional symptoms
2.	To detect somatic presentations of depressive and anxiety syndromes
3.	To avoid reinforcing inappropriate disease conviction and avoidance behaviour
4.	To give simple psychological and rehabilitative treatments
5.	To prescribe appropriate psychotropic medication
6.	To act as a gatekeeper for access to secondary care services
7.	To care for patients with chronic functional syndromes

The general hospital

Hospital doctors see large numbers of patients with functional somatic symptoms. They are therefore in an excellent position to provide clinical services for such patients (see Chapter 22). Thus, the gastroenterology department could offer a comprehensive service for irritable bowel syndrome (see Chapter 14), the infectious disease clinic a service for 'post-viral fatigue' (see Chapter 16), and the surgical unit a service for functional pain syndromes (see Chapter 11).

In practice there are very few such services. The failure to recognize the problem of functional somatic symptoms and to tackle it constructively has important consequences. Patients with functional somatic symptoms consume considerable resources (Fink 1992*a*), are typically regarded as difficult and frustrating to treat (Lin *et al.* 1991), and are more likely to be over-investigated, inappropriately treated, or simply returned to the primary care physician, than to receive more effective management as described in this book (Fink 1992*b*). The role of hospital services is summarized in Table 4.2.

Table 4.2 The role of hospital medical and surgical services

1.	To exclude treatable disease
2.	To give the patient a clear message about the absence of disease
3.	To provide specialist treatment for chronic severe functional syndromes
4.	To coordinate management with the primary care physician

General psychiatry

Patients with functional somatic symptoms are likely to refuse referral to traditional psychiatric services, particularly if these are based in a mental hospital. Clinical experience indicates that even if they attend general psychiatry clinics, the psychiatrists' emphasis on psychological and emotional symptoms, together with a relative neglect of somatic complaints and disease beliefs, frequently results in the patient rejecting this form of help.

Specialist psychiatric clinics

Psychiatric services are more likely to be acceptable to patients with functional somatic symptoms if they are based either in the general hospital or in primary care. The psychiatrist providing these services must also possess special skills (see Chapter 5). The best example of these clinics are those run by consultation–liaison psychiatrists and specialist psychologists (Sharpe and Hawton 1990). These are widespread in the USA and some European countries but sparse in others, including the UK (Mayou 1991).

Most specialist clinics see only a small proportion of the patients with functional somatic symptoms who pass through the general hospital and are rarely able to offer anything like a comprehensive service for those whom they do see. None the less, these services can provide important opportunities for educating both primary care and hospital physicians and for developing and evaluating treatment interventions (Table 4.3; see also Chapter 22).

Table 4.3 The role of specialist services

---
1. To provide a service for the management of severe functional somatic symptoms
2. To advise other doctors on patient management
3. To provide education for doctors
4. To conduct research into the nature and treatment of functional somatic symptoms
---

Specialist multidisciplinary clinics

Perhaps the ideal tertiary referral service is a combined medical-psychiatric 'one-stop clinic' where the patient can receive a comprehensive assessment on a single visit. There are few of these. Combined clinics do exist for patients with chronic pain syndromes (see Chapter 11) and provide a useful model for the management of patients with all types of chronic functional illness (Sullivan 1993).

Specialist in-patient units

The specialist in-patient unit is rare. Such units provide an opportunity to offer more intensive treatment (Lipowski 1988) and can have an important role in the treatment of the small minority of very disabled patients and others who are unable to attend for out-patient treatment.

How should patients be treated?

General aspects of care

Listening to the patient All patients want their doctor to listen sympathetically and to take their complaints seriously (Armstrong 1991). Although this is obviously an essential part of 'good doctoring', it is all too often skimped or badly done when the patient's symptoms are thought to be functional. Failure to listen or dismissal of the patient's complaints as 'non-existent' or 'all in the mind' is likely damage the doctor–patient relationship (see Chapter 5).

The patients' concerns Patients may be troubled by a perceived threat to life or health, by the effect of the illness on their functioning, or by psychosocial stressors unrelated to the symptoms. Most want a diagnosis or an explanation of their symptoms and help to get better. Some have other aims including the validation of illness for the purpose of claiming compensation or insurance benefits, or as an excuse for personal failure. Others may not really know what they want except that they expect the doctor to help. Whatever the patient's concerns and expectations it is essential that patient and doctor agree on the aims of treatment (Sharpe *et al*. 1994).

Assessment

Wherever the patient is seen, adequate assessment is the *sine qua non* of management. The specific aims of assessment are outlined in Table 4.4, the overall aim of the assessment being to produce an adequate formulation of the problem.

Table 4.4 The aims of assessment

---
1. To clarify the nature of the patient's complaints
2. To understand what the patient wants
3. To elicit the patient's fears and beliefs about their illness
4. To exclude organic disease
5. To identify emotional disorder and distress
6. To identify relevant psychological and social stressors

Formulation

Diagnosis alone is inadequate to determine the treatment of the patient with functional somatic symptoms. Rather each patient should be assessed individually and a simple formulation produced. A useful formulation should consider multiple aetiological factors. These can be conveniently divided into biological, psychological, and social realms (Lipkin *et al.* 1966). It should also distinguish between those factors that may have *predisposed* the person to develop the illness, those that *precipitated* it, and those that are acting to *perpetuate* it. Treatment must focus on the perpetuating factors. The formulation may be represented as a grid (see Table 4.5 for an example).

Table 4.5 Organization of aetiological factors into a tabulated formulation

	Predisposing factors	Precipitating factors	Perpetuating factors
Biological	Genetics	Trauma	Pathophysiological processes
	Temperament	Infection	
Psychological	Habitual modes of thinking	Life stress	Belief in disease
		Failure to cope with change	Fear of disease
	Experience of illness		Failure to resolve problems
Social	Quality of relationships	Conflict	Reinforcement of sick role
		Employment stress	
	Chronic life difficulties		Ongoing stress
		Relationship problems	

General aspects of treatment

There are a number of general aspects of treatment that must be implemented before more specific measures are considered. These are listed in Table 4.6. A full account is given by Bass and Benjamin (1993).

The doctor–patient relationship A satisfactory doctor–patient relationship is essential for treatment success. It is particularly important in the case of patients with functional somatic symptoms who are likely to have experienced disbelief, or even dismissal of their symptoms by other doctors

Table 4.6 General measures in the management of patients with functional somatic symptoms

1. Make the patient feel understood
2. Establish a positive collaborative relationship
3. Correct misconceptions about disease and give a positive explanation of symptoms
4. Avoid unnecessary investigation and treatment
5. Negotiate a formulation and treatment plan with the patient

(Ware 1992). Not infrequently an impasse develops in the doctor–patient relationship as a consequence of a mismatch between the patient's expectations (usually of precise diagnosis and definitive treatment) and what the doctor is able to provide (Sharpe *et al.* 1994). We have found that this situation is best managed by shifting the emphasis of the doctor–patient relationship from the traditional pattern, in which the doctor provides all the answers, to a collaborative exploration of the problem and it's treatment. This type of therapeutic relationship is central to the practice of cognitive behaviour therapy (see Chapter 7) and has been termed 'collaborative empiricism' (Beck *et al.* 1979).

Giving an explanation of the illness   Patients want an explanation of the origin of their symptoms. Before attempting to do this the doctor should elicit the patient's own theory. This may be close to the doctor's own medical understanding, but may on occasion be idiosyncratic and even bizarre (Wright and Morgan 1990).

The first step in the explanation is to try to correct the patient's erroneous beliefs. This often requires sensitivity if the patient is not to feel misunderstood or even humiliated (for example, see Chapter 16). The second step is to provide as clear and unambiguous a statement as possible about the absence of a sinister physical disease. The next step is to educate the patient about the actual cause of their symptoms. This explanation should be in positive terms and, if possible, should start from the patient's own theory and be consistent with their own experience.

Whenever possible, explanation should include physiological as well as psychological factors (Sharpe and Bass 1992). In some cases (irritable bowel syndrome, pelvic pain, and atypical chest pain) plausible mechanisms of symptom production, for which there is reasonable evidence (see Chapters 14, 17, and 18) are available; in others the mechanisms are less well understood. We believe that the physician should only offer explanations for which there is reasonable empirical evidence and that it is unethical and potentially harmful to suggest hypothetical or frankly incorrect mechanisms. In such cases it may be better to admit ignorance.

The explanation offered will be most convincing to the patient when a demonstration reproduces their symptoms in the clinic. An example is the role of over-breathing in non-cardiac chest pain (Salkovskis 1992), which can be demonstrated by voluntary over-breathing. Such explanations may lead logically to treatment, in this case re-evaluation of the significance of the symptoms and the practice of breathing control (Cluff 1984).

Avoiding inappropriate investigation Another important aspect of the management of the patient with functional somatic symptoms is limiting the seeking of further medical opinions, examinations, and investigations unless these are likely to offer new and useful information (Todd 1984b). This issue is discussed in Chapter 9 on hypochondriasis.

Providing treatment The treatment offered will depend both on the formulation of the patient's problems and on what clinical resources are available to the doctor. Whatever the treatment, compliance is likely to be better if the doctor and patient have successfully negotiated a shared explanation of the patient's illness, and if the treatment proposed follows logically from this.

Specific treatments

Over and above the general measures outlined above, a number of more specific strategies are described in the following chapters of this book (see Table 4.7). Clinical experience would suggest that these should rarely, if ever, be applied without first paying careful attention to the general measures.

Behavioural and life-style change There is considerable evidence for the benefits of simple behavioural and life-style changes in the management of functional somatic symptoms. The main targets for such changes are

(1) stress and life-style;

(2) activity and physical fitness.

Many functional somatic symptoms have their origin in anxiety and tension (Sainsbury and Gibson 1954; Tyrer 1976). Therefore, helping the patient to be aware of tension, to identify sources of 'stress', and to manage these effectively, are important therapeutic techniques. Clinical experience suggests that many patients with functional somatic symptoms suffer stress because of maladaptive coping strategies. These include excessively high standards, lack of assertiveness, and avoidance of interpersonal conflict. Some may be helped by simple advice about these

Table 4.7 Specific treatments for patients with functional somatic symptoms

Behavioural and life-style change	Occupational and social interventions
Life-style advice	Liaise with employer
Graded increases in activity	Occupational counselling
Relaxation	Problem solving for social problems
Pharmacological	
Antidepressant drug therapy	
Other drugs	
Specific psychological interventions	
Dynamic psychotherapy	
Cognitive behaviour therapy	
Group therapy	
Family therapy	

issues, others will benefit from more specific instruction in relaxation and breathing control, often combined as anxiety management programmes (Butter *et al.* 1991), whilst yet others may require more specialized psychotherapeutic interventions (see below).

Increased activity and improving physical fitness are of benefit in patients with fatigue and musculoskeletal pain and are a component of the treatment programmes for many functional somatic symptoms (McCain 1991; Dubbert 1992). Activity programmes should start at a reasonable level and progress slowly. Initial increases in activity can aggravate symptoms and consequently, lead to poor compliance. The patient may therefore need encouragement and help to attribute any increase in symptoms to the physiological effects of activity, rather than to worsening of disease (see, in particular, Chapter 16).

Drug therapy A large number of pharmacological agents have been advocated for the treatment of various functional somatic symptoms (see for example, Gantz and Holmes 1989). Most are symptomatic remedies, few are of proven efficacy, and some may even be harmful. The prescribing of pharmacological agents may also have psychological effects. On the one hand the patient may benefit from a placebo effect (Shepherd 1993), while on the other a prescription may serve to reinforce the patient's conviction that they have disease and to undermine any verbal reassurance given to the contrary (Todd 1984*a*). In particular, the use of analgesics may actually perpetuate rather than relieve chronic pain (Pither 1989); opiates present their own special problems of addiction (see Chapter 11). Polypharmacy risks dangerous drug interactions and, in general, should be avoided.

Probably the most useful currently available agents for use in functional somatic symptoms are the antidepressant drugs. The rationale for their use is fully discussed in Chapter 6. Their applicability extends beyond the treatment of depressive syndromes and includes anxiety and panic, poor sleep, and pain. There is particularly good evidence of their efficacy in the treatment of chronic pain syndromes (see Chapter 6), fibromyalgia (Goldenberg 1989) and irritable bowel syndrome (Whitehead and Crowell 1991). There is also some evidence to support their use in other functional somatic symptoms such as chronic fatigue (Lynch *et al.* 1991). The relative usefulness of the newer agents such as the selective serotonin reuptake inhibiting (SSRI) antidepressants such as fluoxetine and the reversible manoamine inhibitors oxidase (MAO) such as moclobamide remains to be established, but they may be found to have specific advantages for certain functional somatic syndromes.

One of the principal problems in using antidepressant drugs in patients with functional somatic symptoms is compliance with treatment. This may be maximized by fully discussing the reason for prescribing the drug, its possible side-effects, and likely benefits with the patient and by careful follow-up (see Chapter 6).

Specific psychological therapies   The initial assessment and explanation given to the patient is a *general* psychological treatment of great importance and potential efficacy. It is a skill that should be possessed by all doctors. A variety of *specific* psychotherapies have been employed in the management of patients with functional somatic symptoms. The most commonly practised are cognitive behavioural (see Chapter 7) and brief dynamic psychotherapies (see Chapter 8). Ingredients common to both these types of psychotherapy include helping the patient to make sense of their symptoms, shifting their focus of concern from somatic symptoms to relevant psychological and social issues, and actively coping with relationship and life-style problems. There are also differences between them; cognitive and behavioural therapies focus more on practical methods of managing symptoms in the present and dynamic therapies on their historical origins and on relationships, including that of the patient with the therapist (Altshuler and Rush 1984).

There is currently considerable evidence for the efficacy of cognitive and behavioural therapies in the treatment of functional somatic symptoms (see Chapter 7). Although there has been less systematic evaluation of the efficacy of dynamic psychotherapy, it has been shown to be useful in patients with 'treatment resistant' irritable bowel syndrome (see Chapter 8). In practice these relatively sophisticated therapies will only be necessary for a minority of patients.

Although usually administered on a one-to-one basis, psychotherapy may also be given in a group setting (Melson and Rynearson 1986; Stern and Fernandez 1991) with a potential saving of skilled therapist time. Therapeutic groups for patients with functional somatic symptoms can be difficult to conduct, however, and the need for careful preparation of each session may mean that less time is saved than might be anticipated.

Family interventions   It is important not to neglect the patient's family and other relationships. These may be relevant to their illness in a variety of ways. First, they may be a major cause of stress. Second, the patient's family may hold strong beliefs about the nature of the patients illness. Third, the behaviour of others may shape the patient's adoption of the sick role (Benjamin *et al.* 1992). Where the assessment indicates that they are relevant, these interpersonal factors must be addressed.

Perhaps the simplest measure is to arrange a joint interview with patient and spouse in order to explain the nature of the patient's illness and the intended treatment. More formal family therapy (Bloch *et al.* 1991) has also been advocated for the treatment of functional somatic symptoms (Griffith *et al.* 1989), although it has not been systematically evaluated for this purpose. The family is of particular importance in the management of children and adolescents with functional somatic symptoms (Rikard-Bell and Waters 1992) (see Chapter 19).

The management of occupational and social factors   The workplace may be a source of both psychological and physical stress and changes in working practice may be important in the management of musculoskeletal pain (Brooks 1993). Problems with return to work because of dissatisfaction with employment and reluctance on the part of the employer to permit a gradual return to full duties, are major potential obstacles to rehabilitation. Negotiation with occupational physicians or with the patient's employers can therefore be important in achieving a return to work (Peel 1988).

Social factors appear to shape functional illnesses and may also give rise to 'fashions' in the form of such illness (Shorter 1992). The role of the media is discussed below and in Chapter 16. Compensation payments and state benefits can influence the course of functional illness and can be difficult for the individual doctor to influence (Lucire 1988). These issues are discussed more fully in Chapter 12.

Practical treatment strategies

Faced with a patient whose symptoms are functional how should management be planned and organized?

Treatment specificity   The available evidence suggests that there is, in fact, little specificity in the relationship between a certain functional somatic symptom and a given treatment. This means that the pharmacological, psychological, and social interventions outlined above may be useful across the range of functional syndromes. The choice of intervention should therefore be more greatly influenced by the formulation of the patient's illness and by practical considerations than by the specific symptom presented.

Plan of approach   We recommend a stepped care approach to treatment. This means starting with the most simple treatments and only employing more complex and expensive therapies for those who do not respond to simpler measures.

After assessment all patients should be given education and advice and where possible the patient's spouse or partner should also be interviewed. Care should be taken to avoid iatrogenic harm by not making presumptive diagnoses of disease, ordering excessive investigation or prescribing in appropriate treatment.

If there is evidence of depression or if there is evidence that the syndrome may respond to an antidepressant, then a trial of an appropriate drug should be considered. The practitioner who feels able to give a brief psychological therapy may use this as an alternative to, or in combination with, drug treatment.

If these measures prove to be ineffective, referral for specialist treatment and assessment may be considered. Review by a specialist physician or surgeon may be useful in reassuring both the patient and the referring doctor that the problem is not one of occult organic disease and in facilitating referral for psychological assessment and treatment. Alternatively the doctor may choose to refer the patient for psychological treatment directly. The choice of specific therapy will be dependent both on the availability and on the patient's preference. In most cases we would favour a cognitive behavioural approach, but for patients treated outside research studies it may be more effective to adopt an eclectic stance (Murphy 1993). Treatment can almost always be administered on an out-patient basis, but for patients who are severely disabled in-patient treatment may be required.

Treatment combinations   Treatment should be kept simple and targeted at the factors that the assessment indicates are perpetuating the illness. In practice, as with all chronic illness, multiple factors may be important. Combined treatments may include a biological intervention (for example, an antidepressant), a psychological intervention (for example, re-attribution of symptoms from disease to functional syndrome), and an interpersonal component (for example, education of the spouse how to respond to patient's complaints).

Which patients should be treated?

Clearly not every patient who presents with a functional symptom requires specific treatment. The decision to treat must be based on the degree of distress, disability, and the duration of the symptoms. Patients who were well adjusted before becoming ill are more likely to respond to reassurance and other brief treatments. Aims should be less ambitious for those patients who have exhibited lifelong difficulty in social and occupational adjustment (see Chapter 10).

Who should treat the patient?

Most patients will be treated by their primary care doctor or by a hospital physician. However, many doctors feel they lack the necessary skills and time to treat such patients effectively. How is this clinical problem to be tackled in practice?

Training

Neither physicians nor psychiatrists are well trained for the task of managing patients with functional somatic symptoms. Non-psychiatric physicians often lack psychological assessment skills. Psychiatrists are often unable to negotiate treatment with patients whose concerns are somatic. Training can help doctors to be more effective in the management of functional somatic symptoms and is discussed in Chapter 21.

The role of non-physicians

Whilst the physician must continue to play a key role in treatment, other professions may make an important contribution. In primary care counsellors may be trained in simple psychological treatments. There is also an important role for nurses, physiotherapists, and occupational therapists (see Chapter 22). One such initiative has recently commenced in Oxford for patients with non-cardiac chest pain. Following their coronary angiogram, patients with negative results receive counselling by one of the unit's nursing staff aimed at minimizing the persistent fear of disease and chronic disability which often occurs in such patients (see Chapter 18).

Some physicians may feel that these patients are best treated by alternative and complementary practitioners. Whilst such treatment can undoubtedly be helpful in certain cases, it is often ineffective and not without hazard and we cannot recommend it as a general strategy (see Chapter 23).

Services

The ideal care of patients with functional somatic symptoms would be based on skilled management by primary care physicians who would assess and treat the majority. Those patients who could not be effectively managed in primary care would be further assessed in the out-patient clinic of the appropriate speciality, their fears discussed, and education given about how to cope with their symptoms. Patients with persistent or severe problems would be seen in specialist clinics run jointly by physicians and specialist psychiatrists or psychologists. These clinics would have ongoing treatment programmes for patients with severe functional somatic symptoms. A small in-patient rehabilitation unit would also be available. Clearly most services currently fall far short of this ideal.

What can go wrong?

In practice the treatment of patients with functional somatic symptoms, whilst often rewarding, frequently runs into difficulties. Many of these difficulties can be anticipated and some can be avoided (see Table 4.8).

Table 4.8 What goes wrong

The patient	The doctor–patient relationship
Feels disbelieved or humiliated	Becomes over-involved
Does not respond to treatment	Becomes hostile
Seeks multiple treatments	Breaks down
The doctor	
Acts on feelings of frustration	
Omits to assess the mental state	
Does not address the patient's fears and beliefs	
Orders excessive investigations	

What not to do

Imply that the symptoms are 'all in the mind' This is easy to do by the inadvertent use of psychological terminology or by poor preparation of the patient before telling them of a referral to a psychiatrist. Pressing psychological explanations onto a reluctant patient is not only likely to reduce their trust and compliance, but may also make them angry. Furthermore, it may have the paradoxical effect of strengthening their conviction in disease.

Neglect assessment of the patient's mental state Whilst there are many pitfalls for the unwary, perhaps the principal one is to neglect the assessment of the patient's emotional state. A rare but important consequences of this omission is the patient's death by suicide.

Fail to address the patient's fears and beliefs If the patients fears are not elicited and addressed, or their beliefs about their illness not heard, the doctor's explanation and reassurance is unlikely to be effective and the patient may feel rejected. Subsequent attempts at management are unlikely to go smoothly.

Use excessive investigations as reassurance A limited amount of investigation may be necessary to exclude possible organic disease. Using investigation to reassure the patient is an expensive and hazardous strategy. Whilst some neurologists use magnetic resonance imaging scans to reassure patients with headache this investigation may be equally likely to raise new fears of disease in the patient's mind.

The doctor's own feelings and beliefs

The doctor will often find him/herself frustrated or even angry with patients whose illness is unexplained by physical assessment (Lin *et al.* 1991). It is more useful to examine why this is, than to act out the frustration by overtreating the patient or by discharge with the simple aim of getting rid of them. Such negative feelings will often result from the doctor's awareness of their own inadequacy in diagnosing and treating the patient's illness (Corney *et al.* 1988; Goldberg *et al.* 1992).

Difficult patients

Patients with multiple chronic symptoms A proportion of patients with functional somatic symptoms will not respond to any of the treatments described. Many of these patients will have lifelong problems in functioning, associated with multiple and changing somatic symptoms (see Chapter 10). In such cases, the physician has an important role in limiting iatrogenic damage and unnecessary health care expenditure. Infrequent but long-term follow-up can limit the patient's use of other medical services (Smith 1991) and the physician who adopts this policy will often be rewarded by slow but definite improvement in the patient.

Patients with very strong fears or beliefs about disease There are number of special issues in the care of patients with unusually strong but inaccurate fears or beliefs about organic disease. Patients who are very fearful may be regarded as hypochondriacal. Their management requires special measures which are considered in more detail in Chapter 9. A small minority of patients have extremely strong beliefs about their health (which may sometimes be of delusional of near-delusional intensity) and the effective management in such cases may require specialist psychiatric treatment.

Patients who manufacture complaints Patients with manufactured or 'factitious' complaints are uncommon but can be very difficult to manage. In extreme form, this clinical presentation has been referred to as Munchausen's syndrome (Gattaz *et al*. 1990). Such patients will usually require confrontation about their behaviour. One approach is 'confrontation with support', which is carried out by both physician and psychiatrist (Bass and Murphy 1994). It is always easier to confront patients when there is tangible evidence of fabrication, for example a supply of syringes or 'illicit' medication in the patient's locker. The doctor should acknowledge the seriousness of the patient's physical problems and how he/she has felt compelled to aggravate these, then should shift the focus of management onto the patient's psychological problems and psychological care.

How do we know what works?

Any review of the relevant medical literature will reveal a large number of anecdotes, case studies, and uncontrolled case series. The 'gold standard' by which we usually judge clinical efficacy, randomized controlled trials, are much fewer. There has, however, been a welcome increase in research in recent years so that most of the therapies described in this book are supported by the results of controlled clinical trials.

Special issues in the design of clinical trials

It has proved possible to conduct clinical trials of various types of therapy for patients with functional somatic symptoms. However, there are frequently problems in the interpretation of the results of these studies. These problems include the observed variability in patient response, doubts about the generalizability of the findings, and the degree of improvement actually achieved. All reflect basic methodological problems in the design and conduct of such trials.

Patient selection One of the major factors hindering the evaluation of treatment is the problem of defining the patient population. Most studies have selected the patient sample on the basis of the principal functional symptom reported by the patient or on a diagnosis of one of a number of loosely defined and overlapping functional syndromes (see Chapter 3). This strategy results in a sample that is heterogenous in terms of psychiatric diagnosis, beliefs, coping behaviours, and personality. We would suggest that future studies need to define and recruit more homogenous sample and to exclude or stratify patients with lifelong problems in functioning.

Treatments The treatments evaluated are usually highly specialized therapies. There is a shortage of studies that evaluate the simpler, often combined interventions, more commonly used in clinical practice. There is a need for the systematic evaluation of simple and feasible treatment packages.

Comparison treatments Most trials of treatment of functional somatic symptoms find a large 'placebo' effect (Shepherd 1993). It is therefore essential that the evaluation of a specific treatment is made against an appropriate comparison condition. It is usual in drug trials to use a placebo treatment and in psychological studies a waiting list or non-specific psychological therapy. We suggest that in trials evaluating the treatment of patients in general medical settings, it may be of more practical use to use 'standard medical care' as the comparison condition (Goldberg 1992).

Outcome measures There is a lack of agreement about how best to measure outcome. It seems clear that not only symptoms but also quality of life, disability, and consumption of medical care should be evaluated. Simple measures for these variables are being developed such as the Hospital Anxiety and Depression scale (HAD) (Zigmond and Snaith 1983) and the 36-item Short Form Scale (SF-36) (Ware and Sherbourne 1992) for disability, but greater standardization is required so that the true clinical significance of patient responses can be judged. There is also a potential role for objective outcome measures such as the electronic recording of activity (Tryon 1991).

Prevention

A challenge for all those working in the area of functional somatic symptoms is prevention. What public health measures would minimize the morbidity and health care consumption associated with functional somatic symptoms? Many of the aetiological factors appear to lie more in the social and political realm than in the strictly medical and are therefore considered to be outside the control of the physician. These factors include increasing public expectation of health (Barsky 1988), dissatisfaction with modern work practices, and the availability of compensation and state benefits (see Chapter 12). Doctors do, however, have a role in advising employers, in giving evidence in compensation cases, and in educating the public. They also have an important task in attempting to further destigmatize psychiatric illness and psychological treatments.

Conclusions

Patients with functional somatic symptoms are poorly served by existing health services. They consume considerable resources but are frequently dissatisfied with their care. Physicians find them frustrating to treat. The causes of this unsatisfactory state of affairs lie in our lack of understanding of functional somatic symptoms, in current medical training and practice, and in the organization of clinical services. Although major improvements in all these areas are clearly desirable, substantial improvements in the management of patients could probably be achieved without major reorganization or increased funding, if doctors only followed a number of simple guidelines. These are listed below.

1. Assessment should always include a brief psychosocial history and mental state assessment and should lead to a formulation, as well as to a diagnosis.

2. All patients require a clear statement about the absence of physical disease, together with a positive explanation of their symptoms.

3. Patients' fears and beliefs about symptoms and illness should be elicited and, where necessary, re-examined by doctor and patient in a spirit of collaboration.

4. Significant depression and anxiety should be effectively treated.

5. Excessive medical and surgical investigation and treatment should be avoided.

6. Specialist assessment and treatment should be obtained for patients who do not respond to basic measures.

References

Altshuler, K.Z. and Rush, A.J. (1984). Psychoanalytic and cognitive therapies: a comparison of theory and tactics. *American Journal of Psychotherapy*, **38**, 4–17.

Anderson, R., Anderson, O.W., and Smedby, B. (1968). Perception of and response to symptoms of illness in Sweden and the United States. *Medical Care*, **6**, 18–30.

Armstrong, D. (1991). What do patients want? *British Medical Journal*, **303**, 261-2.

Barsky, A.J. (1988). The paradox of health. *New England Journal of Medicine*, **318**, 414-18.

Bass, C. and Benjamin, S. (1993). The management of chronic somatization. *British Journal of Psychiatry*, **162**, 472-80.

Bass, C. and Murphy, M. (in press). Somatization, somatoform disorders and factitious illness. In *Textbook of liaison psychiatry*, (ed. F. Creed and E. Guthrie). Royal College of Psychiatrists, London.

Beck, A.T., Rush, A.J., Shaw, B.F., and Emery, G. (1979). *Cognitive therapy of depression*. Guilford Press, New York.

Benjamin, S., Mawer, J., and Lennon, S. (1992). The knowledge and beliefs of family care givers about chronic pain patients. *Journal of Psychosomatic Research*, **36**, 211-17.

Bloch, S., Sharpe, M., and Allman, P. (1991). Systemic family therapy in adult psychiatry. *British Journal of Psychiatry*, **159**, 357-64.

Brooks, P. (1993). Repetitive strain injury: does not exist as a separate medical condition. *British Medical Journal*, **307**, 1298.

Butler, G., Fennel, M., Robson, P., and Gelder, M. (1991). Comparison of behavior therapy and cognitive behavior therapy in the treatment of generalized anxiety disorder. *Journal of Consulting and Clinical Psychology*, **59**, 167-75.

Cluff, R.A. (1984). Chronic hyperventilation and its treatment by physiotherapy: discussion paper. *Journal of the Royal Society of Medicine*, **77**, 855-62.

Corney, R.H., Strathdee, G., Higgs, R., King, M., Williams, P., Sharp, D., and Pelosi, A.J. (1988). Managing the difficult patient: practical suggestions from a study day. *Journal of the Royal College of General Practitioners*, **38**, 349-52.

Dubbert, P.M. (1992). Exercise in behavioural medicine. *Journal of Consulting and Clinical Psychology*, **60**, 613-18.

Eisenberg, D.M., Kessler, R.C., Foster, C., Norlock, F.E., Calkins, D.R. and T.L. Delbanco (1993). Unconventional medicine in the United States—prevalance, costs and pattern of use. *New England Journal of Medicine*, **328**, 246-52.

Escobar, J.I. and Canino, G. (1989). Unexplained physical complaints. Psychopathology and epidemiological correlates. *British Journal of Psychiatry*, Supple. 24-7.

Fink, P. (1992a). The use of hospitalizations by persistent somatizing patients. *Psychological Medicine*, **22**, 173-80.

Fink, P. (1992b). Surgery and medical treatment in persistent somatizing patients. *Journal of Psychosomatic Research*, **36**, 439-47.

Gantz, N.M. and Holmes, G.P. (1989). Treatment of patients with chronic fatigue syndrome. *Drugs*, **38**, 855-62.

Gattaz, W.F., Dressing, H., and Hewer, W. (1990). Munchausen syndrome: psychopathology and management. *Psychopathology*, **23**, 33-9.

Goldberg, D.P. (1992). The treatment of mental disorders in general medical settings. *General Hospital Psychiatry*, **14**, 83-5.

Goldberg, R.J., Novack, D.H., and Gask, L. (1992). The recognition and management of somatization. What is needed in primary care training. *Psychosomatics*, **33**, 55-61.

Goldenberg, D.L. (1989). Treatment of fibromyalgia syndrome. *Rheumatic Diseases Clinics of North America*, **15**, 61-71.

Griffith, J.L., Griffith, M.E., and Slovik, L.S. (1989). Mind-body patterns of symptom generation. *Family Process*, **28**, 137-52.

Kleinman, A., Eisenberg, L., and Good, B. (1978). Culture, illness and care. *Annals of Internal Medicine*, **88**, 251-8.

Lin, E.H.B., Katon, W.J., Von Korff, M., Bush, T., LIpscomb, P., Russo, J., and Wagner, E. (1991). Frustrating patients: physician and patient perspectives among distressed high utilizers of medical services. *Journal of General Internal Medicine*, **6**, 241-6.

Lipkin, M., Almy, T.P., and Kirkham, F.T. (1966). The formulation of diagnosis and treatment. *New England Journal of Medicine*, **19**, 1049-52.

Lipowski, Z.J. (1988). An inpatient programme for persistent somatizers. *Canadian Journal of Psychiatry*, **33**, 275-8.

Lucire, Y. (1988). Social iatrogenesis of the Australian disease 'RSI'. *Community Health Studies*, **12**, 146-50.

Lynch, S., Seth, R., and Montgomery, S. (1991). Antidepressant therapy in the chronic fatigue syndrome. *British Journal of General Practice*, **41**, 339-42.

McCain, G.A. (1991). Role of physical fitness training in the fibrositis/fibromyalgia syndrome. *American Journal of Medicine*, **18** (Suppl. 3a), 73-7.

Mayou, R.A. (1991). What should British consultation-liaison psychiatry be doing? *General Hospital Psychiatry*, **13**, 261-7.

Melson, S.J. and Rynearson, E.K. (1986). Intensive group therapy for functional illness. *Psychiatric Annals*, **16**, 687-92.

Murphy, M. (1993). Psychological management of somatization disorder. In *Psychological treatment in disease and illness*, (ed. M. Hodes and S. Moorey), pp. 65-87. Gaskell, London.

Peel, M. (1988). Rehabilitation in postviral syndrome. *Journal of Social and Occupational Medicine*, **38**, 44-5.

Pither, C.E. (1989). Treatment of persistent pain. *British Medical Journal*, **299**, 1239-40.

Rikard-Bell, C.J. and Waters, B.G.H. (1992). Psychosocial management of chronic fatigue syndrome in adolescence. *Australian and New Zealand Journal of Psychiatry*, **26**, 64-72.

Sainsbury, P. and Gibson, J.G. (1954). Symptoms of anxiety and tension and the accompanying physiological changes in muscular system. *Journal of Neurology, Neurosurgery and Psychiatry*, **17**, 216-24.

Salkovskis, P.M. (1992). Psychological treatment of noncardiac chest pain: the cognitive approach. *American Journal of Medicine*, **92** (Suppl. 5A), 114S-21S.

Sharpe, M.C. and Bass, C. (1992). Pathophysiological mechanisms in somatization. *International Reviews in Psychiatry*, **4**, 81-97.

Sharpe, M.C. and Hawton, K.E. (1990). Liaison psychiatry and psychological sequelae of physical disorders. *Current Opinion in Psychiatry*, **3**, 199-203.

Sharpe, M.C., Hawton, K.E., Seagraott, V., and Pasvol, G. (1992). Patients who present with fatigue: a follow up of referrals to an infectious clinic. *British Medical Journal*, **305**, 147–152.

Sharpe, M.C., Mayou, R.M., Seagroatt, V., Surawy, C., Bulstrode, C., Dawber, R., and Lane, D. (1994). Why do doctors find some patients difficult to help? *Quarterly Journal of Medicine*, **87**, 187–93.

Shepherd, M. (1993). The placebo: from specificity to the non-specific and back. *Psychological Medicine*, **23**, 569–78.

Shorter, E. (1992). *From paralysis to fatigue: a history of psychosomatic illness in the modern era.* Free Press, New York.

Smith, G.R., Monson, R.A., and Ray, D.C. (1986). Psychiatric consultation in somatization disorder — a randomized controlled study. *New England Journal of Medicine*, **314**, 1407–13.

Smith, R.C. (1991). Somatization disorder: defining its role in clinical medicine. *Journal of General Internal Medicine*, **6**, 168–75.

Stern, R. and Fernandez, M. (1991). Group cognitive and behavioural treatment for hypochondriasis. *British Medical Journal*, **303**, 1229–31.

Sullivan, M.D. (1993). Psychosomatic clinic or pain clinic — which is more viable? *General Hospital Psychiatry*, **15**, 375–80.

Todd, J.W. (1984a). Referrals to hospital. *The Lancet*, **ii**, 1089.

Todd, J.W. (1984b). Investigations. *The Lancet*, **ii**, 1146–7.

Tryon, W.W. (1991). *Activity measurement in psychology and medicine.* Plenum Press, New York.

Tyrer, P. (1976). *The role of bodily feelings in anxiety.* Institute of Psychiatry Maudsley Monograph 23. Oxford University Press, Oxford.

Ware, J.E. and Sherbourne, C.D. (1992). The MOS 36-item short-form health survey. *Medical Care*, **30**, 473–81.

Ware, N.C. (1992). Suffering and the social construction of illness: the delegitimation of illness experience in chronic fatigue syndrome. *Medical Anthropology Quarterly*, **6**, 347–61.

Whitehead, W.E. and Crowell, M.D. (1991). Psychologic considerations in the irritable bowel syndrome. *Gasteroenterological Clinics of North America*, **20**, 249–67.

Wright, A.L. and Morgan, W.J. (1990). On the creation of 'problem' patients. *Social Science in Medicine*, **30**, 951–9.

Zigmond, A.S. and Snaith, R.P. (1983). The hospital anxiety and depression scale. *Acta Psychiatrica Scandinavica*, **67**, 361–70.

PART 2 TREATMENT METHODS

5 The patient with medically unexplained symptoms: making the initial psychiatric contact

Allan House

Dr House points out that the patient's initial contact with a psychiatrist has to be very carefully managed. He stresses the importance of eliciting the patient's attitudes to psychiatric referral, as well as exploring the beliefs and assumptions that influence each patient's understanding of his or her illness.

The importance of acknowledging the reality of the patient's physical symptoms during the assessment interview is emphasized, as is the need for a flexible, empathic style of interviewing. In tandem with the 'illness history' Dr House encourages the adoption of a developmental approach, during which those experiences that might lead the patient to express distress in somatic terms are explored. Finally, the key role of family attitudes and beliefs is described and the importance of interviewing family members emphasized.

Introduction

Patients with medically unexplained symptoms are usually referred to a psychiatrist by another doctor. The questions being asked are almost invariably: do you think there is a psychological explanation for this person's presentation? and do you think that a psychiatric intervention might improve his or her well-being?

Once such a referral has been made, the psychiatrist's task is to answer those questions and when the answer is 'yes', to engage the patient in therapy. It is a common complaint of our medical colleagues that psychiatrists fail to grasp this basic point, but instead behave as if their task were solely to determine the presence or absence of diagnosable mental disorder. This chapter outlines an approach to the psychiatric assessment of somatic presentations, which aims to meet the needs of patient, referring physician, and psychiatrist.

The purposes of the initial psychiatric contact

The primary purpose of the assessment is to identify the patient's psychological and social problems and the various mediating mechanisms through which these are producing the symptoms. Associated aims are to determine aetiology, the presence of any relevant pathophysiological mechanisms, the resources available to the patient, and the extent of their handicap.

The psychiatrist assessing a patient with unexplained physical symptoms needs to obtain a considerable amount of information. The illness itself comprises not just symptoms but also associated handicap. Understanding the psychological processes which underlie the illness will require an understanding of the individual's developmental history and recent experiences. Identifying mediating (psychophysiological) mechanisms is usually a matter of inference from the symptoms but may involve special investigations.

In addition patients with unexplained physical symptoms pose a particular problem in assessment as they may not recognize the value of seeing a psychiatrist. It is not that they do not regard themselves as ill; rather that they do not see themselves as suffering from a psychiatric illness. Unless these concerns are addressed, the patient will not find the interview therapeutic and will not accept further psychiatric involvement even if it is appropriate (House 1989). The initial contact therefore has to be more than fact-finding; grinding through an orthodox psychiatric history with a few extra questions about medical contacts simply will not do.

There is very little written about the problem of resistance to psychiatric contact among patients with unexplained somatic symptoms. This makes it difficult to evaluate research studies because it is hard to judge how patients were recruited. For example in Kellner's (1983) influential report of a successful treatment outcome following psychotherapy for hypochondriasis, the problem of resistance to treatment is simply not mentioned. Resistance is, of course, also of great importance in the individual contact. Because of the paucity of the literature, much of what I have to say is based on clinical experience and not on research studies.

It is worth pointing out that resistance to psychiatric involvement may be a two-way affair. Patients with unexplained physical symptoms are often unpopular (Groves 1978). They are seen as neither physically ill nor mentally ill, but simply complaining as a means of avoiding life's responsibilities (Goldberg and Bridges 1988). Overcoming these negative attitudes is a matter for proper training of doctors and education of medical students (Smith 1984). I will not discuss this factor further in this chapter, but it must be remembered that the negative countertransference is a potent cause of poor treatment outcomes in psychiatry and medicine and is ignored at one's peril.

I have taken as my focus the first psychiatric interview rather than the psychiatric referral, although of course resistance to referral prevents many patients getting even as far as the first contact. None the less much of what I have to say can be transferred one step back down the clinical line as a guide to physicians in their discussion of unexplained symptoms (Sapira 1972) and in facilitating patient acceptance of psychiatric referral (Bursztajn and Barsky 1985).

This chapter is principally concerned with the chronic patient and the approach may be modified for patients with less severe illnesses of shorter duration, who may be less entrenched in their attitudes and behaviour.

Initiating the assessment process

Eliciting attitudes to psychiatric referral

The major initial problem presented to the psychiatrist by the patient with unexplained physical symptoms is that although there may be a number of potentially useful interventions available, the patient is not interested in exploring them. The first psychiatric consultation should therefore always start by addressing the patient's attitude to psychiatric referral (Bass 1992). My own practice is to open the interview by asking the patient what they have been told by the referring doctor about the reasons for coming to see a psychiatrist. Responses to this question usually fall into one of a number of categories and the patient may have been told any of the following.

1. Either nothing at all or that coming to see a psychiatrist 'might help'. When asked directly the patient may agree that stress or depression (or whatever is mentioned in the referral letter) was discussed, but not always.

2. That he/she was 'depressed', either with or without an explanation of how that might be related to the physical symptoms.

3. That the condition he/she suffers from is due to stress.

4. That I have (or psychiatrists in general have) some specific — but usually unspecified — treatment for pain, chronic fatigue, or whatever the main symptom is.

The second question I ask is how the patient feels about psychiatric referral. Responses to this question can be classified according to their emotional tone.

1. The commonest emotional responses are neutral. Patients express themselves as either indifferent or mildly sceptical but open-minded. They present themselves as rather passively referred from one depart-

ment to another in the hospital and therefore simply turning up to find out what happens next.

2. A few people say they are positively enthusiastic about referral; in fact some have suggested it themselves. Such enthusiasm usually arises when the patient has high levels of personal distress or when he or she feels the illness may be stress related. Neither attitude precludes a belief that the illness is itself based on organ disease.

3. Hostile responders usually develop some variation on the following themes. They are resentful because it has been implied that there is nothing wrong with them; their symptoms are not imaginary or made up; they know when they are ill or in pain; and they are not insane and they can see no reason, therefore, why they should see a psychiatrist.

Sometimes hostile views are expressed openly, but often they are not because of social convention. Such covert hostility will just as surely undermine the therapeutic process and needs to be explored, especially if there are non-verbal clues to its presence. Overt or covert antipathy must be addressed — at least to some extent — before any other aspect of the assessment interview is broached. Anger is an important theme in the psychodynamics of somatizing (Wahl 1963; Lipsitt 1974). It is not elicited with the intention of explaining the symptoms but in order to allow the establishment of a therapeutic relationship between psychiatrist and patient (Bursztajn and Barsky 1985).

Exploring attitudes to psychiatric referral

Four themes constantly recur when feelings about psychiatric referral are discussed, especially with the hostile patient.

Facing the limits of medicine   Patients visit doctors hoping to be diagnosed and relieved of their illnesses. When they are the subject of repeated investigation — perhaps in many different departments — it is tolerable if they have a rare or complicated condition and there is an end in sight. For the somatizer investigation and treatment is intolerable because it is endless; the condition is not amenable to the usual investigative or therapeutic manoeuvres. Patients feel this acutely and it affects their attitudes to referral. They may regard psychiatric referral as a hand-washing exercise and feel bitter or resentful. Surprisingly, some patients feel a sense of failure and they may even apologize for being so difficult to sort out. In my experience very few take any real pleasure in having defeated the medical system.

It is important to acknowledge this failure of the health care system to alleviate the patient's suffering and to help the patient appreciate that continued medical consultations will be fruitless. By acknowledging the negative implications of a return to the medical clinic, it is possible to introduce the idea of the psychiatric contact as a positive new avenue to explore.

Acknowledging the reality of the patient's illness Being told that the medical system can neither diagnose nor treat you should not be the same as being told there is nothing wrong with you. Unfortunately many patients (and doctors) think it is. The psychiatrist needs to 'clear the way for an informative talk by emphasizing unreservedly that the complaints are of real and by no means of an imaginary character' (Leonhard 1961).

In clarifying this point it is helpful to make the distinction between disease (organ pathology) and illness (symptoms and handicap) and to discuss how they can occur independently of each other. This distinction is discussed in Chapter 1. Most people understand that it is possible to have organ disease without symptoms or handicap; asymptomatic infection or cancer are widely recognized examples. Once this point is established, it is possible to introduce the idea of the reverse — illness without disease. Everyday examples such as tension headache, phantom limb pain, fainting through fear, or hypnotic anaesthesia, will illustrate the possibility of symptoms without organ pathology. The accuracy of the analogy or the degree to which it is accepted is relatively unimportant. The examples are a means for discussing the general issue and illustrating *the psychiatrist's* belief in the reality of the patient's experience despite the absence of identifiable organ pathology.

Understanding the reasons for seeing a psychiatrist Most people have no idea what psychiatrists do for a living. If pressed they usually subscribe to one of two views: psychiatrists either look after insane people or they try by more or less devious means to understand deep aspects of a person's personality. It is surprising how uncommonly psychiatrists are seen as people who might assess symptom states, have at their disposal symptom-relieving techniques, or be able to help an 'ordinary' person improve his or her quality of life by looking at how they cope with illness.

It is important therefore to make clear to the patient that the psychiatrist's function in seeing them is not to prove that the presentation is based on insanity (that the illness is imaginary) or that it is due to some deep-seated psychological disturbance. I usually start to discuss this point around the idea that all illness (as opposed to disease) has an emotional component and that sometimes focusing on that emotional component can be of benefit.

Acknowledging the fear of labelling and stigma   It is extremely helpful to discuss negative public attitudes to psychiatry. Patients find this openness reassuring, especially coming from the very person in whose company they most wish not to be. Once this issue is out in the open I often find that the patients themselves are not bothered about seeing a psychiatrist but they fear the response of other people. Since seeing a psychiatrist has now become part of their illness experience, the fear of stigma has to be faced. Confidentiality of medical notes and letters needs to be mentioned. One of the benefits of undertaking clinics in the general hospital is that it is thereby easier to reassure patients that they are not barred forever from access to medical care by virtue of seeing a psychiatrist.

Developing the assessment interview

By this stage a number of points should have been established: physical medicine has failed to relieve the patient's suffering, in such situations experience tells us that psychiatrists can sometimes help, and most people don't like the idea of being referred to a psychiatrist but the idea is worse than the reality.

The patient may remain sceptical or frankly rather hostile but as long as they are at least participating and fairly cooperative it is worth moving on. Further apprehensions may be overcome by a demonstration that the questions asked, the areas explored, and the suggestions made later in the interaction are not particularly peculiar and may be positively sensible and beneficial. Lipowski (1988) points out that patients who have accepted referral in the first place will usually be willing to explore further aspects of their illness even when they do not accept the *centrality* of psychosocial factors.

The stance during this subsequent phase of the assessment should be neutral, open-minded, and exploratory for a number of reasons. First, because that is the most useful way of conciliating hostility. Second, because part of the damage done to somatizers by the health system is due to repeated contact with experts who will claim to elucidate and remove the symptoms and then fail to do so. Third, every so often (albeit rarely) the diagnosis does not prove to be a psychiatric one. The areas which need review are:

(1) physical symptoms — their history and present status;

(2) the patient's experience of illness and the medical system — his or her illness career;

(3) the personal, developmental, and biographical history and mental state examination;

(4) the family perspective.

At least the first two of these are greatly assisted by a prior reading of all the patient's clinical records.

Physical symptoms The patient's illness consists — sometimes exclusively — of physical symptoms. Frequently patients have only been asked to describe their symptoms in so far as they allow a doctor to make or exclude a given diagnosis. The greater the quantity of symptoms, the more inconsistently they are described and the more unusual they are in quality, the more likely it is for the history to have been interrupted or curtailed. No doubt this contributes to patients' common feeling, even if they have consumed enormous amounts of medical time and resources, that they have been dismissed or not had a fair hearing.

For the psychiatrist, physical symptoms should not represent a barrier to be got through so as to move on as quickly as possible to more important psychological matters. They are the essence of the patient's experience of illness and for that reason they should be elucidated clearly, specifically, and in as much detail as the patient wishes to give (Ladee 1966; Aldrich 1981; Brown and Vaillant 1981). Actually probing and encouraging physical complaining therefore has a therapeutic effect (Lowy 1975). It may be the first time the patient has felt listened to. It is a demonstration of the psychiatrist's previous claim to be interested in physical illness. The sharing of bizarre or unusual symptoms without dismissal may be a great relief.

From a more analytical point of view the psychiatrist may also be able to gain some insight into the psychophysiological mechanisms mediating the symptoms. For example, somatic symptoms of tension, hyperventilation, or anxiety can be elicited by breath-holding or hyperventilation tests or by searching for areas of muscle tenderness (Bass 1992).

Elucidation of the origin of symptoms may justify the physical examination favoured by some psychiatrists (Kellner 1983; Pilowsky 1983). If the only purpose of examination is to offer reassurance that the patient is seeing a 'proper doctor' who will take them seriously, my own view is that it is best omitted.

One area of uncertainty is the degree to which physical symptoms should be discussed or attempts made at reattribution, as they are elicited. There are three broad approaches. The first is to make no attempt at all at 'psychologizing' the patient's presentation, simply accepting the symptoms without interpretation. The second is to promote deliberately a state of ambiguity about the meaning of the symptoms, trading on the multiple meanings of words like pain, tension, feeling tired, or weak. The third is to make explicit interpretations about the physical symptoms and their possible mechanisms, indicating that they are the somatic accompaniments of states which are primarily psychological or emotional. The approach adopted is a matter of personal style — given that there are no research data upon which to base a decision.

My own experience is that early and explicit attempts at reattribution work best when the presentation is an acute one and when the symptoms are based on some obvious physiological or autonomic mechanism. Examples might include tension headache, anxious tachycardia, or certain types of irritable bowel syndrome. When such a patient can accept a psychological or psychophysiological explanation of physical symptoms, then early interpretation can be rapidly effective. When the immediate mechanism of symptom production is obscure or there is not a 'single syndrome' presentation, such an approach may be less successful. I find that negative reactions to attempts to 'explain' symptoms can be a major problem with chronic and severe somatizers, who cannot tolerate an early or over-zealous attempt to interpret symptoms. The result is tension and a feeling on the patient's part that they are simply presenting symptoms to have them explained away.

The history of the evolution of the symptoms needs to be elicited, including their onset and the timing of any exacerbations or changes in their character. When they are giving this part of their history, patients very often offer an explanation for changes in their symptoms over time. These observations give valuable insights into the inner representation that the patient has of his or her own illness (see below). From the psychiatrist's perspective, changes in the illness may also be linked (although not necessarily by explicit interpretation to the patient) to life events and difficulties.

The patient's experience of illness   The patient's experience of illness is not the same thing as the history of the progression of their symptoms. A review of the 'illness career' entails obtaining a history of the interactions the patient has had with the health service and the way those interactions have shaped the patient's attitudes (to symptoms, investigations, diagnosis, and doctors) and behaviour.

Attitudes to symptoms   Attitudes to symptoms lie on a continuum. At one end is a vague perhaps barely formulated idea that physical symptoms always represent physical disorder. This idea can be formed into a more definite concern that certain physical symptoms are likely to represent disease in certain organs. For example, symptoms in the chest are likely to represent heart or lung disease, headache or 'funny turns' is likely to represent neurological disease, and so on. Further along the spectrum is worry about specific disorders such as stroke, heart attack, or multiple sclerosis. Only occasionally does one encounter a patient who has a fixed belief about having a specific named disorder.

Attitudes to investigation and diagnosis   Attitudes to investigation and diagnosis also vary considerably. Some people regard investigation and diagnosis as an essential prerequisite of treatment. They find it difficult to believe that symptoms can be relieved without a clear idea of their cause. They find it even more difficult to believe that the majority of all medical investigations draw a blank. On the other hand, some people are indifferent to investigation and unimpressed by descriptive diagnostic statements. A good illustration is the variability among patients with chronic fatigue in the degree to which they think that having a diagnosis of myalgic encephelomyelitis (ME) explains (as opposed to describes) their state (see Chapter 16).

In research or clinical practice, it will be possible to recruit for treatment only those patients who have accepted that further investigation is unnecessary or can be deferred. How else, for example, could a patient enter group treatment for hypochondriasis introduced as providing an educational 'course on the perception of bodily symptoms' (Barsky *et al.* 1988)? Gaining acceptance of such a belief must be via a sort of 'pre-treatment' which is unfortunately rarely described and yet which is pivotal to successful treatment in this setting.

Attitude to doctors   Attitudes to doctors are often highly ambivalent. On the positive side doctors are perceived as the best people to help with physical symptoms; they are powerful figures, with a near-magical understanding of the inner workings of the body. By contrast patients often express quite negative attitudes to the medical care they have received. Doctors are perceived as rude, bored, or dismissive: 'You never see the same doctor twice and if you do they usually tell you there is nothing wrong or repeat a test you have had before.' It is difficult to spend any time working in a large hospital and not acknowledge the reality of some of these complaints.

It is important to recognize the ambivalence which lies behind both positive *and* negative expressions towards doctors and medical care. It is not always easy to see why somatizing patients speak highly of doctors when their actual experience of medical contact has been so negative. Repeated attendance and contact with doctors has not led to recovery. It has revolved around what isn't present and has been constantly confusing because of inconsistent or half-understood exchanges about symptoms. None the less it is only through hospital contact that many patients seem able to pursue attribution of their experiences or acknowledgement of their suffering. In this respect the chronic somatizer is very like the chronic litigant. Both are caught in a system which is very unlikely to meet their needs, while it captures them in a repetitive cycle of invalidation and humiliation.

Attitudes to treatment   Attitudes to treatment are no less diverse. Some people have a child-like faith in the ability of drugs or machines to alleviate their symptoms. Others have faith in psychological therapies, which they can accept uncritically while criticizing an orthodox biological medicine which has much stronger scientific foundations. Beliefs about treatment do not need to match beliefs about the cause of illness or disease. For example, most people who believe that alternative therapies improve the prognosis of cancer do not regard cancer primarily as a psychogenic disorder.

Attitudes to doctors, to treatment, and to investigation can be illogical and mutually incompatible. Together they constitute what is sometimes called by health psychologists the illness representation (see, for example, Murray 1991). Such representations or internal schemata of illness are acquired by internalization of a whole range of family, medical, and social experiences which are assimilated into an internal set of beliefs about illness.

The importance of exploring these various attitudes to illness and the experience of being a patient cannot be over-emphasized. They cannot be inferred readily from the patient's behaviour. One of the characteristics of somatizers is that they are active agents in pursuing medical care for their condition. A great deal of time is wasted by assuming that the patient understands his or her interaction with the health service as having the same purposes as does the doctor. Too often what the patient wants (a diagnosis, more tests, a dramatic treatment, and reassurance) is simply assumed or their explanation of what they want is taken at face value without full exploration of the contradictoriness, illogicality, or ambivalence of the beliefs that underlie their presentation.

Illness behaviours   Illness behaviours are manifest in two spheres which I call consulting behaviour and social behaviour. *Consulting behaviour* can be readily identified in the details of the patient's illness career: thick case-note folders revealing numerous futile attendances, contact with multiple hospital specialists, and repeated requests for drugs which are complained of as ineffective but are taken none the less. Consulting behaviour is also manifest in the individual clinical contact, although relatively few patients are histrionic or dramatic in this context. More often, they present an ambivalent mixture of behaviours well captured in the medical expression 'presenting complaints'. Complaints can be symptoms; an array of experiences of illness which elicit caring behaviour. Complaints can be challenging, assertive expressions of dissatisfaction which lead to an uncomfortable desire to placate.

Social illness behaviour manifests in life away from the medical arena. It is interesting to note how the patient lives the life of an invalid in the family. For example, Hodgson Burnett's (1982) story *The secret garden* is a marvellous evocation of the invalid child as a tyrant. Adults can of course play the same part. Abnormal social illness behaviour is often associated with protracted unemployment and the receipt of benefits dependent upon invalidity.

Evaluating illness behaviour is important in understanding the patient's dilemma as an ill person. The assessment of the degree to which illness behaviour influences various social functions is also an important part of making a decision about intervention, since the more areas of social function that are affected, the less likely is a purely individual (biological or psychological) intervention to be effective.

The personal history and mental state examination   Taking a personal and biographical history is most like that part of the assessment undertaken with any other patient referred for a psychiatric opinion. It usually represents an obvious departure from the rest of the physical illness-oriented interview undertaken so far and it therefore needs a little introduction. I usually say that I want to get a wider view of the patient as a person, of the sort of life they have led and are leading, and, therefore, of the effect that illness has had on their life.

In some ways the developmental history is the mirror of the history of the illness career. It is designed to uncover the experiences which might lead the patient to express distress in somatic terms in later life or to develop the sort of intractable and ambivalent relationships which are so typical of those which the severe chronic somatizer has with health care professionals (see, for example, Benjamin and Eminson 1992).

The more recent personal and biographical history is designed to elucidate those factors which might have determined the onset of symptoms. The key players in the patient's social network are central both in relation to provoking life events and in the construction of social illness behaviour which sustains chronicity.

Some somatic presentations are associated with other mental disorders, especially mood disorders. This point has been so overstated by psychiatrists who do not work in general hospital settings — and, therefore, see biased samples — that it is easy to dismiss it in reaction. At the initial interview it may not be feasible to undertake a full formal mental state examination, but some attempt must be made to elicit as many of the major symptoms of psychiatric disorder as the patient will tolerate.

The family perspective   The work of the Bedford College team on life events and illness is useful in helping to understand how recent and past experiences can explain the onset and shape the presentation of a whole range of disorders (Brown and Harris 1989). Since most life events also involve key relationships, the intervention to which life events research points most obviously is some form of assessment of the family, social network, and interpersonal relationships of the patient. There is no doubt that family interviewing is an underused part of the assessment of adult patients in general psychiatric practice. Occasionally contact with family or significant others is resisted by the patient, but often it is encouraged. The commonest reason for which it is neglected in British practice is that most psychiatrists do not receive even basic training in family interviewing techniques unless as part of a child psychiatry experience.

For the patient with unexplained physical symptoms, the attitudes and behaviour of the immediate family may be a crucial factor in understanding the presentation and in planning intervention (Benjamin *et al.* 1992). How and when family members are involved is a matter of personal preference, but they always should be unless the patient actively declines permission, in which case this itself should be a subject for exploration.

Conclusion

Using an analogy from chess, the procedures outlined above could be compared with the opening moves. The opening should develop the main pieces and establish the themes for the rest of the game. In this context the main themes are the patient's symptoms and their natural history, the patient's illness career and its manifestation in the illness representation and illness behaviour, and the personal and social experiences which have preceded the onset of symptoms and run parallel and intertwined with the illness career. The advantage of the approach I have outlined is that opening moves will be relatively familiar to the other player — involving as they do the physical illness as he or she experiences it. The patient will be reassured that even the rules of engagement are discussed as part of the preamble.

The initial contact must necessarily address a number of issues related to attitudes and illness behaviour. This can be beneficial both in engaging the patient and perhaps in obtaining improvement with a short-term and relatively superficial intervention. However, I do not believe that a cognitive or cognitive-behavioural approach can alone form the basis for managing most patients with chronic or recurrent unexplained physical symptoms. The initial psychiatric contact must keep several therapeutic options open by looking at the origins of the presentation from more than one perspective.

A strength of the 'opening' outlined above is flexibility; as the middle game develops, any one of a number of strategies can be adopted with an equal chances of success. Subsequent management may be *symptom oriented* as in, for example, the use of relaxation for tension pain, the behavioural treatment of anxiety, or the use of antidepressants. If so, the symptoms have already been well elucidated. Treatment may be *behaviourally oriented*; directed towards modifying consultation behaviour through an intervention aimed at reducing inappropriate health service resource use (Smith *et al.* 1986). A management plan may be *function oriented* as in many pain management programmes or the types of graded activity programme used in chronic fatigue. The initial assessment must have outlined the relevant functional deficits and illness behaviours. Management may be more *aetiologically oriented* as in the psychodynamic or interpersonal therapies which aim to understand and resolve personal dilemmas and conflicts which lie behind symptom onset or persistence, or cognitive therapies aimed at re-attributing experiences and reducing maladaptive illness behaviours. Finally the approach may be one of *containment and support* with the main focus being limitation of the unreasonable expectations of the patient and doctor (Adler 1981; Strain 1986).

Details of these various therapeutic approaches are reviewed in other chapters; I hope the approach to initiating those therapies which I have outlined here will be regarded as flexible enough to be compatible with any of them.

References

Adler, G. (1981). The physician and the hypochondriacal patient. *New England Journal of Medicine*, **304**, 1394–6.

Aldrich, C.K. (1981). Severe chronic hypochondriasis 1. A practical method of treatment 2. An intervention technique for prevention. *Postgraduate Medicine*, **69**, 139–56.

Barsky, A., Geringer, E., and Wool, C. (1988). A cognitive-educational treatment for hypochondriasis. *General Hospital Psychiatry*, **10**, 322–7.

Bass, C. (1990). The frequent attender in general practice. *Postgraduate Update*, 494–501.

Bass, C. (1992). Patients who somatize: what can the psychiatrist offer? In *Practical problems in clinical psychiatry*, Vol. 2, (ed. P.J. Cowen, and K. Hawton), pp. 105–17. Oxford University Press, Oxford.

Benjamin, S. and Eminson, D. (1992). Abnormal illness behaviour: childhood experiences and long-term consequences. *International Review of Psychiatry*, **4**, 55–70.

Benjamin, S., Mawer, J., and Lennon, S. (1992). The knowledge and beliefs of family care givers about chronic pain patients. *Journal of Psychosomatic Research*, **36**, 211–17.

Brown, G. and Harris, T. (1989). *Life events and illness*. Guilford, New York.

Brown, H. and Vaillant, G. (1981). *Archives of Internal Medicine*, **141**, 723–6.

Bursztajn, H. and Barsky, A. (1985). Facilitating patient acceptance of a psychiatric referral. *Archives of Internal Medicine*, **145**, 73–5.

Goldberg, D. and Bridges, P. (1988). Somatic presentations of psychiatric illness in primary care settings. *Journal of Psychosomatic Research*, **32**, 137–44.

Groves, J.E. (1978). Taking care of the hateful patient. *New England Journal of Medicine*, **298**, 883–7.

Hodgson Burnett, F. (1982). *The secret garden*. Puffin. London.

House, A. (1989). Hypochondriasis and related disorders: assessment and management of patients referred for a psychiatric opinion. *General Hospital Psychiatry*, **11**, 156–65.

Kellner, R. (1983). Prognosis of treated hypochondriasis: a clinical study. *Acta Psychiatrica Scandinavica*, **67**, 69–79.

Ladee, E.A. (1966). *Hypochondriacal syndromes*, Elsevier, Amsterdam.

Leonhard, K. (1961). On the treatment of ideohypochondriac and sensohypochondriac neuroses. *International Journal of Social Psychiatry*, **7**, 123–33.

Lipowski, Z. (1988). An inpatient programme for persistent somatizers. *Canadian Journal of Psychiatry*, **33**, 275–8.

Lipsitt, D. (1974). Psychodynamic considerations of hypochondriasis. *Psychotherapy and Psychosomatics*, **23**, 132–41.

Lowy, F. (1975). Management of the persistent somatizer. *International Journal of Psychiatry in Medicine*, **6**, 277–39.

Murray, M. (1991). Lay representations of illness. In *Current developments in health psychology*, (ed. P. Bennett, J. Weinman, and P. Spurgeon), pp. 63–90. Harwood Academic, London.

Pilowsky, I. (1983). Hypochondriasis. In *Handbook of psychiatry* Vol. 4, (ed. G. Russell, L. Hersor) pp. 319–23. Cambridge University Press, Cambridge.

Sapira, J. (1972). What to say to symptomatic patients with benign diseases. *Annals of Internal Medicine*, **77**, 603–4.

Smith, G.R., Monson, R., and Ray, D.C. (1986). Psychiatric consultation in somatisation disorder. *New England Journal of Medicine*, **314**, 1407–13.

Smith, R.C. (1984). Teaching interview skills to medical students: the issue of 'countertransference'. *Journal of Medical Education*, **59**, 582–88.

Strain, J.J. (1986). The diagnosis, ontogenesis, and management of hypochondriasis. In *Emotional disorders in physically ill patients*, (ed. R. Roessler and N. Decker), pp. 150–65. Human Sciences Press, New York.

Wahl, C. (1963). Unconscious factors in the psychodynamics of the hypochondriacal patient. *Psychosomatics*, **4**, 9–14.

6 Antidepressant treatment of functional somatic symptoms

Wayne Katon and Mark Sullivan

In this chapter Dr Katon and Dr Sullivan review the role of antidepressant drugs in the treatment of patients with functional somatic symptoms. They first review the prevalence and importance of depression and anxiety in the aetiology of functional somatic symptoms and then go on to use their recent research into chronic tinnitus to illustrate the complex relationship between depression and the experience of symptoms. The evidence for the efficiency of antidepressants is reviewed and practical guidelines for treatment outlined.

Introduction

This chapter will examine the role of antidepressant drug therapy in the management of patients with functional somatic symptoms. There are several reasons to believe that antidepressant drugs may have a place in the management of functional somatic symptoms.

1. The importance of depression and anxiety in their aetiology and presentation.

2. The evidence for the efficacy of these drugs in reducing the symptoms, disability, and distress in functional syndromes such as chronic pain, fibromyalgia, premenstrual syndrome, chronic fatigue syndrome, and tinnitus.

3. The need for a cheap, effective readily available treatment for the large number of patients with functional symptoms seen in general medical settings.

Each of these points will be discussed in turn. In order to examine the importance of depression in the aetiology and treatment of functional somatic symptoms, our own research into the treatment of patients with depression, chronic tinnitus, and hearing impairment will be described. Finally, we offer practical guidelines about how to use antidepressant medication in this patient group.

The importance of depression and anxiety in patients with functional somatic symptoms

Depression, anxiety, and somatic symptoms

Studies have consistently shown that patients with high levels of psychological distress report many more functional somatic symptoms then do the general population (Katon and Sullivan 1990). The Epidemiologic Catchment Area Study (ECA) (Escobar and Canino 1989) of a large sample of the general population found that virtually all psychiatric disorders were associated with increased somatic symptom reporting. Studies of clinical populations have also demonstrated a higher level of somatic symptom reporting in patients with major depression or panic disorder than in patients without psychiatric disorder (Katon and Sullivan 1990; Katon 1991*a*). Furthermore, patients who report functional somatic symptoms are likely to be suffering from psychiatric disorders, particularly anxiety and depressive disorders. Among the ECA respondents who reported five or more current medically unexplained symptoms, 63 per cent also reported current psychological symptoms and 50 per cent met criteria for a current psychiatric disorder, compared with 7 and 6 per cent, respectively, of those respondents with fewer current somatic symptoms (Simon and von Korff 1991). The odds ratios for the association of psychiatric disorder with five or more medically unexplained somatic symptoms illustrate the strength of the association: panic disorder (204); schizophrenia (90); mania (24); major depression (17); and phobia (12). Finally, studies of patients with panic disorder and major depression have found that successful pharmacologic treatment of the disorder is associated with a reduction in the reporting of somatic symptoms (Kellner *et al.* 1986; Noyes and Clancy 1986).

At the University of Washington, Division of Consultation-Liaison Psychiatry, we have conducted a series of studies in which we have attempted to elucidate the association between functional somatic symptoms and psychiatric illness. In each of these studies patients with a specific principal functional symptom were compared to a medical control group with a well-defined medical diagnosis. For example, patients with chest pain but negative angiographic studies were compared with patients with chest pain and positive angiographic evidence of coronary artery disease (Katon *et al.* 1988).

In these studies we examined both groups of patients using a structured psychiatric interview, the National Institute of Mental Health (NIMH) Diagnostic Interview Schedule (DIS) (Robins *et al.* 1981). This interview has high inter-rater reliability and is based on the American Psychiatric Association criteria for the diagnosis of psychiatric disorders (DSM-III). Moreover, the interview requires the examiner to enquire about the 33

Table 6.1 Prevalence rates of major depression as related to chronic pain, tinnitus, and fatigue

	Current major depression	Lifetime major depression	Number of episodes	Associated psychiatric and/or medical illness
Back pain	33	57	3	Alcoholism
Chest pain versus controls	35 vs 3	64 vs 16	5	Panic disorder
Pelvic pain versus controls	34 vs 10	66 vs 16	5	Substance abuse Sexual abuse
Tinnitus versus controls	60 vs 7	75 vs 15	3.5	Mild sensori-neural hearing loss
Fatigue versus controls	15 vs 3	76.5 vs 42	2	Somatization disorder
Irritable bowel syndrome versus controls	21 vs 5.5	61 vs 17	2.5	Panic disorder Somatization disorder
Dizziness versus peripheral ear	12 vs 5	42 vs 18	2	Panic disorder

physical symptoms which make up the diagnosis of somatization disorder and thereby elicits both functional somatic symptoms and a history of the patient's use of medical services.

Table 6.1 demonstrates the similarity of the findings from this series of studies. In each case, patients with functional somatic symptoms had a significantly *higher* prevalence of both current and lifetime depression than the comparison group with proven disease. Other important psychiatric and psychosocial differences between the groups were found. For instance, patients with non-cardiac chest pain (Katon *et al.* 1988) and irritable bowel syndrome (Walker *et al.* 1990), were significantly more likely to meet DSM-III criteria for panic disorder and generalized anxiety disorder than patients with proven cardiac and bowel disease, respectively. Patients with irritable bowel syndrome (Walker *et al.* 1990) and chronic fatigue (Katon *et al.* 1991) were also significantly more likely to meet DSM-III criteria for somatization disorder than their comparison patients with physical disease. Finally, women with functional chronic pelvic pain were significantly more likely to have been a victim of childhood and adult sexual abuse compared to controls with proven pelvic disease (Walker *et al.* 1988).

The principal conclusion to emerge from these studies is that patients with functional somatic symptoms are more likely than patients with demonstrable physical disease to have a history of major depressive and anxiety disorders, multiple medically unexplained somatic symptoms, and/or somatization disorder (Katon 1991*b*). Many of these patients were also high utilizers of medical care and had undergone extensive costly and often invasive medical investigations (such as angiography, laparoscopy, or electronystagmogram). We also noted that many of the patients had, over the course of their illness, gradually developed considerable psycho-social disability and maladaptive illness behaviour, given up significant work-related and household duties, become more socially withdrawn, and experienced a deterioration in relationship with their partner with reduced sexual activity.

A recent study of 285 patients with medically unexplained chronic fatigue demonstrated further interesting connections between anxiety and depressive disorders and the tendency to experience and report multiple somatic symptoms (Katon and Russo 1992). Based on previously published data, patients with fatigue were divided into four groups, each having a progressively greater number of lifetime functional somatic symptoms. The prevalence of both current and lifetime anxiety and depressive diagnoses was found to increase linearly with the number of lifetime physical symptoms. The extent of impairment in activities of daily living was also noted to increase linearly with the number of medically unexplained physical symptoms reported.

Depression, anxiety, and functional impairment

When psychiatric disorders co-exist with minor somatic symptoms such as chronic tinnitus (Sullivan *et al.* 1988), dizziness (Linzer *et al.* 1992), irritable bowel syndrome (Drossman *et al.* 1982), and migraine headaches (Stewart *et al.* 1992) the patient has significantly more disability. This co-morbidity with anxiety and depressive disorders probably explains why patients with functional symptoms *and* depressive symptoms are as disabled (in terms of decrements in vocational and social function, pain complaints, and a tendency to see their physical health as impaired), as patients with chronic disease (such as hypertension, diabetes, arthritis, and coronary artery disease) (Wells *et al.* 1989).

Depression, anxiety, and utilization of medical services

Studies in primary care have shown that patients with psychiatric disorders have a high utilization rate for non-psychiatric medical services (Hankin and Oktay 1979). Recent studies that have focused on the psychiatric epidemiology of high utilizers (McFarland *et al.* 1985; Katon *et al.* 1990) have found that these patients had both more functional somatic symptoms and a greater prevalence of psychological distress and recurrent affective illness than low utilizers.

In a large health maintenance organization (HMO) study, from which pregnant women and persons with terminal illness were excluded, over half of 767 high utilizers identified scored in the distressed range on one or more self-report measures (Katon *et al.* 1990). Although the high utilizers in this HMO study represented only 10 per cent of patients in two large primary care clinics, over a 1 year period they used 29 per cent of all outpatient primary care visits, 52 per cent of out-patient specialty visits, 48 per cent of all in-patient hospital days, and 26 per cent of all prescriptions. When they were interviewed it was found that these high utilizers had a high rate of depressive disorder with approximately two-thirds suffering from recurring, relapsing major depressive illness (Katon *et al.* 1990). The psychiatric morbidity was not confined to depression: anxiety disorders, somatization disorder, and alcohol abuse were also prevalent.

Recent data from the ECA Study have confirmed the tendency of respondents with mental illness who are living in the community to have a significantly higher usage of general medical services, as well as of mental health services (Simon 1992). In this study, patients with panic disorder and somatization disorder had the highest number of medical visits although the number was also high for those with major depression, phobia, and alcohol and drug abuse (Simon 1992). This study of medical care utilization found a strong association between high utilization (defined as six or more visits to general medical services over a 6 month period) and presence of psychiatric disorders. The odds ratios for these associations were as follows: somatization disorder (males 3.3, females 2.5), panic disorder (males 8.2, females 5.2), major depression (males 1.5, females 3.4), phobias (mates 2.7, females 1.6), alcohol abuse (males 1.6, females 1.6), and drug abuse (males 1.8, female 1.2) (Simon 1992).

When psychiatric disorders co-occur with minor somatic symptoms, health care utilization is increased (Drossman *et al.* 1982; W. Katon and E.A. Walker 1993). For instance, respondents in the community with chronic fatigue who also had a co-morbid anxiety or depressive disorder had significantly higher medical utilization rates than respondents with chronic fatigue alone. Patients with irritable bowel syndrome and co-morbid psychiatric disorder have also been shown to be much more likely to visit physicians with gastrointestinal complaints than patients with irritable bowel alone (Drossman *et al.* 1982; see Chapter 14).

Antidepressant treatment of functional somatic symptoms — theoretical considerations

The example of chronic tinnitus

Our recent research into the problem of chronic tinnitus has implications for our understanding of the role of depression and the place of antidepressant treatment in patients with all types of functional somatic symptoms. Both Swedish and British population studies have found that 15 per cent of adults experience constant or nearly constant tinnitus Medical Research Council Institute of Hearing Research 1981; Coles 1984; Meikle *et al.* 1984; Axellson and Ringdahl 1987). However, only one-sixth of this group with constant tinnitus found it to be severe or disabling (Meikle *et al.* 1984; Axellson and Ringdahl 1987). This difference in severity is poorly understood. The prevalence of tinnitus, but not the severity, increases with age and the degree of high-frequency sensorineural hearing loss (Coles 1984; Meikle *et al.* 1984; Axellson and Ringdahl 1987). Acoustic properties of the tinnitus sound, such as loudness, frequency, and number of sounds, do not account for reported differences in tinnitus severity (Meikle *et al.* 1984; Axellson and Ringdahl 1989).

The role of depression   An increased incidence of psychopathology in tinnitus patients has been documented in studies based on self-report measures (Stephens and Hallam 1985). In addition, the pattern of symptoms and disability (for example, insomnia, dysphoria, and decreased concentration and socialization) is similar to that seen in major depression (Stephens and Hallam 1985; Sullivan *et al.* 1989). In a recent study, using the NIMH Diagnostic Interview Schedule, we confirmed the high prevalence of major depression in patients presenting with tinnitus compared with a control group of persons with equal or greater hearing loss; 60 per cent of the tinnitus patients had current major depression, compared with only 7 per cent of the hearing loss control group (Sullivan *et al.* 1988). The functional disability of depressed tinnitus patients was also more severe than patients with hearing loss and patients with tinnitus who were not depressed. This finding suggests that the disability often attributed by both patient and physician to tinnitus, may be more directly linked to the co-morbid depression.

Antidepressant drug treatment and tinnitus   To further assess the role of depression in tinnitus, a single-blind, placebo-washout pilot study of nortriptyline was performed in 19 patients with both tinnitus and current major depression (Sullivan *et al.* 1990). Those who did not respond to 2 weeks of placebo were titrated up to a therapeutic nortriptyline serum level and maintained there for 6 weeks. At the end of the study 14 patients considered their tinnitus improved, and 12 of those chose to continue taking nortriptyline after the end of study. Depressive symptoms decreased by a mean of 64 per cent. Significant decreases were also found in tinnitus severity, tinnitus loudness, psychological symptoms, and in psychosocial disability attributed to tinnitus. These results suggested that antidepressant treatment reduced the severity of the tinnitus by reducing the severity of the depression.

However, it is not possible to assess the role of placebo response and regression to the mean in a single-blind, placebo-washout design. A randomized, double-blind, placebo-controlled trial using nortriptyline to treat severe chronic tinnitus was therefore conducted. This study included 38 subjects with current DSM-IIIR major depression and 54 subjects with subsyndromal depressive symptoms and significant disability due to tinnitus (Sullivan *et al.* 1993). This latter group included subjects distressed by tinnitus, with depressive symptoms but not meeting DSM-IIIR criteria for major depression (hereafter called the depression–NOS group), were also included. Depression–NOS subjects had a mean baseline Hamilton Depression Score of 10.3 and 1.5 current depressive symptoms on the DIS (69 per cent had sleep disturbance and 51 per cent had decreased concentration). Twenty-eight per cent of this group had a history of major depression.

Analysis of the post-treatment depression severity as defined by the score on the Hamilton depression scale (HAM-D) indicated that, after adjusting for baseline depression by analysis of covariance, subjects receiving nortriptyline were significantly less depressed at follow-up than those receiving placebo. Patients with major depression given nortriptyline had the greatest decrease in depression. There was a similar reduction in disability. The change in audiometric tinnitus variables was assessed by multiple analysis of covariance and a significant drug treatment effect was found. The significance of this effect was due to differences in tinnitus loudness. The nortriptyline group matched their tinnitus to an external source of the same frequency at a level over 5 dB quieter than the placebo group. More simply, when asked 'Has the medication helped you?', 67 per cent of patients on nortriptyline answered 'yes' compared to 39 per cent on placebo.

The results of this study generally replicate those of our previous single-blind pilot study and provide evidence that nortriptyline treatment produces greater improvement in depression, functional disability, and tinnitus loudness in patients with chronic, severe tinnitus than treatment with placebo.

Implication of studies of tinnitus   Otolaryngologists have long noted that tinnitus patients are often depressed. Conventional clinical wisdom has considered that this depression occurs in response to the aversive tinnitus sensation. This study, as well as our previous studies, suggest that the causal relationship between tinnitus and depression may be acting in both directions. Tinnitus (like pain) may prompt a depressive episode. Depression, in turn, may impede habituation to the aversive sensation and thereby increase the severity of the tinnitus experienced. This insight is clinically important because it suggests that antidepressant treatment may be useful for those persons with the most severe tinnitus whom otolaryngologists have felt that they had nothing to offer.

Chronic tinnitus, once established, tends to be a lifelong condition. Disability associated with tinnitus has therefore been assumed to be irreversible in nature and medical in origin. The present study demonstrates that while the illness may be lifelong, the associated disability need not be. In the case of tinnitus and associated disability, what appears to be an irreversible and medical disability may be better regarded as reversible and psychiatric.

Antidepressant treatment of functional somatic syndromes — the evidence of efficacy

There is evidence for the efficiency of antidepressant drugs not only in the treatment of depression, anxiety, and panic disorders, but also in a variety of functional syndromes. This evidence is reviewed below.

Chronic pain syndromes

The management of patients with chronic pain is reviewed in Chapter 11. Depression is particularly common in patients with a complaint of pain. Dworkin *et al.* (1990) have found that patients with one pain complaint were no more depressed than controls, but patients with two pain complaints were six times more likely to be depressed and patients with three pain complaints were eight times more likely to meet depressive criteria. However, the nature of the aetiological relationship between pain and depression remains uncertain. Some researchers have advocated the term 'depression pain syndrome' with the implication that chronic pain and depression are linked biologically and respond to similar treatments (Lindsay and Wyckoff 1981).

A number of placebo-controlled double-blind trials have demonstrated pain relief with antidepressant treatment (Onghena and Van Houdenhove 1992). Studies have demonstrated the efficiency of antidepressant drugs in relieving chronic pain both in depressed and in non-depressed patients. Furthermore, the reduction in pain sometimes occurs more quickly than the relief of depression. Tricyclic antidepressants may therefore have *direct* as well as depression-mediated effects on pain. A recent meta-analysis documented that 28 out of 39 placebo-controlled studies demonstrated analgesic efficacy for antidepressant treatment (Onghena and Van Houdenhove 1992), with a mean of 58 per cent of patients showing a 50 per cent reduction in pain. This reduction in pain was not restricted to patients with major depression or dependent on a reduction in depression severity.

The tricyclic antidepressants produced a greater effect in the meta-analysis than the heterocyclic agents. While amitriptyline was the most studied, doxepin showed the largest effect size (Onghena and Van Houdenbove 1992). It is worth noting that the predominantly serotonergic agents showed no benefit over the predominantly noradrenergic agents (Gourlay *et al*. 1986; Max *et al*. 1992; Onghena and Van Houdenhove 1992). In fact, those drugs with *mixed* action showed the largest effect size. A recent, well-designed double-blind randomized cross-over study comparing amitriptyline, desipramine, fluoxetine, and placebo in diabetic neuropathy bears out this conclusion (Max *et al*. 1992). In terms of pain reduction amitriptyline and desipramine were equally effective but fluoxetine was no better than placebo for pain. The only patients for whom fluoxetine appeared to work were those who were depressed. Furthermore, this advantage of mixed action drugs may be even more marked in the treatment of the myofascial pain syndromes where antidepressant responsiveness is closely correlated with the presence of depressive vegetative symptoms (Pheasant *et al*. 1983).

Theories about the mechanism of the antidepressant analgesic effect refer to the role played by biogenic amines in the endogenous pain modulation system. Two experimental paradigms have been used to activate and investigate this system in animals.

(1)   stimulation-induced analgesia (Richardson and Akil 1977);

(2)   stress-induced analgesia (Terman *et al*. 1984)

The first relies upon direct electrical stimulation of brain regions such as the midbrain raphé nuclei to produce analgesia. The second relies upon the imposition of environmental stressors such as pain or forced swims. With different stimulation locations or stressers, each paradigm can produce opiate (blocked by naloxone) and non-opiate analgesia. Serotonin and noradrenaline are thought to play central roles in the non-opiate branch of the endogenous pain-modulation system (Yaksh 1979). There is evidence of extensive interdependence between the opiate and non-opiate branches of this system. It has been demonstrated that depletion of serotonin or destruction of serotonin neurons will interfere with analgesia produced by endogenous or exogenous opiates (Yaksh 1979). Interdependence of the serotonin and noradrenaline systems has also been demonstrated. For example, intraperitoneal desipramine potentiates the analgesia produced for the rat on a hot plate test by intrathecal noradrenaline, serotonin, and morphine (Sawynok and Reid 1992). There is therefore a clear role for antidepressant drug treatment in patients with chronic pain, irrespective of whether they are also depressed.

Headache   There have been ten double-blind, placebo-controlled studies of the effect of antidepressants on headache. Six of these studies included patients with tension, psychogenic, or mixed headaches (Lance and Curran 1964; Okasha *et al*. 1973; Mørland *et al*. 1979; Sjaastad 1983; Fogelholm and Murros 1985; Martucci *et al*. 1985) and four included patients with migraine only (Gomersall and Stuart 1973; Couch and Hassanein 1979; Martucci *et al*. 1985; Monro *et al*. 1985). Antidepressant treatment of patients with pain in the head region have been found in a meta-analysis to have a significantly higher mean effect size than pain in other regions of the body (Onghena and Van Houdenhove 1992).

The six studies of antidepressant treatment of tension or mixed headache showed a mean effect size of 1.11 and the four studies of antidepressant treatment of migraine patients showed a mean effect size of 0.82. In studies reporting the percentage of patients that had a decrease in pain of 50 per cent or more, 56–80 per cent of tension headache patients and 55–80 per cent of migraine patients reported such a decrease (Onghena and Van Houdenhove 1992).

Chronic facial pain   Chronic facial pain is an important health problem, estimated to affect between five and seven million Americans. Various descriptive categories have been used, such as atypical facial pain, atypical odontalgia, psychogenic pain, and, more recently, somatoform pain disorder. Antidepressants are the most successful and widely evaluated drugs used to treat these types of 'psychogenic' facial pain and their benefits seem to be independent of any antidepressant action (Feinmann and Harris 1984). There is no good evidence to support the use of one drug over another or for particular dosage regimens, although most trials have used dosage over the equivalent of 100 mg amitriptyline a day. Treatment needs to be persisted with for several months (Pilowsky and Barreau 1990). Enhancement of the analgesic effects of antidepressants with low dose neuroleptics has been advocated, but recent evidence suggests that there is no benefit from this addition (Zitman *et al*. 1991).

Fibromyalgia

Fibromyalgia is a syndrome characterized by diffuse, widespread musculo-skeletal aches and pains and stiffness, multiple tender points, and non-restorative sleep. The symptoms overlap with those of chronic fatigue syndrome (see below and Chapter 16). There have been three recent double-blind, placebo-controlled antidepressant trials in patients with fibromyalgia. Carette *et al*. (1986) found that 50 mg amitriptyline was significantly better than placebo in improving morning stiffness, pain, sleep, and patient and physician global assessments in patients with fibromyalgia. Goldenberg *et al*. (1986) found that patients with fibromyalgia improved significantly more with either 25 mg amitriptyline alone or 25 mg amitriptyline combined with 500 mg naproxen (a non-steroidal anti-inflammatory medicine) than with placebo. Naproxen did not add significantly to the improvement seen with amitriptyline. The improvement in the amitriptyline-treated groups was evident on both patient and physician global assessment, as well as ratings of pain, sleep, fatigue, and tender point score.

Bennett *et al.* (1958) compared cyclobenzeprine hydrochloride, a tricyclic compound, in dosages of 10–40 mg/day to placebo in patients with fibromyalgia. They found that compared with controls, patients treated with the tricyclic responded significant improvement in local pain, sleep, and tender points. Russell *et al.* (1991) studied the effect of ibuprofen and alprazolam in 78 patients with fibromyalgia. Patients were randomized into four groups: ibuprofen alone, alprazolam alone, ibuprofen and alprazolam, and double placebo. Clinical improvement in patient rating of disease severity and in the severity of tenderness upon palpation was most apparent in the subgroup of patients receiving both ibuprofen and alprazolam. Antidepressant drugs therefore appear to be of some benefit in the treatment of fibromyalgia.

Premenstrual syndrome

Premenstrual syndrome (PMS) or late luteal phase dysphoric disorders (LLPDD) is a cluster of cyclical emotional and behavioural symptoms experienced only during the late luteal phase of the menstrual cycle. It occurs in an estimated 2–10 per cent of menstruating women. Several studies have demonstrated an increased prevalence of affective disorders in women with LLPDD (see Chapter 15). A recent trial of 20 mg fluoxetine found that fluoxetine significantly decreased symptoms of PMS (Stone *et al.* 1991). The women in the study were treated with either 20 mg fluoxetine or placebo in a double-blind manner for two complete menstrual cycles. When compared with controls, patients treated with fluoxetine showed significant decreases on the physician-rated global assessment scales, as well as patient-rated daily assessment forms.

Three studies have measured the therapeutic effects of alprazolam in LLPDD. Harrison *et al.* (1987) found that alprazolam (0.25–4 mg/day) was significantly more effective than placebo on both patient and physician global symptom index scores. Medication was always begun at the first symptom appearance in the luteal phase and taken daily until the onset of menses, at which time it was tapered by 25 per cent daily to avoid withdrawal. In a second study, Smith *et al.* (1987) found that alprazolam (0.75 mg per day) was significantly more effective than placebo in lowering daily diary scores of nervous tension, mood swings, irritability, anxiety, depression, fatigue, forgetfulness, crying, craving sweets, abdominal bloating, cramps, and headache. Subjects took medication three times daily from cycle day 20 through to day 2 of menses, then tapered medication by one tablet per day to prevent withdrawal. In another study, Harrison *et al.* (1990) found alprazolam (up to 4 mg/day and begun at first symptom and tapered by 25 per cent of the dosage daily at menses onset) to be more effective than placebo in reducing physicians' global ratings of illness, as well as depression, anxiety, irritability, labile mood, impulsivity, fatigue, hysteroid features, and 'organic mental features'. Finally Rickels *et al.* (1989) found that buspirone (25 mg given during the last 12 days of three consecutive menstrual cycles) was significantly more effective than placebo in relieving aches and pains, fatigue, cramps, and impaired social functioning in women with LLPDD.

Irritable bowel syndrome

In a study comparing 150 mg desipramine with placebo, Heefner *et al.* (1978) found that only one of the outcome measures (the degree to which symptoms interfere with daily activities) was significantly improved by desipramine. In another study, however, Greenbaum *et al.* (1987) found measures of physical symptoms decreased more during treatment with desipramine than during treatment with placebo or with atropine. The response was unrelated to the desipramine blood levels and several of the favourable responses occurred with unusually low levels.

Chronic fatigue syndrome

To date, there are no reported placebo-controlled blind trials of antidepressants in patients with chronic fatigue syndrome, apart from their successful use in patients with 'fibromyalgia' (see above). Jones and Straus (1987) reported 'clinical improvement' in 70 per cent of patients with 'low doses of doxepin'. Manu *et al.* (1989) reported that 83 per cent of 24 patients with chronic fatigue and depressive illness reported 'significant improvement of their symptoms of fatigue, as well as of their depressive disorder' with antidepressant drug therapy, most commonly with desipramine.

Antidepressant treatment of functional somatic syndromes — practical considerations

As described in Chapter 3 the size of the clinical problem dictates that an effective, cheap, and readily available treatment is required for patients with functional somatic symptoms. With adequate explanation (see the guidelines below) many patients are willing to try drug therapy. Furthermore, this type of treatment can be readily prescribed by general physicians with only limited special training. Drug therapy therefore has an important role in the treatment of patients presenting with functional somatic symptoms in a variety of medical settings.

Practical guidelines

Indications

When assessing patients with functional complaints it is essential to screen for treatable major psychiatric illnesses such as major depression, dysthymic disorder, panic disorder, and generalized anxiety disorder. If the patient has a functional somatic symptom *and* an affective or anxiety disorder, biological treatment of the psychiatric disorder will often lead to alleviation of the functional somatic symptom, as well as a reduction in disability and health care utilization. Even in the absence of depressive or anxiety disorder, treatment with an antidepressant may result in symptom reduction. Tricyclic antidepressants in particular appear to have an analgesic effect that is independent of their effect on mood. Antidepressant drugs may be usefully combined with psychological aspects of management (see Chapter 4).

Explanation to the patient

If the patient is to comply with antidepressant therapy it is essential that he/she has confidence in the doctor, understands why the drug has been prescribed, and accepts the treatment as helpful and appropriate. The first step therefore (after clinical history and examination) is to acknowledge the patient's somatic symptoms and the reality of their suffering. It is then necessary to elicit the patient's own explanatory model of illness in order to provide an acceptable justification for the prescription of drugs.

There are two principal ways of justifying the use of an antidepressant drug to patients who see depression as a secondary complaint. The first is to explain how they are caught in a vicious cycle of problems. Thus, if the symptom is pain and the patient has depression, the clinician can explain how the pain has led to a disturbance in sleep, that the disturbed sleep has led to the development of low energy and fatigue, and that the lack of energy and fatigue caused the patient to stop participating in enjoyable activities. The pain, insomnia, poor energy, and lack of activities had all caused the patient to be more depressed and irritable, which in turn exacerbated the pain. The usefulness of an antidepressant in breaking the vicious cycle and thereby improving sleep, energy, and mood and reducing sensitivity to pain perception can then be pointed out. The second method is to explain that so-called 'antidepressant' drugs act on neurotransmitters and have a wide variety of effects other than the alleviation of depression. One of these effects is the alleviation of pain.

Whatever the explanation that the patient is given, it must be accompanied by an account of likely adverse effects. Careful follow-up to ensure compliance and monitor possible side-effects is an essential component of successful treatment.

Dosage and compliance

A useful strategy is to start the patient on a low dose, such as 25 mg imipramine or desipramine and to gradually increase it by 25 mg over 3 days. The dose aimed for will depend on both the patient's response and the diagnosis. For patients who have functional somatic symptoms and affective or anxiety disorders, antidepressant medications are usually required at the dosage needed to treat that disorder (that is, for major depression 150–300 mg tricyclic antidepressants). However, in patients with a pain symptom such as headache and perhaps one vegetative sign such as insomnia, lower dosages are often effective.

The dosage should be increased only gradually in order to avoid the occurrence of severe adverse effects and subsequent non-compliance. The patient should be advised to increase the dose as directed (for example, every 3 days), but also told that if problematic side-effects occur they can slow down the rate of increase. It is particularly important to obtain their agreement that they will contact the prescriber by telephone before stopping treatment, so that the side-effects and dosage regimen can be discussed.

Choice of drug and side-effects

All tricyclic antidepressants have side-effects. Many of these result from their anticholinergic action which produces a dry mouth, constipation, blurred vision, urinary retention, sinus tachycardia, and memory dysfunction. Should a serious anticholinergic effect occur, then it might be more appropriate to switch to a tricyclic with a low anticholinergic action such as desipramine. Sedation can also be a problem, especially with amitriptyline, doxepin, trimipramine, and trazodone. Should this occur, then switching to a non-sedating tricyclic such as desipramine may be helpful. Other less common adverse effects of the antidepressant drugs are weight gain and sexual dysfunction. Among the tricyclics, lofepramine is probably the least likely to cause these effects.

Some patients experience stimulant-like effects with imipramine or desipramine. If this occurs, then it may be more appropriate to decrease the dosage to 25 mg and then to increase it again but by only 10 mg increments every 3 days. If the patient still has stimulatory effects, then a change to a less noradrenergic drug, such as 25 mg nortriptyline is indicated. Orthostatic hypertake is another problem which may lead to in tolerance of antidepressants and may be minimized by using nortriptylene. Fluoxetine and the other serotonin-specific reuptake inhibitors (SSRIs) have less propensity to cause either anticholinergic side-effects or orthostatic hypertension but can interfere with sleep and cause nausea. Because of the alerting effect a particularly useful combination is that of an SSRI in the morning, and a sedating tricyclic drug such as trazodone in the evening. To date there have been few studies of the efficacy of SSRI antidepressants in patients with functional somatic symptoms, although several are in progress.

Conclusion

The so-called antidepressant drugs have an important role in the treatment of patients with functional somatic symptoms. Depression and anxiety are important factors in determining the degree of disability and health care utilization of patients with functional somatic symptoms. Furthermore, these 'antidepressant' drugs may also have a direct action on symptoms such as pain, regardless of whether or not the patient is depressed.

There is evidence for the efficacy of antidepressants in a range of functional symptoms and syndromes. Their availability and low cost favour their use. Although many patients have difficulty tolerating them, this problem can be minimized by careful attention to drug choice, dose, and patient follow-up. Despite their obviously important role, antidepressants neither suit, nor help all patients with functional somatic symptoms and many patients will also require specialized psychological management.

References

Axellson, A. and Ringdahl, A. (1989). Tinnitus: a study of its prevalence and characteristics. *British Journal of Audiology*, **23**, 53–62.

Bennett, R.M., Gatter, R.A., Campbell, S.M., Andrews, R.P., Clark, S.R., and Scarola, J.A. (1988). A comparison of cyclobenzaprine and placebo in the management of fibrositis. *Arthritis and Rheumatism*, **31**, 1535–42.

Carette, S., McClain, G.A., Bell, D.A., and Fam, A.G. (1986). Evaluation of amitriptyline in primary fibrositis. *Arthritis and Rheumatism*, **29**, 655–9.

Coles, R.R.A. (1984). Epidemiology of tinnitus, I: prevalence. *Journal of Laryngology and Otology*, Suppl. 9, 7–15.

Couch, S.R. and Hassanein, R.S. (1979). Amitriptyline in migraine prophylaxis. *Archives of Neurology*, **36**, 695–9.

Drossman, D.A., Sandler, R.S., McKee, D.C. and Lovitz, A.J. (1982). Bowel patterns among subjects not seeking care. *Gastroenterology*, **83**, 529–34.

Dworkin, S.F., Von Korff, M.R., and Le Resche, L. (1990). Multiple pains and psychiatric disturbance: an epidemiologic investigation. *Archives of General Psychiatry*, **47**, 239-45.

Escobar, J.I. and Canino, G. (1989). Unexplained physical complaints. Psychopathology and epidemiological correlates. *British Journal of Psychiatry*, **154**, Suppl. 4, 24-7.

Feinmann, C., Harris, M., and Cawley, R. (1984). Psychogenic facial pain: presentation and treatment. *British Medical Journal*, **288**, 436-8.

Fogelholm, R. and Murros, K. (1985). Maprotiline in chronic tension headache: a double-blind cross-over study. *Headache*, **25**, 273-5.

Goldenberg, D.L., Felson, D.T., and Dinerman, H. (1986). A randomized, controlled trial of a amitriptyline and naproxen in the treatment of patients with fibromyalgia. *Arthritis and Rheumatism*, **29**, 1371-7.

Gomersall, J.D. and Stuart, A. (1973). Amitriptyline in migraine prophylaxis: changes in pattern of attacks during a controlled clinical trial. *Journal of Neurology, Neurosurgery and Psychiatry*, **36**, 684-90.

Gourlay, G.K., Cherry, D.A., Cousins, M.J., Love, B.L., Graham, J.R., and McLachlan, M.D. (1986). A controlled study of a serotonin re-uptake blocker, zimelidine, in the treatment of chronic pain. *Pain*, **25**, 35-52.

Greenbaum, D.S., Mayle, J.E., Vanegeren, L.E., Jerome, J.A., Mayor, J.W., Greenbaum, R.B. *et al.* (1987). Effect of desipramine on irritable bowel syndrome compared with atropine and placebo. *Digestive Diseases and Sciences*, **32**, 257-66.

Hankin, J. and Oktay, J.S. (1979). Mental disorder and primary medical care. An analytic review of the literature. In *National Institute of Mental Health*, series D, No. 7, DHEW publication number (ADM)78-661. Superintendent of Documents, Government Printing Office, Rockville, MD.

Harrison, W.M., Endicott, J., Rabkin, J.G., Nee, J.C., and Sandberg, D. (1987). Treatment of premenstrual dysphoria with alprazolam and placebo. *Psychopharmacol Bull.*, **23**, 150-3.

Harrison, W.M., Endicott, J., and Nee, J. (1990). Treatment of premenstrual dysphoria with alprazolam: a controlled study. *Archives of General Psychiatry*, **47**, 270-5.

Heefner, J.D., Wilder, R.M., and Wilson, I.D. (1978). Irritable colon and depression. *Psychometrics*, **19**, 540-7.

Jones, J.F. and Straus, S.E. (1987). Chronic Epstein–Barr virus infection. *Annual Reviews of Medicine*, **38**, 195-209.

Katon, W. (1991*a*). *Panic disorder in the medical setting*. American Psychiatric Press, Washington, DC.

Katon, W. (1991*b*). The development of a randomized trial of consultation–liaison psychiatry trial in distressed high utilizers of primary care. *Psychiatric Medicine*, **9**, 577-91.

Katon, W. and Russo, J. (1992). Chronic fatigue syndrome criteria: a critique of the requirement for multiple somatic complaints. *Archives of Internal Medicine*, **152**, 1604-9.

Katon, W. and Sullivan, M. (1990). Depression and chronic medical illness. *Journal of Clinical Psychiatry*, **51** (Suppl.), 3-11.

Katon, W., Hall, M.L., Russo, J. Cormier, L., Hollifield, M., Vitaliano, P.P. *et al.* (1988). Chest pain: Relationship of psychiatric illness to coronary arteriography results. *American Journal of Medicine*, 84, 1-9.

Katon, W., Von Körff, M., Lin, E. Lipscomb, P., Russo, J., Wagner, E. *et al.* (1990). Distressed high utilizers of medical care. DSM-III-R diagnoses and treatment needs. *General Hospital Psychiatry*, 12, 355-62.

Katon, W., Buchwald, D., Russo, J. Mease, P.J. (1991). Psychiatric illness in patients with chronic fatigue and rheumatoid arthritis. *Journal of General and Internal Medicine*, 6, 277-85.

Kellner, R., Fava, G.A., Lisansky, J. Perini, G.L., Zielenzy, M. (1986). Hypochondriacal fears and beliefs in DSM-III melancholia. *Journal of Affective Disorders*, 10, 21-6.

Lance, J.W. and Curran, D.A. (1964). Treatment of chronic tension headache. *Lancet*, i, 1236-9.

Lindsay, P.G. and Wyckoff, M. (1981). The depression–pain syndrome and its response to antidepressants. *Psychosomatics*, 22, 571-7.

Linzer, M., Varia, I., Pontinen, M. Divine, G.W., Grubbe, B.P., Estes, N.A. (1992). Medically unexplained syncope: relationship to psychiatric illness. *American Journal of Medicine*, 92 (Suppl. A), 18-26S.

McFarland, B.H., Freeborn, D.K., Mullooly, J.P., and Pope, C.R. (1985). Utilization patterns among long-term enrollees in a prepaid group practice health maintenance organization. *Medical Care*, 23, 1221-33.

Manu, P., Matthews, D.A., Lane, T.J., Tennan, H., Hesselbrock, V., Mendola, R., and Affleck, G. (1989). Depression among patients with a chief complaint of chronic fatigue. *Journal of Affective Disorders*, 17, 165-72.

Martucci, N., Manna, V., Porto, C., and Agnoli, A. (1985). Migraine and the noradrenergic control of vasomotricity: a study with alpha-2 stimulant and alpha-2 blocker drugs. *Headache*, 25, 95-100.

Max, M.B., Lynch, S.A., Muir, J., Shoaf, S.E., Smoller, B., and Dubner, R. (1992). Effects of desipramine, amitriptyline, and fluoxetine on pain in diabetic neuropathy. *New England Journal of Medicine*, 326, 1250-6.

Medical Research Council Institute of Hearing Research (1981). Epidemiology of tinnitus: In *Tinnitus: CIBA Foundation Symposium 85*, (ed. D. Evered and G.I. Lawrenson), pp. 16-34. London.

Meikle, M.B., Vernon, J., and Johnson, R.M. (1984). The perceived severity of tinnitus: some observations concerning a large population of tinnitus clinic patients. *Otolaryngology Head and Neck Surgery*, 92, 689-96.

Monro, P., Swade, C., and Coppen, A. (1985). Mianserin in the prophylaxis of migraine: a double-blind study. *Acta Psychiatrica Scandanavica*, 72 (Suppl. 320), 98-103.

Mørland, T.J., Storli, O.V., and Mogstad, T.E. (1979). Doxepin in the prophylactic treatment of mixed "vascular" and tension headache. *Headache*, 19, 382-3.

Noyes, R. and Clancy, J. (1986). Reduction in hypochondriasis with treatment of panic disorder. *British Journal of Psychiatry*, 149, 631-5.

Okasha, A., Ghaleb, H.A., and Sadek, A. (1973). A double-blind trial for the clinical management of psychogenic headache. *British Journal of Psychiatry*, 122, 181-3.

Onghena, P. and Van Houdenhove, B. (1992). Antidepressant-induced analgesia in chronic non-malignant pain: a meta-analysis of 39 placebo-controlled studies. *Pain*, **49**, 205–20.

Pheasant, H., Bursk, A., Goldfarb, J., Azen, S.P., Weiss, J.N., and Borelli, L. (1983). Amitriptyline and chronic low back pain: a randomized double-blind crossover study. *Spine*, **8**, 552–7.

Pilowsky, I. and Barrow, C.G. (1990). A controlled trial of psychotherapy and amitriptyline used individually and in combination in the treatment of chronic intractable "psychogenic" pain. *Pain*, **40**, 3–19.

Richardson, D.E. and Akil, H. (1977). Pain reduction by electrical brain stimulation in man. *Journal of Neurosurgery*, **47**, 178–89.

Rickels, K., Freeman, E., and Sondheimer, S. (1989). Buspirone in treatment of premenstrual syndrome. *Lancet*, **i**, 777.

Robins, L.N., Helzer, J.E., Groughan, J., and Ratcliff, K.S. (1981). National Institute of Mental Health Diagnostic Interview Schedule. *Archives of General Psychiatry*, **38**, 381–9.

Russell, J., Fletcher, E.M., Michalek, J.E., McBroom, P.C., and Hester, G.G. (1991). Treatment of primary fibrositis/fibromyalgia syndrome with ibuprofen and alprazolam. A double-blind, placebo-controlled study. *Arthritis and Rheumatism*, **34**, 552–60.

Sawynok, J. and Reid, A. (1992). Desipramine potentiates spinal antinociception by 5-hydroxytryptamine, morphine and adenosine. *Pain*, **50**, 113–18.

Simon, G. (1992). Psychiatric disorder and functional somatic symptoms as predictors of health care use. *Psychiatric Medicine*, **10**, 49–59.

Simon, G. and Von Korff, M. (1991). Somatization and psychiatric disorder in the NIMH Epidemiologic Catchment Area Study. *American Journal of Psychiatry*, **148**, 1494–500.

Sjaastad, O. (1983). So-called "tension headache" – the response to a 5-HT uptake inhibitor: femoxetine. *Cephalalgia*, **3**, 53–60.

Smith, S., Rheinhardt, J.S., Ruddddock, V.E., and Schiff, I. (1987). Treatment of premenstrual syndrome with alprazolam: results of a double blind, placebo controlled randomized crossover clinical trial. *Obstetrics and Gynaecology*, **70**, 37–42.

Stephens, S.D. and Hallam, R.S. (1985). The Crown–Crisp Experiential Index in patients complaining of tinnitus. *British Journal of Audiology*, **19**, 151–8.

Stewart, W.F., Scheter, A., and Liberman, J. (1992). Physician consultation for headache pain and history of panic: results from a population-based study. *American Journal of Medicine*, **92** (Suppl. A), 355–405.

Stone, A.B., Pearlstein, T.B., and Brown, W.A. (1991). Fluoxetine in the treatment of late luteal phase dysphoric disorder. *Journal of Clinical Psychiatry*, **52**, 290–3.

Sullivan, M., Katon, W., Dobie, R., Sakai, C., Russo, J., and Harrop-Griffiths, J. (1988). Disabling tinnitus: association with affective disorder. *General Hospital Psychiatry*, **10**, 285–91.

Sullivan, M.D., Dobie, R.A., Sakai, C.S., and Katon, W. (1990). Treatment of depressed tinnitus patients with nortriptyline. *Annals of Otology, Rhinology and Laryngology*, **98**, 867–72.

Sullivan, M.S., Clark, M.R., Katon, W.J., Fischl, M., Russo, S., Dobie, R.A., and Voorhees, R. (1993). Psychiatric and otologic diagnoses in patients complaining of dizziness. *Archives of Internal Medicine*, **153**, 1478–84.

Sullivan, M., Katon, W., Russo, J., Dobie, R., and Sakai, C. (1993). A randomized trial of nortriptyline for severe chronic tinnitus. Effects on depression, disability, and tinnitus symptoms. *Archives of Internal Medicine*, **153**, 2251–59.

Terman, G.W., Shavit, Y., Lewis, J.W., Cannon, J.T., and Liebeskind, J.C. (1984). Intrinsic mechanisms of pain inhibition: activation by stress. *Science*, **226**, 1270–7.

Walker, E., Katon, W., and Harrop-Griffiths, J. (1988). Chronic pelvic pain: the relationship to psychiatric diagnoses and sexual abuse. *American Journal of Psychiatry*, **145**, 75–80.

Walker, E.A., Roy-Byrne, P.P., Katon, W.J., Li, L., Amos, D., and Jiranek, G. (1990). Psychiatric illness and irritable bowel syndrome: a comparison with inflammatory bowel disease. *American Journal of Psychiatry*, **147**, 1656–61.

Wells, K.B., Stewart, A., Hays, R.D. Burnham, A., Rogers, W., Daniels, M. *et al.* (1989). The functioning and well-being of depressed patients. *Journal of the American Medical Association*, **262**, 914–19.

Yaksh, T.L. (1979). Direct evidence that spinal serotonin and noradrenaline terminals mediate the spinal anti-nociceptive effects of morphine in the periaqueductal grey. *Brain Research*, **160**, 180–5.

Zitman, F.G., Linssen, A.C., Edelbroek, P.M., and Van Kempen, G.M. (1991). Does addition of low-dose flupentixol enhance the analgetic effects of low-dose amitriptyline in somatoform pain disorder? *Pain*, **47**, 25–30.

7 Cognitive behavioural therapies in the treatment of functional somatic symptoms

Michael Sharpe

In this introductory chapter, Dr Sharpe outlines the historical development of cognitive and behavioural treatment and then discusses the cognitive behavioural model of aetiology. He applies this model to the understanding of functional somatic symptoms and discusses the efficacy of this approach. He concludes with practical guidelines for the treatment of patients with functional somatic symptoms using cognitive behavioural psychotherapy.

Introduction

Psychotherapy, both implicit and explicit, has long been used in the treatment of patients who complain of medically unexplained or functional somatic symptoms. For physicians this has usually meant common-sense methods of explanation directed at changing inaccurate or unhelpful beliefs the patient may hold about the nature and significance of their symptoms and advice on how to cope with them. More recently the systematic techniques of cognitive and behavioural psychotherapy, originally designed for the treatment of anxiety and depressive disorders, have been applied to patients presenting with functional somatic symptoms. This chapter offers an overview of this method of treatment.

What are cognitive and behavioural psychotherapies?

History

The historical roots of cognitive behaviour therapy can be traced back to the scientific study of animal learning and to techniques developed in clinical practice in the early years of this century. The early treatments concentrated on changing behaviour and were called behaviour therapy. Although such therapies clearly altered how the patients thought about their problems, their thoughts and beliefs were not directly addressed. Later developments incorporated efforts to change the patient's thoughts and beliefs directly, using a form of psychotherapy which has been called cognitive therapy. Modern cognitive behaviour therapy combines these techniques (Hawton *et al.* 1989).

Behaviour therapy Behavioural therapies have been informed by behavioural science. Experiments in animal behaviour delineated two types of learning, autonomic and emotional. 'Classical conditioning' of autonomic nervous responses was described by Pavlov and other Russian physiologists. They demonstrated that something associated with one stimulus could become associated with another, initially neutral stimulus, if the two occurred together. Hence, an animal would salivate at the sound of a bell if this was paired with food. The learned behaviour tended to diminish or was extinguished if the neutral stimulus was repeatedly presented alone.

'Operant conditioning' of voluntary behaviour was described by Thorndike and other American psychologists. The nature of this type of learning was summarized in the 'law of effect' which stated that responses followed by satisfying consequences tended to be repeated while behaviours followed by unpleasant consequences tended to diminish in frequency.

These theories of how simple learning took place were applied to the understanding of clinical problems. For example, Mowrer (1960) proposed that both types of learning operated in the development of phobias in humans; an initially neutral stimulus became associated with anxiety and its aversive quality resulted in a tendency to avoid the stimulus. More recently Seligman (1975) and others have demonstrated that the repeated occurrence of unavoidable aversive stimuli produces depressed mood and inactivity.

Clinicians have used these experimental observations to sharpen existing therapeutic technique and to develop new ones. As a result the technique of systematically employing exposure to feared stimuli, and the use of reward to increase desired behaviours, became standard components of a therapy called behaviour therapy. This behaviour therapy was remarkably effective for certain clinical problems and has became an important treatment, especially for phobic anxiety disorders.

Cognitive therapy The more recent development of cognitive therapy has several roots, but can be attributed largely to the work of Beck during the 1970s (Beck *et al.* 1979). Beck, a psychoanalyst, became interested in the idea that the thoughts and beliefs (cognitions) of his patients might not merely be a consequence of their emotional state, but might actually *cause* it. This idea has been developed in clinical research studies that have demonstrated the role of thoughts in perpetuating depression. It has also given rise to the development of a type of therapy which aims to help patients recover from emotional problems by changing the way that they think.

This new approach was well received by many practitioners of behaviour therapy. There are two likely reasons for this: firstly, experimental psychology was moving on from the study of simple animal learning to the investigation of human cognitive processes and secondly, the clinical limitations of a therapy that did not explicitly address patients' thoughts and beliefs had become apparent to all but the most dogmatic practitioners. The resulting combination of psychological and behavioural techniques offered an attractive and potentially powerful therapy for the treatment of patients with a variety of neurotic problems.

The cognitive behavioural model

Research into the nature and treatment of neuroses has indicated that they might be better understood if they are broken down into the separate, although inter-related, components of cognition, emotion, behaviour, and physiology (Hodgson and Rachman 1974). Central to the cognitive theory is the view that a patient's cognitions are of primary importance in determining their behaviour and their emotional and physiological state. It therefore follows that neurotic syndromes could be most effectively treated by helping patients to re-evaluate the types of thinking that led to the unhelpful behaviours, the undesirable emotional state, and the associated physiological changes that comprise the syndrome they are suffering from. Thus, a person who is phobic of spiders may overestimate the likelihood of being bitten, consequently tend to avoid spiders, feel anxious when they see a spider or think about them, and suffer from symptoms associated with autonomic nervous system activity such as sweating, palpitations, and shaking. A simple outline of such a cognitive behavioural perspective on anxiety is illustrated in Fig. 7.1. Treatment would consist of helping the patient to gain a more accurate appraisal of the risk of handling spiders. A discussion of the actual risk would be followed by a behavioural experiment in which the patient tests out their exaggerated fear by actually approaching spiders, rather than avoiding them.

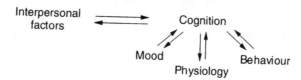

Fig. 7.1 A simple cognitive model illustrating the central role of cognitions and reciprocal relationships between the components

This model of neurosis and the approach to treatment that follows from it, can, with only minor modifications, be applied to patients complaining of functional somatic symptoms. This is because patients with functional somatic symptoms and patients with emotional disorders have many similarities. Both are ill with similar disturbances in cognition, emotion, behaviour and physiology, and both lack the major pathological changes that are present in patients who have organic disease. There are, however, important differences between patients attending attending psychological treatment services with neurosis and patients presenting to medical clinics with functional somatic symptoms. In particular patients with functional somatic symptoms tend to be more concerned about their somatic symptoms, to have more salient beliefs about physical disease, and to exhibit a greater antipathy to psychological explanations of their illness and, consequently, to a psychotherapeutic approach (Sharpe *et al.* 1992). Another complication is that the beliefs and behaviour of patients with functional somatic symptoms may have been further influenced by their contact with the health care system (both conventional and alternative).

The cognitive model of neurosis and the associated cognitive behaviour therapy, therefore require modification if they are to be successfully applied to patients with functional somatic symptoms. The components of this model and the modifications required are described below.

Cognition This term may be used to encompass a number of aspects of the patient's mental life. It includes simple *thoughts*, and also more fundamental *beliefs* and *assumptions* about themselves and about the world. The most basic of these underlying beliefs are called *schema*. These basic beliefs have their origin in the patient's earlier life and are further shaped by cultural and family beliefs, as well as the patient's own previous personal experience.

For any given person some cognitions may be regarded as *functional*, in that they tend to lead to the effective resolution of problems and to mental and physical health. Others may be regarded as *dysfunctional*, in that are less effective in solving life problems and tend to perpetuate excessive and undesirable behavioural, emotional, and physiological responses.

For example, the thinking of patients with depressive disorders is typically dysfunctional in that it tends to a distorted and excessively negative view of the self, the world and the future (for example, 'I am a bad person, the world is a bad place, the future is hopeless') (Beck *et al.* 1979). In the case of patients with anxiety disorders there is typically a tendency to make excessively frightening predictions about the self and the world (for example, 'I will fail', 'other people will reject me') (Beck and Emery 1985). This thinking although exaggerated and inaccurate, tends to be self-perpetuating.

This self-perpetuating nature of dysfunctional cognitions at first appears puzzling. Why do such persons not learn from experience that their thinking is distorted? The most likely reason is that deeply held beliefs exert an ongoing influence on perception and behaviour, such that the world is seen as consistent with those beliefs. Thus, a person who believes they are a failure is likely to notice and remember every possible example of failure and to ignore or discount their successes. They may also tend to avoid opportunities for success, in case they fail.

Patients with functional somatic symptoms commonly hold similar dysfunctional beliefs. In addition they may also have specific fears and beliefs about their *physical health and functioning* (for example, 'I am prone to illness', 'bodily sensations mean disease'). They therefore tend to *attribute* bodily sensations to physical disease, rather than to emotional or trivial causes (Robbins and Kirmayer 1991). Such cognitions can also be self-perpetuating. The more one believes that one has a disease, the greater is the focus of attention on the body and more symptoms are perceived (Skelton and Pennebaker 1993). The resulting behavioural and physiological changes may contribute to this process (see below) and provide further evidence that one does indeed have a disease. This preoccupation with disease may also be associated with a reluctance to consider psychological explanations for the symptoms and to accept a psychotherapeutic approach. This reluctance clearly has important practical implications for treatment.

Behaviour   Like thinking, behaviour may also be regarded as either functional if it is helpful in resolving problems, or dysfunctional if it tends to perpetuate them. Dysfunctional behaviours include the inactivity typical of depressive states and the avoidance and excessive checking associated with anxiety states.

Patients with functional somatic symptoms may also employ dysfunctional behaviours that arise from either an excessive fear of, or an inaccurate belief in, physical disease. For example, they may avoid activities that they fear might exacerbate their 'disease' and seek physical medical, rather than psychological help. They may continually ask for reassurance that they do not have disease or request repeated medical investigations (see also Chapter 5). This way of coping is usually dysfunctional in that it is unlikely to result in the resolution of psychological or social problems. On the contrary it is likely to increase any pre-existing preoccupation with disease and may even exacerbate the pathophysiological processes that are underlying the symptoms (see below).

Emotional distress   Central to the syndromes of emotional disorder seen in psychiatric practice is the patients report of anxiety and of depression.

Patients with functional somatic symptoms, almost by definition, do not usually present with complaints of emotional distress but with somatic symptoms. In practice however, emotional distress can often be elicited by direct enquiry (see Chapter 5) and the somatic symptoms then seen as physiological concomitants of the emotional state (see below). Even if emotional distress is not reported the cognitive model can still be applied, but with less emphasis placed on the emotional component.

Pathophysiology Patients who present with emotional distress commonly exhibit associated physiological changes. Anxiety is particularly associated with activity of the sympathetic nervous system and is associated with tachycardia, shaking and sweating (Tyrer 1976). Anxiety-associated hyperventilation may produce other somatic symptoms including breathlessness, dizziness, paraesthesia, and chest pain (Salkovskis and Clark 1990). Depression is also associated with physiological changes. Abnormalities in brain function, particularly of the hypothalamic pituitary axis, can be demonstrated. These may give rise to a long list of somatic symptoms including reduced energy or fatigue and pain (Mathew *et al.* 1981).

When applying the cognitive model to patients with functional somatic symptoms, emphasis has to be put on those physiological processes which are of central concern to the patient. Furthermore the patient's behavioural response to somatic symptoms can result in further physiological changes, for example excessive rest can produce loss of fitness and changes in the muscular, cardiovascular, and respiratory responses to exertion (Sharpe and Bass 1992).

Interpersonal factors Interactions with other persons are of major importance in giving rise to the cognitions that shape and trigger anxiety and depressive disorders.

Clinical experience suggests that specific interpersonal factors are also important in patients with functional somatic symptoms. The behaviour of relatives, friends, and medical practitioners may cause not only emotional distress, but may also reinforce preoccupation with disease and symptom-maintaining behaviours (Benjamin *et al.* 1992). Repeated reassurance about the absence of disease may actually maintain such morbid concerns in some anxious hypochondriacal patients (Warwick and Salkovskis 1985) (see also Chapter 9).

An additional complication in the understanding and management of patients with functional somatic symptoms is their interaction with the health care system. Doctors can generate and unintentionally perpetuate patients' distorted views of their symptoms (Bergman and Stamm 1967). Their advice may be ambiguous or contradictory (for example, 'I'm sure that there is nothing wrong, but I'll order another test, just to make sure'), may fail to address the patient's particular worries ('He told me that it wasn't a stroke, but I am worried that it might be a brain tumour'), or may contribute towards the patient's avoidance behaviour ('go home and rest until you feel better').

The cognitive behavioural model of functional somatic symptoms

The components described above can be combined to form a cognitive behavioural model of functional somatic symptoms. An outline model is

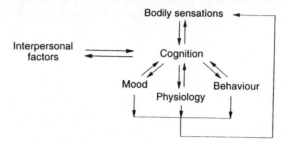

Fig. 7.2   A simple cognitive model of functional somatic symptoms

illustrated in Fig. 7.2. The precise nature of the cognitive, emotional, behavioural, and physiological components varies between functional syndromes. Examples are shown in Table 7.1.

How is cognitive behavioural therapy applied to patients with functional somatic symptoms?

Patient assessment and treatment

Cognitive behavioural therapy is usually a brief psychotherapy which is principally concerned with overcoming identified problems and attaining specified targets. Adequate assessment is an essential preliminary to treatment. The stages of treatment are shown in Table 7.2.

Table 7.2 Stages in a programme of treatment

1. Assessment
2. Discuss formulation of problem and targets for therapy
3. Review thoughts and beliefs about problem – consider alternatives
4. Review coping behaviours – try new ones
5. Review other causes of distress – examine assumptions
6. Problem solving – for practical difficulties
7. Review what has been learned

NB: each stage may require several sessions and different stages may run concurrently.

Treatment is usually delivered as an individual therapy over 5–20 sessions, but can also be used in groups (Davis 1989). A typical treatment session is oulined in Table 7.3. The application of cognitive behavioural therapy to a patient with functional somatic symptoms will be illustrated using the example of a patient with non-cardiac chest pain (see also Chapter 18). For reasons of clarity the components of therapy will be described in sequence. In practice they may need to be applied together.

Table 7.1 Common presentations and commonly associated cognitions, emotions, and physiological mechanisms

Symptoms	Cognitions	Emotion	Physiology	Behaviour
Chest pain	Heart attack	Anxiety, panic	Minor chest wall pain, oesophagitis, hyperventilation	Avoidance
Palpitations	Heart stops beating	Anxiety	Excessive awareness of cardiac rhythm	Focus attention on heart
Breathlessness	Stop breathing	Anxiety	Hyperventilation	Avoidance
Abdominal pain	–	Anxiety	Sympathetic activity	Focus attention
Fatigue	Cannot perform	Depression	Loss of fitness, hyperventilation	Inactivity avoidance
Dizziness	Collapse	Panic	Hyperventilation	Hold on Avoid
Headache	Stroke, tumour	Depression, tension	–	Focus attention Avoid
Chronic pain	Damage	Depression	–	Inactivity avoid, focus attention

Table 7.3 General session outline

1. Agree agenda
2. Review homework
3. Elicit and examine thoughts and beliefs about symptoms and illness by education, discussion, behavioural experiments, and review of experience
4. Agree homework assignments
5. Session review

Therapist–patient relationship   The successful practice of cognitive behavioural therapy requires that the therapist cultivates a special type of relationship with the patient. This is different from the usual doctor–patient relationship and is more like that between a student and tutor. It is referred to as 'collaborative empiricism' (Beck *et al*. 1979). Rather than giving didactic instructions, the therapist and patient work together to discover how the patient's current thinking and behaviour may be perpetuating the problem and how positive change may be brought about.

Cognitions and behaviour   The main focus of cognitive behavioural therapy is on changing the patient's cognitions and behaviour. An assessment of relevant cognitions and behaviour is therefore the first step in treatment. The techniques used include diary keeping, discussion, and the identification of thoughts occurring during the treatment sessions.

Example. The assessment of a man with chest pain revealed that he was fearful that his pain indicated undetected ischaemic heart disease. His evidence for this belief was that his father had died at the same age of a heart attack after being told by his doctor that it was 'indigestion'. The pain came on when he was under stress at work. When he felt the pain he thought 'it's a heart attack' and became very distressed and increasingly aware of irregularities in his heart beat.

This patient's assessment diary is shown in Fig. 7.3.

The patient and therapist then discussed the likely causes of the symptoms. The patient suggested a simple explanation in terms of insufficient oxygen getting to the heart. The therapist helped the patient to develop an alternative formulation based on the assessment. According to this alternative hypothesis the pain resulted from benign stress-related physiological processes and was amplified by the patients excessive, although understandable, fear of cardiac disease and further exacerbated by the physiological consequences of anxiety.

In order to help the patient to choose which was the most accurate formulation of their problem, the patient and therapist reviewed the available evidence. This evidence included education by the therapist, other information (for example, from books), and from trying things out — so-called behavioural experiments.

Record of symptoms, feelings and thoughts   Name ....Smith, P.....................

Date	Symptoms (how bad; 0–10) Situation (what were you doing or thinking about)	How did you feel? (how bad; 0–10)	What were you thinking? (how much did you believe each of the thoughts? 0–10)
4/6/94 11 am	Pain in chest bad (8) (also short breath, palpitations) At work - criticized by boss, not keeping up	Anxious (9)	Its my heart, I'm having a heart attack — I'm going to die (7)

Fig. 7.3 A patient's diary showing symptoms, emotions, and associated cognitions

Example. After discussion with the therapist the patient agreed to consider the alternative formulation that the pain came from the muscles of the chest wall and was aggravated by anxiety and hyperventilation, although he initially though this was unlikely. Two behavioural experiments were planned to obtain new information about the problem.

1. In order to assess the effect of hyperventilation the patient voluntarily hyperventilated — this exercise reproduced the pain.

2. In order to assess the effects of different types of activity on the pain the patient carefully monitored his activity and its relation to pain.

It was hypothesized that if the pain resulted from ischaemic heart disease it should occur with all vigorous activity, whereas if it arose from joints and muscles of the thorax it would be more related to exercise of this part of the body. He discovered that vigorous exercise not involving the arms often did not result in pain, whereas light exercise using the arms often did.

The therapist discussed this evidence with the patient who consequently thought it much less likely that the chest pain was a result of heart disease and more likely that chest wall discomfort and hyperventilation were a possible alternative explanation. The patient subsequently recorded his thoughts about the pain and practised writing down the alternative 'benign' explanation whenever he became concerned about his heart.

Emotional distress   Emotional distress is managed principally by helping the patient to become aware of and to change dysfunctional cognitions that underline the distress. However, psychotherapeutic techniques of ventilation, empathy, and offering hope for recovery are also important ingredients (Frank 1971). Although the patient may present the symptoms as being the only problem, careful assessment usually reveals areas of concern other than symptoms and disease. These concerns include relationship problems, employment difficulties, and life changes. The initial formulation may consequently have to be broadened to incorporate these more general issues.

Example. As he became less worried about his heart the patient's anxiety lessened. However, is diaries showed that the anxiety increased whenever he returned to work. It emerged that he could not keep up with the demands on him at work, but thought 'if I say anything they will think I'm weak'. Fear of being considered weak emerged as a lifelong concern or assumption. After discussion and a review of the evidence which revealed the inaccurate and unhelpful nature of this belief, he talked to his supervisor about his pattern of working and was able to negotiate changes. His anxiety subsequently subsided.

Thus a more general problem of lack of assertiveness and fear of being seen as weak emerged. Such problems are common in patients with functional somatic symptoms. Cognitive behavioural therapy can also be employed to tackle these more basic assumptions. Some problems such as financial debts are based more on external difficulties than on distorted thinking. In these cases problem-solving techpiques can be incorporated within the collaborative self-help-oriented approach of cognitive behavioural therapy (Hawton and Kirk 1989).

Behaviour   The aim of this component of therapy is to help the patient to stop dysfunctional behaviours and to attain targets for more functional behaviour. Careful recording and assessment of behaviour is the starting point.

Example. Behavioural assessment revealed that when the patient experienced chest pain he lay down on the floor. At home he stopped digging in his garden and sat indoors repeatedly taking his pulse and attending closely to his heart beat to check it was regular. The patient was persuaded to try to change these behaviours as an 'experiment' and agreed not to lie down in response to pain or to check his pulse. He rated his concern about his heart and found it diminished a week after changing to this new coping behaviour. He was then encouraged to gradually return to gardening and although this temporarily resulted in increased concern about his heart, it was dealt with by encouraging him to challenge the dysfunctional thoughts as described above.

Pathophysiology Cognitive and behavioural techniques can also be used to modify pathophysiological processes. Relaxation has been widely used in the management of anxiety in order to reduce sympathetic arousal and muscle tension (Ost 1987).

In patients with functional somatic symptoms techniques have been used to enable the patients to control somatic symptoms. Relaxation may reduce headache and muscle pain (Linton 1986) and breathing exercises the symptoms of hyperventilation (Cluff 1984).

Example. After demonstrating that voluntary hyperventilation could reproduce the chest pain, the patient was taught breathing exercises. He practised these four times each day as part of his therapy homework. By using the technique when he started to get chest pain he was able to control his symptoms.

Hypnosis (Kornfeld 1984) and biofeedback (Blanchard *et al*. 1990*b*) can also be used for this purpose. The patient's physiology may also be affected by his or her behaviour, for example by excessive resting and sleeping (Sharpe and Bass 1992) and can often be normalized simply by changing these behaviours (see also Chapter 16).

Interpersonal factors The behaviour of others will also influence the patient's cognitions and behaviour. Such influences usually need to be considered in therapy.

Example. When the patient became aware of chest pain at work he lay down on the floor and his colleagues called the works doctor who performed repeated electrocardiograms. At home his wife was worried that he might die and would not let him out of her sight.

Other family members may need information about the nature of functional somatic symptoms and it may be appropriate to actually involve them in therapy. The collaboration of other doctors is also of obvious importance. It may be necessary to make a contract with the patient in which he agrees not to pursue further medical consultations whilst he is receiving cognitive behavioural therapy (Salkovskis 1989).

Is cognitive behavioural therapy effective in the treatment of functional somatic symptoms?

The efficacy of cognitive behavioural therapy in emotional disorder

Cognitive behavioural therapy has been demonstrated in controlled clinical trials to be a potent therapy for psychiatric patients with neurosis. Cognitive behavioural therapy is of proven efficacy in the treatment of depression (Beck *et al.* 1985), anxiety (Butler *et al.* 1991), and panic (Gelder 1991).

The efficacy of cognitive behavioural therapy in the treatment of functional somatic symptoms

Recently there has been an increase in the number of randomized controlled trials of cognitive behavioural therapy for the treatment of patients with functional somatic symptoms. Whilst much of this work has been devoted to the problem of chronic pain (Benjamin 1989) there has been increasing interest in applying cognitive behavioural therapy to other functional symptoms (Sharpe *et al.* 1992). This research is summarized in Table 7.4.

It can be concluded that cognitive behavioural therapies are effective in reducing distress, disability, and symptoms and can probably also modify pathophysiological processes in patients with functional somatic symptoms. However, many questions remain. Few studies have adequately controlled for the non-specific factors of therapy. Most versions of cognitive behavioural therapy are multicomponent therapies and the relative importance of each of the ingredients remains uncertain. The efficacy of cognitive behavioural therapy compared with other forms of psychotherapy and with pharmacotherapy has been little studied in the treatment of functional somatic symptoms. Even with these uncertainties, cognitive behavioural therapy offers the clinician a practical approach based on a plausible theoretical rationale which is generally acceptable to both clinicians and patients. The adoption of a collaborative relationship with the patient can be especially useful in overcoming disagreement when managing the patient with functional somatic symptoms (Sharpe *et al.*, 1994).

Practical guidelines for treatment

I will not attempt here to provide a comprehensive guide to cognitive behavioural pschotherapy. The interested reader should refer to a relevant texts (for example, Hawton *et al.* 1989). However, several issues are of particular importance in the management of patients with functional somatic symptoms and are highlighted below.

Special issues in the application of cognitive behavioural therapy to functional somatic symptoms

Starting therapy   Patients who present to physicians with somatic complaints are commonly concerned that their symptoms are caused by organic disease. It is therefore unreasonable to expect all such patients to take readily to cognitive behavioural therapy, particularly if it is couched in psychological terminology and administered in a psychiatric clinic. However, clinical experience suggests that if care is taken in engaging the patients in psychological therapy these obstacles can be overcome (see also Chapter 5).

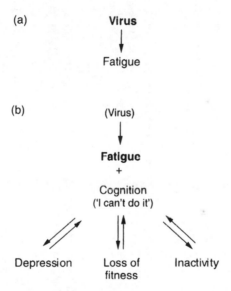

Fig. 7.4   (a) Patients initial model of the cause of their fatigue. (b) The negotiated revision of the model including cognitions, multiple factors, reciprocal relationships, and a less certain role for the initial virus infection

Developing a shared formulation   If therapy is to make sense to the patient, it must be based on a formulation of the problem that is acceptable to both doctor and patient. The patient's own initial formulation is first elicited. This varies in sophistication but is often simple. An example of the initial formulation of a patient with chronic fatigue syndrome is shown in Fig. 7.4(a). Using discussion and the patient's own history, an afternative model is then constructed. This new model aims to introduce four new concepts:

Table 7.4 Cognitive behavioural therapy for functional somatic symptoms

Symptoms and syndromes	Descriptions of treatment	Controlled trials and reviews	Comments
Non-cardiac chest pain	Cott et al. (1992), Salkovskis (1992a)	Klimes et al. (1990)	Cognitive behavioural therapy of proven efficacy
Headache	Blanchard (1992)	Martin et al. (1989), Holroyd et al. (1991), Blanchard et al. (1990a and b)	Behavioural methods effective, but value of cognitive component uncertain
Chronic pain syndromes	Philips (1988), Keefe et al. (1992), Pearce (1983)	Pitcher (1989), Keefe et al. (1992), Linton (1986), Philips (1987), Skinner et al. (1990)	Behaviour therapy and cognitive behavioural therapy of proven efficacy. Treatments commonly complex
Chronic back pain	Kriegler and Ashenberg (1987), Tollison et al. (1985)	Nicholas et al. (1992), Turner and Clancy (1988), Heinrich et al. (1985)	As for chronic pain
Irritable bowel syndrome	Neff and Blanchard (1987), Litt and Baker, (1987)	Blanchard et al. (1992), Corney et al. (1991), Lynch and Zamble (1989), Svedlund et al. (1983)	Controlled trials mixed. Evidence for psychodynamic psychotherapy
Premenstral syndrome	Gath and Iles (1988)	Blake et al. (in press)	Cognitive behavioural therapy effective in recent trials

Hypochondriasis	Warwick and Salkovskis (1990), Stern and Fernandez (1991), House (1989), Visser and Bouman (1992)	Warwick et al. (submitted)	Cognitive behavioural therapy effective in recent controlled trial
Chronic fatigue syndrome	Butler S. et al. (1991)	Lloyd et al. (1993)	Cognitive behavioural therapy effective in case series but not yet more than clinical care in a controlled trial
Fibromyalgia syndrome	Bradley (1989)	Buckelew (1989)	Cognitive behavioural therapy effective in case series
Tinnitus	Sweetow (1986)	Jakes et al. (1992), Scott et al. (1985)	Cognitive behavioural therapy probably helpful
Mixed patients groups	Salkovskis (1992b), Sharpe et al. (1992)	Hellman et al. (1990)	Cognitive behavioural therapy effective in primary care and in reducing costs

(1) the importance of cognitions;

(2) the greater importance of perpetuating factors than precipitating causes;

(3) the multifactorial nature of perpetuating causes;

(4) factors previously seen as simple reactions to symptoms can also act as causes and thereby trap the patient in vicious circles.

The alternative formulation obtained after further discussion with the patient is shown in Fig. 7.4(b). It is not necessary for the patient to accept the alternative wholly, but simply to note that it is worthy of examination; therapy can then be directed towards deciding which is the best.

The focus of treatment Treatment will need to address the patient's dysfunctional cognitions and behaviours. Many of these will be concerned with their functional somatic symptom(s). It is important, however, not to neglect cognitions and behaviours relevant to the person's relationships, occupation, and self-image which may be important and more fundamental causes of distress.

The management of interpersonal and iatrogenic factors The ways in which the behaviour of others perpetuates the symptoms may be apparent at the initial assessment. Those who may be most concerned include family, friends, and fellow sufferers but it may also be necessary to consider the role of employers, lawyers, and insurance companies, as well as that of other doctors and therapists. The patient may seek diagnostic opinions, investigations, or treatments from other doctors whilst receiving cognitive behavioural therapy. Two options are open to the therapist who encounters this problem. He can negotiate a contract with the patient in which they desist from such contact for the duration of therapy. Alternatively, he can seek the collaboration of the other doctors and therapists that the patient is in contact with. It may sometimes be preferable to defer therapy until outstanding claims and litigation are settled.

Conclusions

The cognitive behavioural model of functional somatic symptoms offers a plausible, scientifically testable model that enjoys a degree of experimental support. It is logical, understandable by physicians and patients alike, and can be readily adapted to the individual patient's problems. Whilst clinical experience suggests that it can be effective in reducing disability and symptoms in a variety of functional somatic syndromes, more controlled trials are required. There is a special need to develop and evaluate simple methods of cognitive behavioural therapy that are suitable for use in routine medical care.

The availability of treatment is currently severely limited by a shortage of skilled therapists. Few general practitioners and physicians have these skills and clinical psychologists and nurse therapists are in short supply. Many, perhaps most, general psychiatrists do not have the interest or the skill necessary to offer this type of psychological management and the number of specialist liaison psychiatrists remains grossly inadequate. Although some economy in treatment time may be possible if treatment is given in groups (Davis 1989) this way of delivering psychological treatment only goes a small way to bridging the gap between need and availability.

Better training and improved facilities for cognitive behavioural treatments (especially for in-patient treatment) would greatly improve patient care. In view of the enormous use of medical resources by these patients such investment may well prove to be not only effective, but also cost-effective. Chapters 21 and 22 consider the ways in which psychological treatments could be effectively delivered in primary care and in the general hospital.

References

Beck, A.T. and Emery, G. (1985). *Anxiety disorders and phobias: a cognitive perspective*. Basic Books, USA.

Beck, A.T., Rush, A.J., Shaw, B.F., and Emery, G. (1979). *Cognitive therapy of depression*. Guilford Press, New York.

Beck, A.T., Hollon, S.D., Young, J.E., Bedrosian, R.C. and Budenz, D. (1985). Treatment of depression with cognitive therapy and amitriptyline. *Archives of General Psychiatry*, **42**, 142–8.

Benjamin, S. (1989). Psychological treatment of chronic pain: a selective review. *Journal of Psychosomatic Research*, **33**, 121–31.

Benjamin, S., Mawer, J., and Lennon, S. (1992). The knowledge and beliefs of family care givers about chronic pain patients. *Journal of Psychosomatic Researh*, **36**, 211–17.

Bergman, A.B. and Stamm, S.J. (1967). The morbidity of cardiac nondisease in schoolchildren. *New England Journal of Medicine*, **18**, 1008–13.

Blake, F., Salkovskis, P., and Gath, D. A controlled trial of cognitive behavioural treatment for women with premenstrual syndrome. Submitted for publication.

Blanchard, E.B. (1992). Psychologial treatment of benign headache disorders. *Journal of Consulting and Clinical Psychology*, **60**, 537–51.

Blanchard, E.B., Appelbaum, K.A., Radnitz, C.L., *et al.* (1990*a*). Placebo-controlled evaluation of abbreviated progressive muscle relaxation and of relaxation combined with cognitive therapy in the treatment of tension headache. *Journal of Consulting and Clinical Psychology*, **58**, 210–15.

Blanchard, E.B., Appelbaum, K.A., Radnitz, C.L. *et al.* (1990*b*). A controlled evaluation of thermal biofeedback and thermal biofeedback combined with cognitive therapy in the treatment of vascular headache. *Journal of Consulting and Clinical Psychology*, **58**, 216–24.

Blanchard, E.B., Schwarz, S.P., Suls, J.M. *et al.* (1992). Two controlled evaluations of multicomponent psychological treatment of irritable bowel syndrome. *Behaviour Research and Therapy*, **30**, 175–89.

Bradley, L.A. (1989). Cognitive-behavioural therapy for primary fibromyalgia. *Journal of Rheumatology*, **16** (Suppl. 19), 131–6.

Buckelew, S.P. (1989). Fibromyalgia: a rehabilitation approach. *American Journal of Physical Medicine and Rehabilitation*, **68**, 37–42.

Butler, G., Fennell, M., Robson, P., and Gelder, M. (1991). Comparison of behavior therapy and cognitive behavior therapy in the treatment of generalized anxiety disorder. *Journal of Consulting and Clinical Psychology*, **59**, 167–75.

Butler, S., Chalder, T., Ron, M., and Wessely, S. (1991). Cognitive behaviour therapy in chronic fatigue syndrome. *Journal of Neurology, Neurosurgery and Psychiatry*, **54**, 153–8.

Cluff, R.A. (1984). Chronic hyperventilation and its treatment by physiotherapy: discussion paper. *Journal of the Royal Society of Medicine*, **77**, 855–62.

Corney, R.H., Stanton, R., Newell, R., Clare, A., and Fairclough, P. (1991). Behavioural psychotherapy in the treatment of irritable bowel syndrome. *Journal of Psychosomatic Research*, **35**, 461–9.

Cott, A., McCully, J., Goldberg, W.M., Tanser, P.H., and Parkinson, W. (1992). Interdisciplinary treatment of morbidity in benign chest pain. *Angiology*, **43**, 195–202.

Davis, D.L. (1989). George Beard and Lydia Pinkham: gender, class, and nerves in late 19th century America. *Health Care and Women International*, **10**, 93–114.

Frank, J.D. (1971). Therapeutic factors in psychotherapy. *American Journal of Psychotherapy*, **25**, 350–61.

Gath, D. and Iles, S. (1988). Treating the premenstrual syndrome. *British Medical Journal*, **297**, 237–8.

Gelder, M.G. (1991). New ways of treating panic disorder. *Annals of Medicine*, **23**, 97–9.

Hawton, K.E. and Kirk, J. (1989) Problem-solving. In *Cognitive behaviour therapy for psychiatric problems*, (ed. K. Hawton, P.M. Salkovskis, J. Kirk, and D.M. Clark), pp. 406–27. Oxford University Press, Oxford.

Hawton, K.E., Salkovskis, P., Kirk, J., and Clark, D.M. (1989). *Cognitive behaviour therapy for psychiatric problems: a practical guide*. Oxford University Press, Oxford.

Heinrich, R.L., Cohen, M.J., Naliboff, B.D., Collins, G.A., and Bonebakker, A.D. (1985). Comparing physical and behaviour therapy for chronic low back pain on physical abilities, psychological distress, and patient's perceptions. *Journal of Behavioural Medicine*, **8**, 61–78.

Hellman, C.J., Budd, M., Borysenko, J., McClelland, D.C., and Benson, H.

(1990). A study of the effectiveness of two group behavioral medicine interventions for patients with psychosomatic complaints. *Behavioural Medicine*, **16**, 165–73.

Hodgson, R. and Rachman, S. (1974). Desynchrony in measures of fear. *Behaviour Research and Therapy*, **12**, 319–26.

Holroyd, K.A., Nash, J.M., Pingel, J.D., Cordingley, G.E., and Jerome, A. (1991). A comparison of pharmacological (amitriptyline HCL) and nonpharmacological (cognitive-behavioral) therapies for chronic tension headaches. *Journal of Consulting and Clinical Psychology*, **59**, 387–93.

House, A. (1989). Hypochondriasis and related disorders: assessment and management of patients referred for a psychiatric opinion. *General Hospital Psychiatry*, **1**, 156–65.

Jakes, S.C., Hallam, R.S., McKenna, and Hinchcliffe, R. (1992). Group cognitive therapy for medical patients: an application to tinnitus. *Cognitive Therapy and Research*, **16**, 67–82.

Keefe, F.J., Dunsmore, J. and Burnett, R. (1992). Behavioural and cognitive behavioural approaches to chronic pain: recent advances and future directions. *Journal of Consulting and Clinical Psychology*, **60**, 528–36.

Klimes, I., Mayou, R.A., Pearce, M.J., Coles, L., and Fagg, J.R. (1990). Psychological treatment atypical non-cardiac chest pain: a controlled evaluation. *Psychological Medicine*, **20**, 605–11.

Kornfeld, A.D. (1984). Hypnosis and behavior therapy: historical relationships. *International Journal of Psychosomatics*, **31**, 22–6.

Kriegler, J.S. and Ashenberg, Z.S. (1987). Management of chronic low back pain: a comprehensive approach. *Seminars in Neurology*, **7**, 303–12.

Linton, S.J. (1986). Behavioral remediation of chronic pain: a status report. *Pain*, **24**, 125–41.

Litt, M.D. and Baker, L.H. (1987). Cognitive-behavioral intervention for irritable bowel syndrome. *Journal of Clinical Gastroenterology*, **9**, 208–11.

Lloyd, A.R., Hickie, I., Brockman, A., Hickie, C., Wilson, A., Dwyer, J., and Wakefield, D. (1993). Immunologic and psychologic therapy for patients with chronic fatigue syndrome: a double-blind, placebo-controlled trial. *American Journal of Medicine*, **94**, 197–203.

Lynch, P.M. and Zamble, E. (1989). A controlled behavioural treatment study of irritable bowel syndrome. *Behaviour Therapy*, **20**, 509–23.

Martin, P.R., Nathan, P.R., Milech, D., and van Keppel, M. (1989). Cognitive therapy vs self-management training in the treatment of chronic headaches. *British Journal of Clinical Psychology*, **28**, 347–61.

Mathew, R.J., Weinman, M.L., and Mirabi, M. (1981). Physical symptoms of depression. *British Journal of Psychiatry*, **139**, 293–6.

Mowrer, O.H. (1960). *Learning theory and behaviour*. Wiley, New York.

Neff, D.A. and Blanchard, E.B. (1987). A multi-component treatment for irritable bowel syndrome. *Behaviour Therapy*, **18**, 70–83.

Nicholas, M.K., Wilson, P.H., and Goyen, J. (1992). Comparison of cognitive-behavioral group treatment and an alternative non-psychological treatment for chronic low back pain. *Pain*, **48**, 339–47.

Ost, L.G. (1987). Applied relaxation: description of a coping technique and review of controlled studies. *Behaviour Research and Therapy*, **25**, 397–410.

Pearce, S. (1983). A review of cognitive-behavioural methods for the treatment of chronic pain. *Journal of Psychosomatic Research*, **27**, 431–40.

Philips, H.C. (1987). The effects of behavioural treatment on chronic pain. *Behaviour Research and Therapy*, **25**, 365–77.

Philips, H.C. (1988). *The psychological management of chronic pain: a manual.* Springer, New York.

Pither, C.E. (1989). Treatment of persistent pain. *British Medical Journal*, **299**, 1239–40.

Robbins, J.M. and Kirmayer, L. (1991). Attributions of common somatic symptoms. *Psychological Medicine*, **21**, 1029–45.

Salkovskis, P.M. (1989). Somatic problems. In *Cognitive behaviour therapy for psychiatric problems*, (ed. K. Hawton, P.M. Salkovskis, J. Kirk, and D.M. Clark), pp. 235–76. Oxford University Press, Oxford.

Salkovskis, P.M. (1992*a*). Psychological treatment of noncardiac chest pain: the cognitive approach. *American Journal of Medicine*, **92** (Suppl 5A), 114S–21S.

Salkovskis, P.M. (1992*b*). The cognitive-behavioural approach. In *Medical symptoms not explained by organic disease*, (ed. F. Creed, R. Mayou, and A. Hopkins), pp. 70–84. Royal College of Psychiatrists and Royal College of Physicians of London, London.

Salkovskis, P.M. and Clark, D.M. (1990). Affective responses to hyperventilation: a test of the cognitive model of panic. *Behaviour Research and Therapy*, **28**, 51–61.

Scott, B., Lindberg, P., Lyttkens, L., and Melin, L. (1985). Psychological treatment of tinnitus. An experimental group study. *Scandanavian Audiology*, **14**, 223–30.

Seligman, M.E.P. (1975). *Helplessness.* Freeman, San Francisco.

Sharpe, M.C. and Bass, C. (1992). Pathophysiological mechanisms in somatization. *International Reviews in Psychiatry*, **4**, 81–97.

Sharpe, M.C. and Hawton, K.E. (1990). Liaison psychiatry and psychological sequelae of physical disorders. *Current Opinion in Psychiatry*, **3**, 199–203.

Sharpe, M.C., Peveler, R., and Mayou, R. (1992). The psychological treatment of patients with functional somatic symptoms: a practical guide. *Journal of Psychosomatic Research*, **36**, 515–29.

Sharpe, M., Mayou, R., Seagroatt, V., Surawy, C., Warwick, H., Bulstrode, C., Dawber, R., and Lane, D. (1994). Why do doctors find some patients difficult to help? *Quarterly Journal of Medicine*, **87** 187–93.

Skelton, J.A. and Pennebaker, J.W. (1982). The psychology of physical symptoms and sensations. In *Social psychology of health and illness* (ed. G.S. Sanders and J. Suls), pp. 99–128. Erlbaum, Hillsdale, NJ.

Skinner, J.B., Erskine, A., Pearce, S., Rubenstein, I., Taylor, M., and Foster, C. (1990). The evaluation of a cognitive behavioural treatment programme in outpatients with chronic pain. *Journal of Psychosomatic Research*, **34**, 13–19.

Stern, R. and Fernandez, M. (1991). Group cognitive and behavioural treatment for hypochondriasis. *British Medical Journal*, **303**, 1229–31.

Svedlund, J., Sjodin, I., Ottosson, J., and Dotevall, G. (1983). Controlled study of psychotherapy in irritable bowel syndrome. *Lancet*, **ii**, 589–92.

Sweetow, R.W. (1986). Cognitive aspects of tinnitus patient management. *Ears, and Hearing*, **7**, 390–6.

Tollison, C.D., Kriegel, M.L., Downie, G.R. (1985). Chronic low back pain: results of treatment at the Pain Therapy Center. *Southern Medical Journal*, **78**, 1291–5.

Turner, J.A. and Clancy, S. (1988). Comparison of operant behavioural and cognitive-behavioural group treatment for chronic low back pain. *Journal of Consulting and Clinical Psychology*, **56**, 261–6.

Tyrer, P. (1976). Institute of Psychiatry Maudsley Monograph 23. *The role of bodily feelings in anxiety*. Oxford University Press, Oxford.

Visser, S. and Bouman, T.K. (1992). Cognitive-behavioural approaches in the treatment of hypochondriasis: six single case cross-over studies. *Behaviour Revearch and Therapy*, **30**, 301–6.

Warwick, H.M.C. and Salkovskis, P.M. (1985). Reassurance. *British Medical Journal*, **290**, 1028.

Warwick, H.M.C. and Salkovskis, P.M. (1990). Hypochondriasis. *Behaviour Research and Therapy*, **28**, 105–17.

Warwick, H.M.C., Clark, D.M., and Cobb, A. A controlled trial of cognitive behavioural treatment for hypochondriasis. Submitted for publication.

8 Treatment of functional somatic symptoms: psychodynamic treatment

Elspeth Guthrie

In this chapter, Dr Guthrie points out that there are many differences between patients with functional somatic symptoms and those who are usually accepted for psychotherapy in the National Health Service. Although patients with functional somatic symptoms are neither actively seeking psychological help nor psychologically minded, it is often possible to engage them in treatment.

Dr Guthrie reviews studies that have used psychodynamic psychotherapy in the treatment of organic disease before providing evidence to support the efficacy of this treatment in patients with functional somatic symptoms. The author's own study of patients with intractable irritable bowel syndrome is described in some detail and strategies for engaging and treating patients with dynamic psychotherapy are outlined. Finally, she emphasizes the service implications of the effectiveness of this form of brief psychological treatment.

Introduction

Psychoanalytic and psychodynamic concepts have played an influential role in the development of aetiological theories of functional somatic symptoms. The application of psychodynamic psychotherapy in the treatment of such patients, however, has been less striking. For many years it was thought that patients with functional symptoms made poor candidates for psychodynamic therapy and that traditional psychoanalytic approaches to the problem were both time-consuming and ineffective (Sifneos 1972; Lipowski 1977).

The term psychodynamic psychotherapy is used in this chapter to refer to psychotherapies in which the following features are fundamental to the treatment process.

1. Emphasis is placed on the development of an intense relationship between the therapist and patient.

2. The nature of this relationship and the thoughts and feelings of the patient towards the therapist are explored.

3. Exaggerated, intense, and inappropriate feelings are understood in terms of the concepts of transference and countertransference.

4. Empathic and interpretive interventions are used by the therapist.

5. The development and persistence of the patients' functional symptoms is understood in terms of underlying psychological focal conflicts, which emerge during the course of therapy.

The problem

Early psychoanalytic ideas in relation to functional somatic symptomatology were derived from Freudian Drive Theory (Breuer and Freud 1895). These authors undertook a search for specific causal factors to explain the development of different kinds of physical symptoms. Specific kinds of intrapsychic conflict or personality type or psychological characteristics were, in turn, suggested as being responsible for the development of specific kinds of physical disorder. But the limitations of this 'neurosis' model for understanding somatic symptoms became apparent in the 1950s when the hoped-for efficacy of psychoanalytic treatment did not materialize.

During the last 30 years there has been a shift in the focus of psychotherapy and psychoanalysis from neurotic states of mind to more primitive mental states. This has resulted in the development of theoretical concepts involving object relations and the development of the self (Greenberg and Mitchel 1983), which are more relevant to the understanding of functional somatic conditions. It is proposed that deficiencies in the early mother–child relationship leave the individual with structural psychic deficits and an inability to use imagination and language to contain distressing and unbearable feelings. This results in a paucity of fantasy life, dream experiences, and emotional responses and an increased susceptibility to somatic complaints.

Patients with functional somatic symptoms are seen to lie on a continuum. At one end are individuals with a history of severe emotional deprivation during childhood, who have great difficulty in making and sustaining mature relationships as adults. The relationships that they form are either chaotic and fragile or more typically symbiotic. In patients with chronic functional somatic symptoms, symbiotic or enmeshed relationships are often characterized by a 'carer' and an 'invalid'. The invalid (or patient) is cared for by an overly sympathetic and dutiful partner. Both have their needs met through the dynamics of the relationship. The physical symptoms are used by the patient as an expression of and a defence against intolerable emotional feelings. They also have a secondary function as a way of enlisting care from the partner or other people/professionals. Any change to the nature of the relationship is usually fiercely resisted.

At the other end of the spectrum, individuals with good enough care during childhood may develop somatic symptoms at certain times in their lives in relation to particular problems, but essentially form healthy and mutually supportive relationships. Recognition and change in the individual results in improvement in the relationship and resolution of the symptoms.

At both extremes of the continuum, patients commonly view their somatic symptoms as having an underlying organic aetiology and seek physical treatments or medication for their 'disease'. They are usually referred to medical clinics other than psychotherapy departments and may be resistant to the idea of psychological treatment for their complaints. For example, Brook and Bingley (1991) found that many patients in a gastrointestinal clinic refused the offer of working with a psychotherapist and insisted instead on further physical investigations. Bassett and Pilowsky (1985) found many patients attending a pain clinic were highly resistant to the offer of psychotherapeutic help, although a small select group did engage in therapy.

These observations suggest that patients with functional somatic symptoms are very different from those who are usually taken on for psychotherapy in the NHS. Most psychotherapy patients are actively seeking psychological help and are attempting to understand the aetiology of their problems within a psychological/psychodynamic framework. Motivation (Bloch 1979) and psychological mindedness (Coltart 1988) are considered important clinical predictors of outcome. Because patients with functional somatic symptoms may have neither of these qualities they are still considered by many psychotherapists to be difficult to engage and treat.

Overview of evidence

Most of the empirical research conducted in this area has been with brief psychodynamic therapy. It is usual in brief therapy to identify, at an early stage, a single conflict underlying the patient's main symptom, which is then made the focus of the subsequent therapy. Brief therapy usually comprises 12–20 sessions, with a maximum of 30.

Although there have been several controlled trials of dynamic psychotherapy or psychoanalysis in patients with the so-called 'traditional' psychosomatic disorders (for example, chronic obstructive airways disease (Rosser *et al.* 1983); diabetes (Moran *et al.* 1991), peptic ulcer (Sjodin 1983), and ulcerative colitis (Grace *et al.* 1954)) there have been very few controlled trials of dynamic therapy in patients with functional somatic complaints. This is partly because the interest in treating these patients with psychodynamic psychotherapy has only developed recently and partly because, in the past, they were considered unsuitable for psychotherapy.

At this point, it is helpful to consider some of the work that has been conducted with patients with traditional 'psychosomatic' disorders, because many of the findings are relevant to patients with functional somatic symptoms. Although these patients have underlying organic illness they have many psychological similarities with patients who somatize.

Milton (1989) has described her work with patients suffering from brittle diabetes. Most of the patients she engaged in therapy were not asking for psychological treatment. In fact, as she highlighted in her paper, asking for help was one of their major difficulties. Her main task in the therapy was to help patients to recognize how their underlying emotions influenced their diabetic control. As an example she described one young woman who had been brought up by an extremely powerful and dominating mother. In all aspects of her life she was dutiful, conscientious, and obedient and always attended her appointments at the diabetic clinic punctually. However, her diabetic control was haphazard and poor. During the therapy, her extremely ambivalent feelings towards her mother were explored and the poor diabetic control came to be understood as a way of secretly rebelling.

Moran *et al.* (1991) have recently published a controlled trial of psychoanalytic therapy in adolescents with brittle diabetes. The study compared two equivalent groups of 11 diabetic children with grossly abnormal blood glucose profiles that required repeated admissions to a hospital. Patients in the treatment group were offered intensive in-patient treatment including psychoanalytic psychotherapy sessions three to four times per week over 15 weeks, which took place on the hospital ward. The intervention proved highly effective in improving the diabetic control of the children and this improvement was maintained at 1 year follow-up.

Psychodynamic psychotherapy may not be as helpful, however, in patients who are severely physically ill and disabled. Rosser *et al.* (1983) found that psychodynamic psychotherapy was relatively ineffective in patients with severe chronic bronchitis and emphysema. Supportive psychotherapy resulted in greater psychological symptom relief and counselling from a nurse led to greater improvements in breathlessness than with dynamic psychotherapy. Many patients in this trial were elderly, struggling with adverse social conditions, and chronically materially and emotionally deprived.

Patients with functional somatic symptoms are often disabled by their symptoms, but are rarely as ill as those Rosser *et al.* (1983) treated in the trial. In an uncontrolled trial of psychotherapy patients with functional abdominal pain, Hislop (1980) explored each patient's emotional responses and the relationship of these to the development of the somatic symptoms. Those patients who were able to express overt distress during the interview did well, whereas those who were unable to express distress did poorly.

It is notable that the vast majority of Hislop's patients accepted an emotional basis for their somatic symptoms at the outset and accepted his form of psychotherapy. In this respect, the patients in Hislop's (1980) study are not typical of most patients with functional symptoms attending outpatient medical clinics.

Because many psychological intervention studies for patients with functional somatic symptoms fail to provide clear descriptions of the patients' characteristics, interpretation of the results is difficult. Furthermore, patients with functional somatic symptoms presenting to out-patient clinics for the first time are very different from those who are long-term or chronic attenders. The former report less severe and disabling symptoms and approximately 60 per cent respond to simple reassurance and explanation of their symptoms (Harvey *et al*. 1987). The latter report disabling and persistent symptomatology and are resistant to conventional medical treatment. The response rates for improvement for these two groups of patients are very different and suggest that the variable 'duration of symptoms' will have a dramatic effect on the outcome of any intervention, whatever type of treatment is being evaluated. The importance of this point was recently illustrated by Corney *et al*. (1991), who reported a controlled trial of behavioural therapy versus conventional treatment in patients with irritable bowel syndrome attending a gastroenterological clinic. Although patients had reported symptoms for at least 6 months, the study criteria did *not* specify length of attendance at the clinic. It is likely, therefore, that relatively few patients in the study sample were chronic attenders. Because the response rate was likely to be high in both trial groups, it is not surprising that little appreciable difference was found between behaviour therapy and conventional medical treatment. The true worth of behavioural therapy for patients with chronic and resistant irritable bowel syndrome still requires evaluation.

There are no methodologically sound trials of dynamic psychotherapy for patients with functional somatic symptoms who are first-time or recent attenders. However, two major trials of dynamic therapy, involving large numbers of patients and employing rigorous methodology have been conducted in patients with chronic functional somatic symptoms. Both involved patients with irritable bowel syndrome.

The first trial was conducted by Svedlund (1983) and the second by Guthrie *et al*. (1991). Svedlund (1983) compared the effectiveness of routine medical treatment combined with dynamic therapy versus medical treatment alone in 101 out-patients with chronic symptoms of irritable bowel syndrome. The patients had all had symptoms for at least 1 year and had been unresponsive to previous medical treatment. They were recruited consecutively from a gastroenterological out-patient clinic and were randomized to treatment conditions. Patients were assessed at the beginning and end of the trial and again at follow-up 15 months later. Self-assessments were used for both psychological and somatic complaints and, in addition, the two therapists rated each other's patients. Both groups of patients improved during the 3 months of the trial in terms of both psychological and somatic symptoms. The patients who received psychotherapy, however, showed significantly greater improvement in abdominal pain and bowel dysfunction. On the whole differences between the two groups in somatic symptoms were more pronounced at 15 months than at 3 months. This was because the patients in the psychotherapy group continued to improve whereas the patients in the control group deteriorated. This is an impressive study which clearly demonstrates the effectiveness of dynamic psychotherapy compared with conventional medical treatment in this group of patients. The inclusion of an independent assessor of the patients' physical symptoms would have further strengthened the study.

Author's own research

Guthrie *et al.* (1991) conducted a study similar to that of Svedlund but the design included an independent assessment of bowel symptomatology by a gastroenterologist who remained blind to the treatment condition. One hundred and two out-patients with chronic symptoms of irritable bowel syndrome and resistant to medical treatment were recruited consecutively from the gastrointestinal clinic. Following randomization, the treatment group received seven sessions of dynamic psychotherapy and the control group five sessions of supportive listening. Both groups continued with their medical treatment unchanged. The control group received supportive sessions from the therapist to control for the so-called non-specific effects of psychotherapy (that is, the therapeutic effect of being seen and listened to by someone who is non-judgemental and supportive). At the beginning of the trial, there was no difference between the treatment and control group on baseline measures of gastroenterological and psychological function. At the end of the 12-week trial period the treatment group showed significantly greater improvement than the control group in terms of both gastroenterological and psychological symptoms.

Like Svedlund's (1983) study, this study confirmed that dynamic psychotherapy is superior to conventional medical treatment in patients with chronic irritable bowel syndrome. In addition, this study went one stage further and demonstrated that psychotherapy has a specific therapeutic effect and that improvement cannot be attributed to the therapist 'just being nice' to the patient. In a further phase of this study, patients who were originally controls and who remained symptomatic at the end of the 12-week trial period were subsequently offered therapy. This group of patients also showed significant improvement in their symptoms following treatment. At follow-up 1 year later the majority of patients who had improved with therapy remained well, whereas those who had dropped out of treatment continued to be symptomatic.

Predictors of outcome

Svedlund (1983) was unable to identify any baseline factors that predicted a good response to therapy. Guthrie *et al.* (1991) found that patients with baseline symptoms of psychological distress (either anxiety or depression) did better than those who reported little psychological disturbance. In addition, those patients who were able to acknowledge, during the first long psychotherapy session, some link between their bowel symptoms and emotional factors, were more likely to improve. Case vignettes will illustrate these points.

A 35 year old woman who agreed to participate in the trial initially saw no connection between her bowel symptoms and her emotional life. She acknowledged feeling miserable and depressed, but attributed these feelings to her bowel symptoms. She gave a history of suffering from abdominal pain and distension for the previous 18 months. There were no obvious precipitants or life events before the onset of her symptoms. She had commenced a new relationship with a man several months before the onset of the irritable bowel syndrome but described this relationship as being very happy, remarking that he was supportive and understanding. Five years previously she had suffered from a depressive illness associated with the break-up of her marriage. She had thought that the marriage was happy and stable only to be told one evening by her husband that he had been having an affair for the previous 2 years and intended to leave her for another woman. She described feeling utterly shattered by this and unable to comprehend how she could have been unaware of her husband's infidelity.

She also revealed that her father had had an affair when she was a little girl, which had resulted in the break-up of her parents' marriage. In the long first psychotherapy session, she described her surprise at being met from school one day by her father, sitting in his car outside the school gates and being told by him that he would no longer be living at home. During the session she was to make a link for the first time between her feelings then and her feelings when her husband had told her of his affair. When the therapist asked about any fears she may have about her new boyfriend, she initially affirmed how wonderful her relationship was, but then in the silence that ensued became more and more distressed. From this point, it became possible for her to acknowledge that although her new relationship was 'wonderful', underneath she had terrible fears that her boyfriend would desert her as both her father and her husband had previously done. She was also able to acknowledge a possible link between the development of her bowel symptoms and the deepening of her emotional attachment to this new man. A focus was agreed in which her feelings and fears about rejection would be explored and her tendency to idealize relationships and deny difficulties would be examined.

Key prognostic factors in this case were, first the woman's *acknowledgement of depressive symptoms*, second her *openness and willingness to discuss her previous emotional problems*, and third her *ability to change her view of the causal relationship between her bowel symptoms and psychological factors*.

The main work of the therapy involved exploring the patient's feelings about the ending of the therapy and the links between this and previous rejections. The idealization of the therapist as a kind and supportive figure who would not let the patient down was also acknowledged and addressed. This enabled the patient to express previously hidden feelings of ambivalence and anger. It also resulted in her being able to view her current relationship in a more realistic fashion. These changes would not have occurred, however, if the patient had been unable to acknowledge the relevance of emotional factors to her bowel symptoms at an early stage of the therapy.

Patients who did not report or acknowledge symptoms of psychological distress in our study had a poor response to psychotherapy. This did not mean that they had to be very psychologically minded to do well, but it did imply that some acknowledgement of a link between psychological and physical factors was important. It is interesting that the type of pain which patients complained of appeared to have a powerful predictive effect. For example, those patients who reported constant, unremitting abdominal pain had a poor response to psychotherapy and a high drop-out rate. In addition, the longer the duration of the patients' symptoms the less likely they were to respond. It must be remembered, however, that by definition all patients entered into the study had chronic, unresponsive symptoms. The author's own clinical experience also suggests that in those patients where the physical symptoms provided both considerable psychological protection and financial and practical advantages, such a brief out-patient intervention was unlikely to produce therapeutic change.

A 50-year-old man reported suffering from severe abdominal pain and diarrhoea for the previous 10 years. He had lived at home all his life and had never had any important relationships outside his family. His father had died when he was 3 years old; he had been brought up by his mother and a sister 10 years his senior. His symptoms began when his mother became seriously ill and had to be admitted to hospital. Despite being 40 years old this was the first time he had been separated from his mother. Although his mother recovered, his bowel symptoms became worse and this resulted in him having to give up work and remain permanently at home. He agreed to participate in the trial but denied any kind of emotional upset or any connection between the onset of his bowel symptoms and his mother's illness.

Poor prognostic factors in this case were his *inability to acknowledge any kind of emotional distress*, his *inability to link emotional factors to the onset of his bowel symptoms*, the *chronicity* of his symptoms, and the complaint of *constant, unremitting pain*.

Patients with chronic pain

Patients whose main or sometimes only complaint is one of severe pain are often extremely difficult to treat. Whale (1992) has recently described her work with patients referred to a pain clinic in the UK. She saw patients for an initial assessment followed by four further sessions of brief dynamic therapy. Follow-up sessions at 6 months and 1 year were also arranged. Over a period of 18 months, she was referred 14 patients for assessment, of whom 11 were offered brief psychotherapy and nine accepted. Of these nine, three showed considerable improvement in their pain following psychotherapy and a further four reported that although the pain was little changed, their ability to cope with it was greatly improved and their level of functioning increased.

In several patients, Whale (1992) discovered a striking association between the development of the pain and unresolved difficulties with grieving and loss. As an example, she described a 50-year-old woman who had suffered with continuous pain in the shoulder and arm for 9 years. She found that the pain had developed shortly after the death of her beloved and idealized father who himself had suffered from intense neck and shoulder pain. The patient had not been able to accept her father's death or acknowledge deep seated feelings of ambivalence and anger towards him. As the therapy progressed, the woman was able to acknowledge her inability to grieve and some of her anger towards her father was expressed directly at the therapist, through the transference relationship. The ability of the patient to become angry with the therapist appeared to be a key element leading to a successful outcome. Whale (1992) stressed that the aim of such a brief therapy was not to 'cure' the patient, but to help them to become aware of a psychological difficulty or problem that had previously been denied. In other words, the therapy acted as a trigger or catalyst to enable the patient to view their painful symptoms from a different perspective.

Indications of a favourable response to Whale's treatment included an expressed motivation to get better, an active desire after the initial session to continue with psychotherapy, and the relationship of onset of the pain to a key life event, such as bereavement.

Although Whale (1992) provides a fascinating account of her work with pain patients, it has not been systematically evaluated. One of the few controlled trials of dynamic therapy with pain patients is that by Bassett and Pilowsky (1985). They described a randomized controlled trial of 12 sessions of dynamic therapy versus six sessions of supportive therapy for patients attending a pain clinic. Twenty-six patients were recruited to the study and although the numbers were too small to show any significant differences between the groups at the end of therapy, there was a trend for the patients who received dynamic psychotherapy to report a better outcome than controls. When followed-up 12 months later, the psychotherapy patients showed significantly greater levels of activity than those who had received a supportive intervention, but were similar to controls on most of the other measures of outcome.

There are many limitations to this study, the chief ones being the small numbers and high drop-out rates. Participation in the therapy and attendance was a significant problem. Only four patients in the control group completed the full number of sessions and many patients refused to participate in the study. This reflects the difficulty of engaging such patients in any kind of psychological treatment. It also highlights the importance of the therapeutic aspects of engagement. In the author's own study only five out of over 100 patients refused to participate in the study. This low figure was achieved by the therapist actually attending the clinic in person and being able to have a long first session with the patient, when any fears or antipathy regarding a psychological treatment approach were explored and confronted.

Key components of therapy

There is little empirical data available to determine the mechanism by which psychotherapy leads to improvement in patients with functional somatic symptoms. Detailed statistical analysis of our own trial suggested that the improvement in patients' symptoms resulted from an improvement in psychological symptomatology which then resulted in improved bowel symptomatology. In other words, psychological change was the key therapeutic factor. Other important components of the therapy, already previously mentioned, include allowing the patient to acknowledge psychological distress, moving the patient from a purely physical aetiological understanding of their symptoms to a model which accommodates psychological factors; helping the patient, through the transference relationship, to recognize difficulties or deficiencies in relationships outside of therapy; making a link between symptom development and relationship difficulties, and, finally, helping the patient to make changes to his/her relationships.

Although there are many studies reporting changes in gut physiology in response to emotional change, there have been no studies of the effect of psychotherapy on physiological measures of bowel function. This, will be a fascinating area for future research.

Comparison with other psychological treatments

There has been no satisfactory trial comparing dynamic psychotherapy with other forms of psychological treatment in patients with functional somatic symptoms. Trials of dynamic or explorative therapy versus cognitive therapy in patients with affective disorders (Shapiro and Firth 1987; Elkin *et al*. 1989) have consistently failed to demonstrate appreciable differences between these therapies. It seems likely therefore that a trial comparing these therapies would not detect any overall difference in patients with functional somatic complaints. This is not to say that, within a large group of patients, some would be more suited to one kind of psychological therapy than others.

Two recent trials of hypnotherapy in patients with irritable bowel syndrome (Whorwell *et al*. 1984; Harvey *et al*. 1987) have demonstrated that gut-directed hypnosis is capable of producing an impressive degree of symptom relief in patients with chronic irritable bowel syndrome. It is interesting to note, however, that patients who complained of severe unremitting constant pain did poorly with hypnotherapy (Whorwell *et al*. 1984). This is the same group of patients who have been found to respond poorly to dynamic psychotherapy. Furthermore, patients without symptoms of psychological distress did well with hypnotherapy, whereas those patients who complain of psychological distress do better with psychotherapy. This finding suggests a different response to dynamic therapy and hypnotherapy, although the improvement of the patient group as a whole may be similar. It seems likely, therefore, that patients who report psychological distress respond more favourably to a psychological approach (psychotherapy) that acknowledges and works with feelings, whereas those who are not psychologically distressed or who are unable to acknowledge feelings respond better to a psychological intervention (hypnotherapy) in which emotions and feelings are not discussed.

Long-term therapy

Controlled trials evaluating the efficacy of a long-term therapy (for example, 24 months of once weekly or twice weekly psychotherapy) are extremely difficult to conduct and to date have not been attempted in patients with functional somatic symptoms. It is clear, however, that some patients do not respond to a short-term approach and require further help. Poor predictors of outcome to short-term treatment have already been discussed. Long-term psychotherapeutic work with patients with functional somatic symptoms often involves a 'damage limitation exercise'. The therapist is not aiming for treatment or cure, but attempts to contain the patient's treatment-seeking behaviour and to prevent deterioration. A knowledge of psychodynamics is helpful to the therapist who may have to tolerate intense countertransference feelings from such patients. The patient will often project a great deal of hostility onto the therapist and make considerable demands for further treatment or investigation. These demands have to be resisted, at the same time as maintaining the patient in therapy. It is not yet possible to accurately predict whether patients will respond to long-term treatment or brief interventions. Some predictive factors have been identified (see above), although the standard psychiatric classification systems are not very helpful. From clinical experience, the few patients who have enough symptoms to acquire a diagnosis of somatization disorder are unlikely to respond to brief therapy and require longer term management.

Practical guidelines

Most psychotherapists working with patients with functional somatic symptoms stress the importance of making certain modifications to the usual practice of psychotherapy.

Brook and Bingley (1991) described the benefits of the psychotherapist attending the out-patient clinic and being involved with the clinical medical team as a whole. Hislop (1980) described the importance of taking a detailed history of the patient's somatic symptoms before enquiring about psychological factors. Guthrie (1991) highlighted the need to engage the patient before embarking upon the therapy itself. Svedlund (1983) emphasized the importance of the therapist's flexibility, in being able to move from a very interpretive style, to one which is more empathic and supportive.

The following practical guidelines are offered for those attempting to engage and treat patients with functional somatic symptoms using dynamic psychotherapy.

1. Attendance at the medical clinic. The psychotherapist's attendance at the medical clinic facilitates referral. Patients who would otherwise refuse to see a psychiatrist can meet the therapist in the clinic, where any fears or misconceptions about psychiatry and psychotherapy can be alleviated. The psychotherapist is also seen by the patient as being an integral member of the medical team, which helps to reduce potential splitting of medical staff involved in the patient's care.

2. Address ambivalent feelings about psychiatry. At a very early stage of the interview the therapist must address any ambivalent feelings the patient has about seeing a psychiatrist or psychotherapist (see

Chapter 5). If these feelings are not openly explored and acknowledged the patient's ambivalence may remain hidden. This may result
in superficial compliance, but covert resistance and anger.

3. Metaphorical use of physical symptoms. Taking a detailed history of
   the patient's somatic complaints is essential for two reasons. First, it
   helps to reassure the patient that the therapist is taking his/her
   physical symptoms seriously and to allay any fears that the symptoms
   'are all in the mind'. Second, in dynamic psychotherapy, it can be
   helpful and illuminating to try to understand the way patients describe
   and convey their experience of physical pain and discomfort as a
   metaphorical expression of their internal emotional world. This is particularly useful for patients who have difficulty in putting their feelings into words. For example, a patient with chronic bowel symptoms
   for many years described her pain as sharp and stabbing; it was ever
   present, twisting inside her like a knife. At first, she was unable to
   make any connection between her physical symptoms and her feelings.
   In time, however, it became apparent that she had been sexually
   abused by her father and the metaphorical meaning of her pain
   became clear.

4. Long first session. A long first session of therapy (3–4 h) allows the
   therapist time to gently encourage and explore possible connections
   between the patient's physical symptoms and their underlying emotional difficulties. If this process is rushed, the patient may disengage
   and drop out of the therapy. The length of the session also enhances
   the development of a strong therapeutic relationship and facilitates the
   appearance of transference material. A long first session with these
   patients is more productive than three separate shorter sessions; with
   short sessions patients have time to rebuild their defences in between
   the sessions, so one then has to spend time covering the same ground.

5. Acknowledge and contain angry feelings. Whale's (1992) work emphasized the importance of dealing with the patient's anger and not
   avoiding it or directing it at someone else. Many patients with functional somatic symptoms are angry at their doctors and at the previous
   treatment they have received. In dynamic psychotherapy it is almost
   inevitable that the patient is going to experience intense anger towards
   the therapist at some point. How this anger is contained and dealt with
   can have an important influence on the outcome of therapy.

6. Focus. It is helpful if a theme can be identified during the first session
   which can then become the focus for the rest of the therapy. Whale's
   (1992) work suggests that the therapist should pay particular attention

to any difficulties the patient has with loss and grieving. It must be remembered, however, that in some cases it is not possible to establish a focus.

7. Address the ending. As with other short-term dynamic therapies, the brevity of the therapy and its ending must be addressed at an early stage. This is particularly important for patients who somatize. Psychodynamic theory suggests that the development of somatic symptoms occurs because of issues related to emotional deprivation and a lack of care. The ending of therapy raises issues related to loss and rejection. If these issues can be addressed in the transference and a link made to the patient's somatic symptoms the potential for change is enhanced. Whale (1992) has graphically described the importance of issues related to loss in general and unresolved grief in particular, when working with patients suffering from chronic pain.

8. Flexible style. Some patients with functional somatic symptoms are psychologically minded and can work in a dynamic way with the therapist, whilst others find it more difficult to appreciate transference issues. The therapist has to be able to adjust his/her style to accommodate these different kinds of patients. With the former, the therapist can work in a more conventional psychotherapeutic mode, using interpretations and addressing the transference directly. With the latter group of patients, this traditional therapeutic style can be perceived as persecutory or irrelevant. The therapist has to work in a more supportive fashion, concentrating on building up the patient's trust and strengthening the therapeutic alliance. Subtle linking comments or hypotheses can then be used to draw together psychological issues and physical complaints. Emphasis is still placed, however, on working in the 'here and now' and drawing attention to the link between the patient's feelings towards the therapist and important others in his/her life. Two styles of explorative psychotherapy that can be used in a flexible way are Hobson's (1985) Conversational Model of Psychotherapy and Ryle's (1982) cognitive analytic therapy. Both have been employed to good effect with patients with functional symptoms or psychosomatic problems (Milton 1989; Guthrie 1991).

9. Follow-up. Patients are very rarely followed-up after the end of therapy, unless it is part of a research study. In the author's own trial, follow-up of all the patients was mandatory 1 year after the end of therapy to assess the long-term outcome. It is striking, however, how many of the follow-up interviews were used as a further session of therapy, for the patients to come to some kind of resolution of their feelings and to explore with the therapist further insights they had had

during the intervening year. As a result of this experience it has now become the author's practice to give all patients seen for brief therapy the opportunity of one further session, several months after the therapy has been completed. In patients with a poor prognosis the aim of treatment may change from symptom relief to 'containment' as discussed above. With these patients, more regular sessions on a long-term basis may be required.

Service implications

For psychological treatment to be adopted as a realistic therapeutic option for patients with functional somatic symptoms, it has to fulfil three basic requirements. First, it should be brief, second, it should be easily learned, and, finally, it should be practised by non-medical professionals. The kind of dynamic psychotherapy used in Guthrie's (1991) trial meets all of these criteria. It is brief and can be taught to junior psychiatrists in training. It has also been used in an MRC trial of psychotherapy where most of the treatment was conducted by psychologists, demonstrating its use by non-medical health professionals (Shapiro and Firth 1987).

These findings imply that all mental health professionals with an interest and aptitude for psychotherapy can learn this particular model of psychotherapy quite quickly. They will however, require close supervision and time to develop skills and confidence. The most severely disabled patients will require care from experienced health professionals. This form of intervention is not cheap, but may turn out to be more cost-effective than frequent hospital admissions and expensive investigations.

Conclusions

Dynamic psychotherapy is a treatment of proven efficacy for patients with functional somatic symptoms who are resistant to conventional medical treatment. The majority of patients can be successfully engaged in therapy if the therapist is prepared to make modifications to his/her usual practice. The therapist needs to be flexible in his/her style of therapy; some patients are suited to a direct interpretive style and others to a less direct and more supportive style with the therapist making subtle linking statements and hypotheses. A small minority of patients, predominantly those with severe and very chronic symptoms, do not respond at all to a brief psycho-therapeutic intervention and may be best managed by the development of a long-term supportive relationship with a physician or psychiatrist who will protect them from further unnecessary investigations and treatment (see Chapters 10 and 21).

References

Bassett D. and Pilowsky, I. (1985). A study of brief psychotherapy for·chronic pain. *Journal of Psychosomatic Research*, **29**, 259–64.

Bloch, S. (1979). Assessment of patients for psychotherapy. *British Journal of Psychiatry*, **135**, 193–208.

Breuer, J. and Freud, S. (1895). *Studies in hysteria*, Vol. 3. The Pelican Freud Library, Pelican Books Ltd. London.

Brook, A. and Bingley, J. (1991). The contribution of psychotherapy to patients with disorders of the gut. *Health Trends*, **23**, 83–5.

Coltart, N.E.C. (1988). The assessment of psychological-mindedness in the diagnostic interview. *British Journal of Psychiatry*, **153**, 819–20.

Corney, R.H., Stanton, R., Newell, R., Clare, A., and Fairclough, P. (1991). Behavioural psychotherapy in the treatment of irritable bowel syndrome. *Journal of Psychosomatic Research*, **35**, 461–9.

Elkin. I, Shea, T., Watkins, J.T., Imber, S.D., Sotsky, S.M., Collins, J.F., *et al.* (1989). NIMH. Treatment of Depression Collaborative Research Program: general effectiveness of treatments. *Archives of General Psychiatry*, **46**, 971–82.

Grace, W.J., Pincksy, R.H., and Wolff, H.G. (1954). Treatment of ulcerative colitis. *Gastroenterology*, **26**, 462–8.

Greenberg, J.R., and Mitchell, S.A. (1983). *Object relations in psychoanalytic theory*. Harvard University Press, Cambridge, MA.

Guthrie, E. (1991). Brief psychotherapy with patients with refractory irritable bowel syndrome. *British Journal of Psychotherapy*, **8**, 175–88.

Guthrie, E., Creed, F.H., Dawson, D., and Tomenson, B. (1991). A controlled trial of psychological treatment for the irritable bowel syndrome. *Gastroenterology*, **100**, 450–7.

Harvey, R.F., Mauad, E.C., and Brown, A.M. (1987). Prognosis in the irritable bowel syndrome: a 5-year prospective study. *Lancet*, **i**, 963–5.

Hislop I.G. (1980) Effect of very brief psychotherapy on the irritable bowel syndrome. *Medical Journal of Australia*, **2**, 620–3.

Hobson, R. (1985) *Forms of feeling*. Tavistock, London.

Lipowski, Z.J. (1977). Psychosomatic medicine in the seventies: an overview. *American Journal of Psychiatry*, **134**, 233–44.

Milton, J. (1989). Brief psychotherapy with poorly controlled diabetics. *British Journal of Psychotherapy*, **5**, 532–43.

Moran, G., Fonaghy, P., Kurtz, A., Bolton, A., and Brook, C. (1991). A controlled study of the psychoanalytic treatment of brittle diabetes. *Journal of the American Academy of Child and Adolescent Psychiatry*, **30**, 926–35.

Rosser, R., Denford, J., Heslop, A., Kinston, W., Macklin, D., Minty, K. *et al.* (1983). Breathlessness and psychiatric morbidity in chronic bronchitis and emphysema: a study of psychotherapeutic management. *Psychological Medicine*, **13**, 93–110.

Ryle, A. (1982). *Psychotherapy: a cognitive integration of theory and practice*. Academic Press, London.

Shapiro, D. and Firth, J. (1987). Prescriptive v. explorative psychotherapy: outcomes of the Sheffield Psychotherapy Project. *British Journal of Psychiatry*, **151**, 790–9.

Sifneos, P.E. (1972). Is dynamic psychotherapy contraindicated for a large number of patients with psychosomatic diseases? *Psychotherapy and Psychosomatics*, **21**, 133–4.

Sjodin, I. (1983). Psychotherapy in peptic ulcer disease: a controlled outcome study. *Acta Psychiatrica Scandinavica*.

Svedlund, J. (1983). Psychotherapy in irritable bowel syndrome: a controlled outcome study. *Acta Psychiatrica Scandinavica*, (Suppl. 306). **67**, 1–86.

Whale, J. (1992). The use of brief focal psychotherapy in the treatment of chronic pain. *Psychoanalytic Psychotherapy*, **6**, 61–72.

Whorwell, P.J., Prior, A., and Faragher, B. (1984). Controlled trial of hypnotherapy in the treatment of severe refractory irritable bowel syndrome. *Lancet*, **ii**, 1232–4.

PART 3 CLINICAL SYNDROMES

9 Treatment of hypochondriasis

Hilary M.C. Warwick

This chapter concentrates on patients who fulfil the criteria for a particular sub-category of somatoform disorder, hypochondriasis. It focuses especially on hypochondrias unaccompanied by other major psychiatric disorder, so-called primary hypochondriasis. The status of this category as a distinct syndrome subgroup remains controversial (Barsky, *et al.* 1992).

Patients with hypochondriasis have always been regarded by physicians and psychiatrists as difficult and unrewarding to treat. Dr Warwick reviews a cognitive behavioural formulation, outlines principles of treatment, and describes a controlled treatment trial. Although the chapter is primarily concerned with cognitive behavioural treatment, Dr Warwick also reviews other treatments and shows that successful treatments have common features.

Dr Warwick emphasizes the importance of clear diagnostic criteria and describes the difficulty of comparing published findings which mainly relate to poorly described clinical series. The criterion for selection for her own trial was DSM-IIIR hypochondriasis. Although the trial subjects reported problems which were less severe than those meeting criteria for somatization disorder, they were a relatively chronic and disabled group of subjects who were therefore more difficult to treat than many of the patients described in the chapters dealing with other syndromes.

Whilst Dr Warwick outlines methods which may require special training and experience, she also emphasizes that understanding of the cognitive behavioural model and of general principles of treatment can be applicable to less specialized management. She emphasizes that early treatment is important and that it is likely to be considerably easier when uncomplicated by ongoing medical treatment. She briefly reports encouraging findings from her own controlled trial of cognitive behavioural treatment. This is not only a well-designed randomized controlled trial of the treatment of hypochondriasis but also an important demonstration of the effectiveness of the psychological treatment of functional symptoms.

The problem

The generally accepted view of the treatment of primary hypochondriasis is well summarized by Kaplan and Sadock (1985): 'Hypochondriasis is notoriously refractory to treatment, and many of the clinicians who have written about the disorder either ignore the subject of therapy entirely, or speak in pessimistic tones about the prognosis. Clinical evidence suggests that, unless hypochondriasis is a part of a depressive disorder with an overt affective disturbance, medications and electroconvulsive treatment are without effect.' In addition to such pessimism about effective treatment, management is made more difficult by the pejorative attitudes of the general public and by hostility and a lack of understanding on the part of professionals. Disabling problems which have not responded to treatment have been attributed to 'secondary gain' in the absence of any good evidence (Warwick and Salkovskis 1990). Prognosis of the disorder has long been regarded as poor and development of new approaches to treatment has been inconsistent and neglected. Such attitudes are still common and must be modified if the real distress of these patients and of their families is to be acknowledged.

Over the years the term hypochondriasis has been used to describe a wide range of conditions. both physical and psychological (Kellner 1986). Although more recently, it has been restricted to a clearly defined subgroup of patients who have unwarranted concerns about their health, the term is still not used consistently. Published studies of hypochondriasis have generally not used standardized diagnostic criteria and the results are therefore difficult to interpret. This situation would be improved by the systematic use of DSM-IV (Diagnostic and Statistical Manual, 4th edition) and ICD-10 (International Classification of Diseases, 10th edition)) criteria (see Chapter 3).

One of the main areas of difficulty has been the distinction between hypochondriasis as a *primary* problem and hypochondriasis occurring as *secondary* to another condition, such as an affective disorder. A good history and phenomenological analysis, including a clear account of the order of onset of the different symptoms is crucial. When considered together with information from a relative or other informant, it will enable the clinician to establish the correct diagnosis. If the hypochondriacal symptoms are secondary to another condition diagnosis, such as DSM-IV major affective disorder, the diagnosis of primary hypochondriasis should not be made. In such cases the appropriate management is that of the primary condition and special treatment of the hypochondriacal symptoms may not be necessary. When the primary diagnosis is hypochondriasis, then the appropriate management is less clear, as neither physical medicine nor psychiatry have been able to offer these patients effective treatment.

The treatment of hypochondriasis

General measures

Supportive treatment is still regarded as the mainstay of routine treatment for primary hypochondriasis (Kaplan and Sadock 1985). There have been few reports of specific treatments for hypochondriasis and no controlled trials. Furthermore, many of the existing studies have methodological limitations. They have not used consistent or comparable diagnostic criteria and have included patients with both primary and secondary hypochondriasis. Comparisons between these earlier studies and more recent research using DSM and ICD criteria are therefore of limited value.

Ladee (1966) studied a series of 23 cases of hypochondriasis treated with psychotherapy or psychoanalysis and reported 'satisfactory to good' improvement in only four. Kenyon (1964) reported a retrospective study of the clinical management of hypochondriasis in a psychiatric hospital, in which a wide range of treatments had been used, including medication, electroconvulsive therapy (ECT), and psychotherapy. Forty per cent of the primary group were rated as 'unchanged or worse' on discharge, compared with 15 per cent of secondary cases. Pilowsky (1968) treated and followed up 147 cases of hypochondriasis over 31 months. He found that 48 per cent had a good outcome, 28 per cent a fair outcome, and 24 per cent a poor outcome. This study was uncontrolled and comprised 'a wide variety of treatments, both physical and psychological' with no less than 28 per cent of the sample receiving electroconvulsive therapy. It is not clear if the cases were of primary or secondary hypochondriasis, but it should be noted that a good prognosis was found in cases having symptoms of anxiety and depression. Kellner (1983) described a study of 36 patients who suffered what was described as 'hypochondriacal neurosis' for 6 months or longer. The study was of long duration and treatments changed as new research emerged. It included individual psychotherapy focused on giving accurate information about symptoms, the role of selective perception, and persuasion. The patients also received repeated physical examinations and reassurance and were given anxiolytic drugs if severely distressed. Sixty-four percent were rated as either recovered or improved. The study was uncontrolled and it is unclear which treatments were responsible for patient improvement.

Cognitive and behavioural approaches in hypochondriasis

Cognitive and behavioural methods have recently been shown to be effective in the treatment of a variety of neurotic conditions, such as obsessive–compulsive disorder. Cognitive (Salkovskis and Warwick 1986) and behavioural correlates (Marks 1981) of hypochondriasis are well documented and cognitive treatments of hypochondriasis are now being reported. Warwick and Marks (1988) described a retrospective case-note study of patients treated with behaviour therapy. Promising results were achieved using techniques such as exposure, response prevention, modelling and prevention of reassurance seeking. In a case series of patients with fears concerning acquired immune deficiency syndrome (AIDS) (Logsdail *et al.* 1991) six patients were improved after behavioural treatments, while a seventh required additional cognitive therapy. Kellner (1985) has put forward a psychological formulation of hypochondriasis and describes treatment strategies derived from this, including explanation, persuasion that the patient does not have a serious physical illness, and repeated reassurance. Barsky *et al.* (1988) reported an uncontrolled group 'cognitive educational' treatment of hypochondriasis, based on the view that somatosensory amplification is an important aetiological factor in the condition. Stern and Fernandez (1991) described an uncontrolled study of similar cognitive educational treatment in a group of six patients. Nine treatment sessions covered education, the effect of focus of attention on the body, relaxation, cognitive therapy, and prevention of reassurance seeking. The results were encouraging and the authors were able to show that this form of group treatment is feasible in a general hospital setting. House (1989) describes the use of cognitive behavioural treatment in a series of 100 patients referred to a general hospital clinic for hypochondriacal concerns. Treatment also included use of antidepressants when appropriate. Of the 80 per cent who completed treatment, 80 per cent were reported to show at least moderate improvement.

A cognitive behavioural formulation of hypochondriasis

Warwick and Salkovskis (1990) proposed a cognitive behavioural formulation of hypochondriasis, describing the psychological processes occurring in patients with this condition and considering factors important in its aetiology and maintenance. They also outlined a cognitive behavioural treatment based on this theoretical formulation (see Salkovskis and Warwick 1986). This section summarizes theoretical concepts and general principles of treatment, together with a summary of the findings from a controlled treatment trial. The core of the formulation is the cognitive error of persistently misinterpreting innocuous physical symptoms as evidence of serious illness. Everyone experiences frequent innocuous physical symptoms but most people are able to make a correct assessment of their significance. In contrast, a hypochondriacal patient does not attribute a headache to tension or eye-strain, but will immediately jump to the conclusion that they have a brain tumour. It is essential to know why some patients persistently make these misinterpretations, whilst others do not. The cognitive behavioural explanation is that hypochondriacal patients are likely to hold faulty general beliefs (dysfunctional assumptions) about health and illness. These assumptions are more firmly held, more extreme, and more erroneous than those of the non-hypochondriacal general population. A trigger stimulus, often a physical symptom, activates these assumptions making misinterpretation of symptoms more likely. For example, a patient who holds the general belief that 'people like me are prone to lung disease' might misinterpret exertional dyspnoea as a sign of serious illness. When a physical symptom is misinterpreted, the patient is likely to experience a series of negative automatic thoughts, for example 'this could be cancer', 'I have a serious illness', 'no-one can help me'. The likelihood of an adverse event, such as a serious illness is overestimated and the likelihood of successful treatment underestimated. The emotion associated with such automatic thoughts is anxiety, which is a prominent feature of primary hypochondriasis.

Anxiety also has an important role in the maintenance of the syndrome. It is associated with a variety of behaviours intended to check current health status, including the repeated seeking after medical consultations, investigations, and reassurance. All of these behaviours, along with avoidance of health-related stimuli, serve to increase anxiety in the long-term, as they both prevent habituation to the symptoms and maintain preoccupation with illness. Direct checking of symptoms can also actually exacerbate them, for example repeated palpation of a small cut will pre-vent healing and lead to further misinterpretation of the significance of the symptom.

It is further suggested that health anxiety may be associated with actual changes in cognitive processing. Hypochondriacal patients selectively attend to and recall information related to health and illness, particularly that which can be construed in a way which provides support for their fears. Their focus of attention on their bodily state means they are more likely to notice and misinterpret further innocuous bodily variations. In addition, anxiety will be associated with the somatic symptoms of auto-nomic arousal, such as palpitations and rapid breathing and these also can be misinterpreted as further evidence of illness. The behavioural, cogni-tive, and physiological changes all serve to increase anxiety and negative thoughts about health. A vicious circle then develops and accounts for the characteristic preoccupations of hypochondriacal patients.

Principles of cognitive behavioural treatment

If this formulation correctly identifies the psychological processes involved in hypochondriasis, it should be possible to show that treatment strategies derived from it are effective. Such cognitive behavioural treatment has been described (Salkovskis 1989; Warwick and Salkovskis 1990) and has been used successfully in case studies (Salkovskis and Warwick 1986). The principal components of this treatment are shown in Table 9.1 and will be discussed in turn.

Explanation The patient may only attend the psychological assessment because of strong pressure from a relative or on the promise of further physical tests from another doctor. Many will want to convince the therapist that their symptoms are not 'all in the mind' and that they are not mentally ill. For this reason it is often difficult to engage them in any

Table 9.1 Principles of cognitive behavioural treatment

1. Explanation of the treatment rationale and engagement
2. Self-monitoring of physical symptoms, health anxiety, negative thoughts, and illness-related behaviours
3. Reattribution — developing alternative explanations of symptoms, using cognitive restructuring, and behavioural experiments
4. Exposure, response prevention, and prevention of repeated reassurance-seeking
5. Recognition and modification of dysfunctional assumptions, using cognitive restructuring

form of psychological treatment. In practice this problem can usually be overcome. A thorough assessment of their somatic symptoms can be of great help; the patient may feel for the first time that they are being given enough time to explore their problem in detail and that the therapist is taking them seriously. The therapist should also take care to show a sympathetic attitude to the patient's difficulties, which is likely to contrast to previous hostile responses. Experienced therapists will ask questions in a manner which suggests that the therapist has met and treated many similar patients in the past.

At the end of the assessment the therapist should have enough information to construct a simplified form of the formulation described above, using the specific thoughts, physical symptoms, and behaviours the patient describes. This formulation should be written down in a way that demonstrates to the patient how the vicious circle could perpetuate their concerns. In practice, patients readily recognize this as a radically different approach to their difficulties and are usually relieved and encouraged by an explanation of what their problems *are*, rather than what they are *not*. They are then offered a course of cognitive behavioural treatment, specifically aimed at correcting the psychological processes highlighted in the formulation.

Self-monitoring At the beginning of treatment, patients are asked to keep records of subsequent episodes of health anxiety and are provided with monitoring sheets for this purpose. For each episode of health concern, they are asked to note the somatic symptom or other trigger, the degree of anxiety experienced, the negative thought associated, and any ensuing illness-related behaviours. For example, a patient developed health anxiety in response to a headache. She noted the thoughts 'I must have a brain tumour', 'I must seek help' and immediately called out her doctor for reassurance. The information on the monitoring sheets provides the therapist with valuable information, which can be used later in treatment and also helps to introduce the concept of negative or dysfunctional thoughts to the patient. In practice, self-monitoring also helps to demonstrate to the patient that the sequence of events postulated in their formulation actually occurs in their daily life and thereby enhances their compliance with treatment. As in cognitive therapy for other disorders, some patients may initially experience difficulty in recognizing and recording their thoughts. It is therefore important to persist with self-monitoring until it is being carried out adequately.

Reattribution

After a period of self-monitoring, reattribution of negative thoughts can begin. Patients are given written information describing the types of thinking errors most commonly experienced in hypochondriasis. Most can readily recognize examples in their own thinking. The most common are 'jumping to conclusions' and 'catastrophizing'. Using examples recorded on their monitoring sheets, patients work with the therapist to construct alternative, non-threatening alternatives to the negative thoughts. This usually involves correction of faulty information about illness and medical practice. It also involves the construction of behavioural experiments relevant to the patient's concerns. For example, a patient who has fears that they have heart disease and who routinely avoids exercise, needs to learn that they can exercise without harm and will benefit from a short run around the hospital. Similarly patients can be asked to induce tingling in their fingers just by thinking hard about the sensation, confirming the powerful effects of attention in magnifying physical symptoms and that such sensations do not necessarily indicate disease. Voluntary hyperventilation can reproduce the physical symptoms which alarm a number of patients and thereby offer a less threatening explanation for them. At the end of treatment, *all* the 'evidence' that the patient feels shows that they are ill must be considered and alternative explanations in terms of psychological and physiological processes proposed. Patients continue with this reattribution of symptoms as they occur between treatment sessions and are provided with recording sheets which are reviewed at the next treatment session.

Exposure, response prevention, and prevention of reassurance seeking

The importance of inappropriate illness-related behaviours in the maintenance of hypochondriasis, has been stressed in the cognitive behavioural formulation. It is also important to consider *avoidance* in the formulation, as this can easily be missed. Patients learn to avoid situations which trigger their health concerns and a programme of graded exposure to these situations must be conducted. Extensive bodily checking for symptoms and signs of illness is common. This includes checking both the appearance and apparent functioning of a part of the body. Thus, a patient who was concerned about throat cancer inspected her throat and swallowed repeatedly.

All these behaviours must be identified and the need to cease them explained.

Reassurance   Salkovskis and Warwick (1986) demonstrated a functional similarity between reassurance seeking and obsessional ritualizing. The similarity provides the rationale for the prevention of all forms of repetitive reassurance seeking. The implementation of this aspect of therapy may involve instructing relatives and other involved professionals how to deal with repeated requests for reassurance.

While the giving of reassurance is one of the most widely used psychotherapeutic strategies throughout medical practice, much can be done to ensure that it is provided effectively. Hypochondriacal patients have characteristically failed to respond to medical reassurance. When hypochondriacal patients seek a consultation, a series of doubts occur which serve to diminish the effectiveness of any reassurance given (Warwick 1992). Soon after and even during their consultations, these patients doubt whether they have explained their symptoms adequately, whether they have shown the doctor all the physical signs they have noticed, and whether normal findings on physical examination are accurate. Ruminating about the results of previous consultations produces increasing doubts about what the doctor *really* meant, with the consequent exacerbation of anxiety, and leads to further requests for consultations and investigation in an effort to obtain yet more reassurance. This pattern should be identified and discussed with the patient. They should then be given only *new* information that they need to deal with their doubts. Repetitive information and examination must be avoided. Relatives can be instructed to respond appropriately to repeated demands for reassurance using role-play. Further research into the education of doctors in the skills needed to reassure patients who have excessive health concerns effectively is required.

Dysfunctional assumptions   During the assessment and the early stages of treatment it should be possible to elucidate dysfunctional assumptions about health. These should then be modified using the techniques of cognitive therapy. In practice, a number of patients report dysfunctional assumptions which extend beyond health issues and to wider aspects of their lives. For example, a patient believed that 'I'm Mrs Jinx, anything bad that can happen will happen to me' and illness was only one of many types of adverse event which concerned her. In such cases, it is necessary to develop cognitive strategies to correct these more basic beliefs.

Whilst earlier studies used extremely diverse treatments, the published cognitive-behavioural treatment approaches have a number of common elements. These include education about the meaning of symptoms and discussion of previous information received from doctors and other professionals. All these treatment approaches describe techniques to correct the patients' false beliefs about their health, for example persuasion (Kellner 1983) and cognitive techniques (Warwick and Salkovskis 1990). They also include behavioural components, such as exposure to feared stimuli, response prevention, and prevention of repeated reassurance seeking. Some authors, for example Kellner (1983), suggest repeated reassurance should be given to these patients. This would, at first sight, appear to be different from the principles outlined above. However, closer examination of the techniques used (Kellner 1992; Warwick 1992) shows that both approaches concentrate on giving the patient *new* information aimed at correcting the false beliefs that they are ill. Neither approach uses repetition of information that the patient already has and, in both, patients are discouraged from seeking further investigations or physical treatments.

A controlled study of cognitive-behavioural treatment for hypochondriasis

A controlled evaluation of cognitive behavioural treatment for hypochondriasis has recently been completed (Warwick, H.M.C. Clark, D. and Cobb, A. to be published). In this study, 32 patients who fulfilled DSM-IIIR criteria for hypochondriasis were recruited. Patients were treated as out-patients in a psychiatric hospital. Half were randomly allocated to individual cognitive behavioural treatment which consisted of weekly treatment sessions over a 4 month period. The other half remained on a waiting list for a 4 month period and were then given identical cognitive behavioural treatment. Subjects were asked to complete a number of ratings using visual analogue scales. These included measures of the belief that they had a physical disease and rating of global problem severity. An independent assessor, blind to whether the patient was receiving cognitive behavioural treatment or was in the waiting list control group, conducted post-treatment assessments. Patients completed the Beck Depression Inventory (BDI) and the Beck Anxiety Inventory (BAI), at weekly intervals throughout the study.

There were no differences between the treatment and control groups on any of the above measures prior to treatment. At 4 months, however, there was a highly significant drop in the treated patients' rating, of the global severity of their problems, compared with the waiting list control group, in whom there was no change. Therapist and independent assessor ratings of global problem severity also revealed highly significant differences between the groups.

The central feature of the cognitive behavioural formulation is the faulty belief in a physical illness and successful treatment should therefore lead to a decrease in this belief. In this study, there was a highly significant drop in the patients' ratings of belief that they were physically ill, compared with the waiting list control group. BDI and BAI scores also showed a highly significant decrease in the treated patients, compared with the waiting list controls.

Guidelines for the non-specialist

There have been no studies of cognitive behavioural treatment of patients with hypochondriasis in primary care. It may be possible to treat less severe cases without referral for specialist cognitive behavioural treatment. The following practical guidelines are intended for those working in primary care (or general psychiatric out-patient clinics).

1. Early recognition of the disorder is important, so that patients do not undergo repeated unnecessary physical examination and investigations, for which there is no clinical indication. These are likely to *maintain* the problem in the long-term.

2. Initial assessment should include a thorough cognitive behavioural analysis so as to clarify the cognitive, behavioural, affective, and physiological factors important in aetiology. It is essential that sufficient time (1 hour or more) is allowed for assessment.

3. The problem should be formulated in cognitive behavioural terms.

4. If no positive psychological processes have been identified, reconsider the possibility of a missed physical disease. If a cognitive behavioural formulation has been achieved, then devise appropriate treatment strategies.

5. The formulation should be explained to the patient, along with treatment rationale and an outline treatment plan. The patient's full understanding of all these points must be checked, along with their willingness to engage in psychological treatment.

6. It is always necessary to provide some education to help allay the patient's concerns. This will include information on the meaning of physical symptoms and the meaning of previous medical information, examinations, and investigations.

7. Therapists with experience of cognitive therapy should try to help the patient to recognize their negative automatic thoughts about their health and to identify cognitive errors. Therapy aimed at correcting these errors should be given.

8. Behavioural guidance will be necessary to deal with avoidance, bodily checking, and reassurance seeking.

9. If patients fail to respond to treatment or refuse to engage in treatment, referral for specialist assessment and cognitive behavioural treatment is indicated. Referral is especially appropriate if:

    (1) the disorder is of long duration;

    (2) there is no decrease in the belief that they have physical disease between bouts of health anxiety;

    (3) there are numerous dysfunctional assumptions about health and also general issues;

    (4) the problems cannot be dealt with in adequate detail in the time available within the particular treatment setting.

Conclusion

The possibility of hypochondriasis as a primary diagnosis should be considered in all clinical settings — the cost of specialist treatment at an early stage of the disorder may be considerably less than repeated physical investigations or lengthy supportive treatment yielding no improvement. It is desirable that both general and child psychiatrists ensure that they have the skills and resources necessary to treat these patients effectively. Further controlled trials of the treatment of hypochondriasis are required. It will be particularly important to define the most effective components of treatment so that it is less time-consuming and, hence, more suitable for non-specialist application. Controlled trials of group treatment are particularly necessary. Future research should include patients with hypochondriasis who present to general hospital clinics and to general practice as well as those seen in specialist psychiatric settings. It may be that these patients are more convinced that they are physically ill than those who can be persuaded to see a psychiatrist and, therefore more resistant to cognitive behavioural treatment.

References

American Psychiatric Association (1987). *Diagnostic and statistical manual of mental disorders*, (3rd edn) (revised). American Psychiatric Association Washington, DC.

Barsky, A.J., Geringer, E., and Wool C.A. (1988). A cognitive-educational treatment for hypochondriasis. *General Hospital Psychiatry*, **10**, 322-7.

Barsky, A.J., Wyshak, G., and Klerman, G.L. (1992). Psychiatric co-morbidity in DSMIII-R hypochondriasis. *Archives of General Psychiatry*, **49**, 101–8.

House, A. (1989). Hypochondriacs and related disorders: assessment and management of patients referred for a psychiatric opinion. *General Hospital Psychiatry*, **11**, 156–65.

Kaplan, H.I. and Sadock, B. (1985). *Modern synopsis of the comprehensive text-book of psychiatry*, (4th edn). Wilkins & Wilkins, Baltimore.

Kellner, R. (1983). The prognosis of treated hypochondriasis: a clinical study. *Acta Psychiatrica Scandinavica*, **67**, 69–79.

Kellner, R. (1985). Functional somatic symptoms and hypochondriasis. *Archives of General Psychiatry*, **42**, 821–33.

Kellner, R. (1986). *Somatization and hypochondriasis*. Praeger, New York.

Kellner, R. (1992). The treatment of hypochondriasis: to reassure or not to reassure? *International Review of Psychiatry*, **4**, 71–5.

Kenyon, F.E. (1964). Hypochondriasis: a clinical study. *British Journal of Psychiatry*, **110**, 478–88.

Ladee, G.A. (1966). *Hypochondriacal syndromes*. Elsevier, New York.

Lesse, S. (1967). Hypochondriasis and psychiatric disorders masking depression. *American Journal of Psychotherapy*, **21**, 607–20.

Logsdail, S.J., Lovell, K., Warwick, H.M.C., and Marks, I.M. (1991). Behavioural treatment of AIDS phobia. *British Journal of Psychiatry*.

Marks, I.M. (1981). *Cure and care of neuroses*. Wiley, New York.

Pilowsky, I. (1968). The response to treatment in hypochondriacal disorders. *Australian and New Zealand Journal of Psychiatry*, **2**, 88–94.

Salkovskis, P.M. (1989). Somatic problems. In *Cognitive behaviour therapy for psychiatric problems: a practical guide*, (ed. K. Hawton, P.M. Salkovskis, J. Kirk, and D.M. Clark). Oxford University Press, Oxford.

Salkovskis, P.M. and Warwick, H.M.C. (1986). Morbid preoccupations, health anxiety and reassurance: a cognitive-behavioural approach to hypochondriasis. *Behaviour Research and Therapy*, **24**, 597–602.

Stern, R. and Fernandez, M. (1991). Group cognitive and behavioural treatment for hypochondriasis. *British Medical Journal*, **303**, 1229–331.

Warwick, H.M.C. (1992). Provision of appropriate and effective reassurance. *International Review of Psychiatry*, **4**, 76–80.

Warwick, H.M.C. and Marks, I.M. (1988). Behavioural treatment of illness phobia. *British Journal of Psychiatry*, **152**, 239–241.

Warwick, H.M.C. and Salkovskis, P.M. (1990). Hypochondriasis. *Behaviour Research and Therapy*, **28**, 105–17.

World Health Organisation (1992). *ICD 10: Classification of mental and behavioural disorders*. World Health Organization, Geneva.

10 Treatment of patients with multiple symptoms

G. Richard Smith Jr

Dr Smith begins by describing the wide range of terms that have been used to describe patients with multiple functional somatic symptoms. The high prevalence of patients with 'chronic somatization' in different medical settings is emphasized and the consequences of failing to identify and treat them is described.

The principles of treatment in this group of patients are outlined and the author's own research, which involves both individual and group treatment, is outlined. The importance of reducing the health care costs incurred by these patients is stressed. A coordinated management approach involving the primary health care team remains the mainstay of treatment, although some patients with more intractable disorders should be managed in the mental health care sector.

Introduction

This chapter addresses the treatment of patients with multiple functional somatic symptoms. The problems of definition and prevalence are presented first, followed by an overview of treatment studies. After this the author's work is described and the chapter concludes with practical guidelines for treatment.

The problem

The terms used to describe patients with multiple functional somatic symptoms can distract the reader. In this chapter the terms 'multiple functional somatic symptoms' and 'somatizer' will be used synonymously to describe this group of patients. 'Somatizer' will refer to patients with a lifetime history of four functional symptoms for men and six functional somatic symptoms for women from the list of symptoms used to diagnose somatization disorder; these definitions are derived from work carried out by Escobar *et al.* (1987) and the author's research group (Smith *et al.* 1995). It is presumed that patients satisfying these operational criteria have had the symptoms adequately evaluated by their physicians.

Patients with somatization disorder are a relatively small subset of the group of patients with multiple functional symptoms (Katon *et al.* 1991). They have a chronic relapsing psychiatric condition characterized by a lifetime history of 12 or more functional somatic complaints from the DSM-IIIR criteria list (American Psychiatric Association 1987). These symptoms are of sufficient severity to cause the patient to:

(1)   consult a physician;

(2)   take medication for the symptom;

(3)   change his or her life-style.

This condition was originally described as a type of hysteria (Purtell *et al.* 1951) and was subsequently called Briquet's syndrome (Guze 1970); it later became known as somatization disorder with the publication of DSM-III (Diagnostic and Statistical Manual, 3rd edition; American Psychiatric Association 1980). The main reason for including somatization disorder in this discussion is that most of the empirical work concerning patients with multiple functional symptoms is about patients with this condition.

Our knowledge of the prevalence of 'somatizers' in the community results primarily from the Epidemiology Catchment Area (ECA) study conducted in the USA. In this project, trained lay interviewers interviewed randomly selected community respondents using the Diagnostic Interview Schedule (DIS) (Robins *et al.* 1981). This instrument tends to under-estimate functional medical symptoms (because interviewers must accept the patient's explanation that a symptom was caused by a medical problem). Nevertheless, the results of the ECA study demonstrate strik-ingly high prevalences. Escobar *et al.* (1987) found a lifetime prevalence of 4.4 per cent from the Los Angeles site of the ECA. Recently, the find-ings on somatization from the entire ECA study were published (Swartz *et al.* 1990). Across all five ECA sites, the prevalence of patients with multiple functional somatic complaints was 11.6 per cent. As both these figures are likely to be underestimates, it is clear that there is a high prevalence of this disorder in the population.

Somatization is even more common in primary care (Katon *et al.* 1984a; Bridges and Goldberg 1985; Bridges *et al.* 1991; Chapter 21). Some primary care studies have the same limitation as community based studies, that is, the DIS was used to identify patients and as a consequence the following figures are also likely to be underestimates. Kessler *et al.* (1985) found that 4 per cent of patients in primary care had somatization disorder. Kirmayer and Robbins (1991) studied patients in two family medicine clinics in Montreal and found that 16.6 per cent of patients could be regarded as 'somatizers' (Kirmayer and Robbins 1991). A similar study was conducted by de Gruy *et al.* (1987) in a family medicine clinic in Mobile, Alabama, USA, and found a lifetime prevalence of somatization disorder of 9 per cent.

Other investigators have reported the prevalence of somatizers or somatization disorder seen by consultation services in general medical hospitals. One study by Katon *et al.* (1984*b*) found that 6 per cent of patients referred to a consultation service in a teaching hospital had somatization disorder.

Somatization is often unrecognized by clinicians and as Katon *et al.* (1982, 1986) have pointed out, misdiagnosis is a major problem. Katon and colleagues (1982) have demonstrated that many somatizers have major depression, but this is not diagnosed because they often minimize the affective and cognitive component of their disorder and emphasize the somatic manifestations. As a result treatment is prescribed for the somatic complaints rather than the underlying depressive disorder.

Even when somatization is recognized, there is frequently a discrepancy between the patient's expectations and the clinician's management. This occurs when the patient believes that the physical complaints suggest an underlying medical problem, while the clinician perceives the patient as having no physical disorder but rather a psychiatric or psychosocial problem. When this mismatch in expectations is poorly handled, both the patient and clinician become frustrated and the patient may then seek another clinician to treat his or her symptoms (see Sharpe *et al.* 1992).

An overview of treatment

There are four components of the treatment of patients who somatize. First, it is essential to make a correct diagnosis, a process which requires a number of basic interviewing skills (Craig and Boardman 1990). Second it is important to manage the chronic form of the disorder, because damage limitation may be a more realistic therapeutic goal than 'cure'. The management approaches cited in the next section are the mainstay of the clinical care of these patients. Third, the conservative management of certain psychiatric symptoms within the overall somatizing syndrome has to be addressed. Finally, it may be possible to provide specialized care in certain circumstances.

Group treatment for somatizing patients has received considerable attention over the past three decades (Mally and Ogston 1964; Schoenberg and Senescu 1966; Kass *et al.* 1972; Kimble *et al.* 1975; Ford and Long 1977; Schreter 1980; Melson *et al.* 1982; Ford 1984; Corbin *et al.* 1988). Generally, authors advocate directed, time-limited group therapy which seeks to help the patients improve their social and coping skills. While uniform in their recommendations none of these authors used an experimental design to test their interventions.

Another even more specialized modality is the in-patient care of somatizing patients. Abbey and Lipowski (1987) have described such a program which includes readmission consultation and screening, comprehensive assessment, multifactorial treatment, discharge planning and follow-up. More recently these authors published the results of in-patient treatment for chronic somatizers (Shorter *et al.* 1992).

The author's own research

Patients with somatization disorder will be used as the principal example in the description of empirical studies of effective management. Until recently it was only assumed that treatments found to be effective for somatization disorder patients would also be effective for those with less severe and chronic forms of somatization. Recent work by the author and his colleagues have confirmed this assumption (Smith *et al.* 1991; Kashner *et al.* 1991, 1992; Rost *et al.* 1994).

The first major study of the treatment of patients with somatization disorder tested the effectiveness of a standard consultation–liaison intervention (Smith *et al.* 1995). Study 1 employed a randomized controlled design of 41 patients with somatization disorder who were cared for by primary care physicians in the central Arkansas area of the USA. The intervention comprised a consultation letter sent to the physicians of each patient in the experimental group. The letter outlined a standard management approach to patients with somatization disorder. The physician was encouraged to:

(1) provide brief, regularly scheduled visits so that the patient need not develop new symptoms in order to see the physician;

(2) establish a strong patient–physician relationship in which only one physician is providing the majority of the care;

(3) perform a physical examination of the area of the body where the symptoms arise;

(4) search for signs of disease instead of relying on symptoms;

(5) understand the somatic symptom as a emotional communication rather than as a harbinger of new disease;

(6) avoid diagnostic tests and laboratory or surgical procedures unless clearly indicated by signs of disease;

(7) gradually move the patient to being 'referral ready'; that is, ready to receive care in the mental health sector.

Table 10.1 Socio-demographic characteristics of somatization disorder patients in study 2

	Experimental ($n = 40$)	Control ($n = 33$)
Female (%)	95.0	72.7
Currently married (%)	72.5	66.7
White (%)	75.0	84.8
Mean age (SD)	44.6 (8.5)	43.4 (10.0)
Mean years of education (SD)	11.5 (2.6)	12.1 (3.5)

The results of study 1, an 18 month single cross-over experiment, showed that patients did not deteriorate. Specifically, there were no changes in physical, social, or mental health, general health perceptions, or disability days. Simultaneously, however, their use of health care decreased over the 18 months, primarily as a result of a reduction in in-patient hospital days. Furthermore, the satisfaction with the medical care they received improved over time.

In study 2, the author and his colleagues (Kashner *et al.* 1992; Rost *et al.* 1994) attempted to replicate these findings with 73 patients cared for by primary care physicians, again in the central Arkansas area, USA. A similar randomized controlled trial design was used except that the intervention was for 1 year instead of 9 months. The socio-demographic characteristics of the study 2 sample are shown in Table 10.1. The same intervention was tested as described above.

The results of study 2 demonstrated a general improvement in health. In particular, physical health was improved by 18 points ($p < 0.05$) on the RAND Physical Capacities Index (range of possible scores 0–100) (Brook *et al.* 1979). No change was found in mental health, general health, social health, or disability days. As in the previous study, health care utilization and health care charges were reduced. Charges were reduced by $466 per year per patient ($p < 0.001$).

In an attempt to further improve the general health of patients with somatization disorder, the author and his colleagues (Kashner *et al.* 1991) undertook a group therapy intervention using a randomized controlled design (study 3). Somatization disorder patients from the primary care setting who had already received the intervention described above in study 2 were the subjects of study 3. Subjects randomized to the group intervention were invited to participate in a small group which met eight times every other week over the course of 4 months. Four groups comprising five subjects each were supervised by masters' level clinicians according to a structured protocol developed before the study. The goals of the group intervention were to promote peer support, to share methods of coping with physical problems, to enable patients to increase their ability to perceive and express emotion, and to enjoy the experience. Both the process and the content of the intervention were tailored to address these goals.

Each session began with a didactic presentation of the topics described below to create the atmosphere of a class and to avoid the threat that the intervention involved 'psychotherapy'. The didactic presentation was followed by a small group discussion to facilitate peer communication. Following this discussion a therapy exercise was used to increase group cohesiveness and also to develop feelings of competence and the ability to take risks. The therapeutic exercise was followed by another group discussion in which the activity itself, feelings during the activity, humour, and self-expression were emphasized. Each session closed with the presentation of a future topic, the appointment of two group members as facilitators for the following week, and a 'brag' session so that group members could make and receive positive statements about themselves.

The content of the eight sessions was as follows:

(1)　goals for the group and procedural rules;

(2)　techniques to use for coping with physical problems;

(3)　assertiveness in dealing with physicians;

(4)　ways in which patients could take more control over their own lives and increase the positive aspects of their day-to-day life;

(5)　structured problem-solving;

(6)　and (7) personal risk-taking;

(8)　helping patients to identify any positive changes they had made during the group and encouragement to continue to implement positive changes after the group ended.

There were no significant differences at baseline in socio-demographic or general health measures between those randomized to the group intervention and those not. Twenty of the 44 subjects (45.4 per cent) randomized to the group intervention participated in one or more sessions. The mean number of sessions attended by subjects randomized to the experimental group was 2.2 (SD = 2.9). Four of the 44 subjects attended one to two sessions, five attended three to four sessions, five attended five to six sessions, and six attended seven to eight sessions. All 70 subjects completed the study.

Subjects who received the group intervention reported significant improvement in general health. Compared to control patients, experimental subjects' perceptions of their physical functioning improved by 3.4 points ($p < 0.05$) on the RAND physical health index (range of possible scores 0–100) (Brook *et al.* 1979). Mental health also significantly improved during and after randomization to group therapy by 7.0 points ($p < 0.001$) on the RAND Mental Health Index (range of possible scores 0–100). As expected, physical and mental health improved even more for subjects who attended the group compared to all non-attenders. The more group sessions a subject attended the greater the improvement in general and mental health and the fewer bed days reported. The total annual health care charges of patients randomized to group therapy decreased $192 in the year during and after the intervention.

Study 4 sought to extend the intervention from somatization disorder patients to somatizers with fewer symptoms (Smith *et al.* 1995), that is, patients with a lifetime history of four (for men) or six (for women) functional somatic complaints from the DSM-IIIR list of 35 symptoms of somatization disorder. We used the same study design as in study 2 namely, a 2-year randomized controlled crossover design involving 56 patients who met criteria for somatization but not somatization disorder. All patients were recruited from physicians in the primary care setting. The intervention was the same as employed in study 2 and concentrated on specific management recommendations identical to those described for patients with somatization disorder. After 1 year the control group was crossed over to the treatment condition by sending the consultation letter with the treatment recommendations to the primary care physician.

The results of study 4 confirmed that the intervention which was successful with somatization disorder patients was also successful with somatizers. After the intervention, patients reported significant improvements in physical functioning, which remained stable during the year following the intervention. The intervention had no effect on emotional health, general health, or social functioning. Patients reported 0.8 fewer bed days per month after the intervention, although this difference was not statistically significant.

During the year after the intervention, annual medical care charges decreased by $289 (32.9 per cent). This reduction in charges remained stable during the year following the intervention and resulted from fewer hospital days. During the year following baseline treatment patients averaged 3.0 hospital days compared to control/crossover patients who averaged 3.6 hospital days. For the same period both groups averaged 2.3 emergency room visits and 11.3 physician visits.

Table 10.2 Practical guidelines for treatment of patients with multiple functional complaints

---

1. The physician should attempt to become the patient's main and if possible only physician
2. Set up regularly scheduled out-patient visits at relatively frequent intervals (every 4–6 weeks)
3. Conduct brief out-patient visits
4. Perform a partial physical examination of the organ system of which the patient has complaints
5. Understand the new symptom as an emotional communication rather than as the harbinger of a new disease
6. Look for signs of disease instead of symptoms
7. Avoid tests and procedures unless indicated by signs of disease

---

Practical guidelines

As a result of studies carried out by the author and others we can now make practical recommendations for the treatment of patients with multiple functional symptoms. These recommendations have been demonstrated to be both effective in improving the health of patients with somatization disorder and in achieving a prudent use of health care resources. The management of patients with multiple functional complaints should include the components listed in Table 10.2.

The recommendation for a physical examination contrasts with procedures described by Warwick (see Chapter 9). This contradiction is understandable since she studied patients with hypochondriasis (a different patient population with different treatment needs). Other important considerations include understanding the symptom as an emotional communication rather than as a sign of new disease, looking for signs of disease instead of being symptom focused, and avoiding diagnostic tests, laboratory evaluation, and operative procedures unless clearly indicated. Finally, although this was not tested in the studies, a goal of primary care management should be to prepare selected patients for referral to the mental health sector, that is, help them to become 'referral ready'.

The cornerstone of successful management of patients with multiple functional symptoms is the establishment of a trusting relationship with a single physician: this person should become the main, if not the only, physician that the patient sees. The constant 'doctor hopping' that frequently occurs in these patients is countertherapeutic. In the author's experience this is more likely to occur when both patient and physician are frustrated with the unsuccessful management of the condition. These patients do very poorly without a coordinated management approach. While it may be possible to provide coordinated management if several physicians are involved, it is much more cumbersome and involves more work for the primary care physician than if he/she alone manages the patient.

Regularly scheduled visits are very important, especially in the first year of managing a new patient or in the period following an exacerbation. In an effort to conserve health care resources (and possibly to avoid seeing difficult patients), physicians inadvertently contribute to their own management problems by telling the patient 'Nothing is wrong; come back and see me only if you need to'. The resulting patient-initiated visits create a situation in which the patient must develop a new symptom in order to see the physician. Since a visit to the physician is of great importance to the patient, the physician who attempts management on an as-needed basis is likely to create many more problems than if a *proactive* approach is adopted, that is, regular, scheduled visits. Conversely, the physician can capitalize on the patient's desire to see them to expedite his or her management strategy.

The optimal interval between visits is unknown. The interval recommended by the studies published to date is every 4–6 weeks and in my clinical experience this seems to be appropriate. Once a patient has established a pattern of regular visits he or she may then look forward to the next consultation and will (hopefully) contain any new complaints until that appointment. When establishing a new patient–physician relationship, either during relapse or during periods of psychosocial distress, 4–6 weeks is too long an interval and the interval needs to be shortened so that the patient does not initiate extra visits or go to the emergency room. It is on these patient-initiated visits that the patient usually presents new symptoms. New symptoms require more diagnostic effort and more of the physician's time. During these periods of new symptoms intervals of 1 or 2 weeks may be required in order for the patient to feel more secure and to stop the patient-initiated consultations. However, once the patient-initiated visits cease, the primary care physician should not lengthen the interval for at least several weeks or possibly months. During the first year of management, it is generally not wise to lengthen the interval beyond 6 weeks, unless, of course, the patient suggests it.

When the patient presents with a new symptom, it is important to physically examine at least the organ system(s) relevant to the complaint(s). This examination serves two purposes:

(1) it reassures the physician that there are no signs of organic disease;

(2) patients receive comfort from the examination, which resembles the symbolic gesture of 'laying on of hands'.

After eliciting a brief history of the symptom and carrying out a physical examination of the appropriate part of the body, the physician should reassure the patient that there is no serious physical disease. Furthermore, the physician should convey the impression that he/she is interested in both the patient and the symptom and wants to follow the patient closely to ensure that the symptom resolves. This reassures the patient that the physician will provide ongoing care. It is important for the physician to communicate concern for the patient and the symptom. It is also important to avoid any suggestion that the symptom does not exist or that it is not substantial. Rather, the physician should acknowledge that the patient 'hurts'. Indeed, it is helpful if the physician understands a new symptom as an emotional communication that says 'I hurt' or 'I am in distress'.

Avoiding diagnostic procedures, laboratory tests, and surgical procedures unless clearly indicated serves three purposes:

(1)   it contains health care utilization;

(2)   it decreases the exposure to iatrogenic complications;

(3)   it decreases false-positive laboratory tests.

Finally, it is beneficial for most of these patients to enter the mental health care sector. Regrettably, for somatizing patients this is much easier said than done: a willingness on the patient's part usually only develops from a long-term patient–physician relationship. The primary care physician should first empathize with the patient's distress; this may be followed by the suggestion that the patient would benefit from someone (from the mental health sector) providing more time for support.

In the author's experience the above strategy is effective in a substantial number of somatizing patients, but it should not be attempted before the physician–patient relationship is well established. Furthermore, it is very important for the patient not to perceive the primary care physician as abandoning him or her; rather, the physician will continue to be available as before. This is similar to the model of 'shared care' described by Bass and Murphy (1991). If the patient accepts psychiatric treatment, then long-term supportive psychotherapy is probably necessary in most cases if any improvement is to be maintained. Successful engagement depends not only on the patient, but also on the therapist's understanding of the patient's beliefs, fears, and experiences. Treatment and engagement should preferably only be undertaken by someone interested in such patients as the job is time-consuming and demands patience, therapeutic skill, and flexibility (see Murphy (1993) for a more detailed description of the skills involved). Psychiatrists working in liaison services are probably best suited to the work.

Summary

There is a high prevalence of patients with multiple functional symptoms in primary care settings. Numerous authors have recommended similar treatment approaches for these difficult patients. Relatively recent work using systematic interventions has demonstrated that these are effective in improving the health of somatizing patients and lead to significant reductions in the use of health care resources.

References

Abbey, S.E. and Lipowski, N.J. (1987). Comprehensive management of persistent somatization: an innovative inpatient program. *Psychotherapy and Psychosomatics*, **48**, 110-7.

American Psychiatric Association (1980). *DSM-III (diagnostic and statistical manual of mental disorders)*. American Psychiatric Association, Washington DC.

American Psychiatric Association (1987). *DSM-III-R (diagnostic and statistical manual of mental disorders*, 3rd edn, revised). American Psychiatric Association, Washington DC.

Bass, C. and Murphy, M. (1991). Somatisation disorder in a British teaching hospital. *British Journal of Clinical Practice*, **45**, 237-44.

Bridges, K.W. and Goldberg, D.P. (1985). Somatic presentation of DSM III psychiatric disorders in primary care. *Journal of Psychosomatic Research*, **29**, 563-569.

Bridges, K., Goldberg, D., Evans, B., and Sharpe, T. (1991). Determinants of somatization in primary care. *Psychological Medicine*, **21**, 473-83.

Brook, R.H., Ware, J.E., Jr, Davies-Avery, A., Stewart, A.L., Donald, C.A., Rogers, W.H. *et al.* (1979). *Conceptualization and measurement of health for adults in the health insurance study:* Volume VII *Overview*. Rand Corporation, Santa Monica.

Corbin, L.J., Hanson, R.W., Hopp, S.A., and Whitley, A. (1988). Somatoform disorders: how to reduce overutilization of health care services. *Journal of Psychosocial Nursing and Mental Health Services*, **26**, 31.

Craig, T.J.K. and Boardman, A.P. (1990). Somatization in primary care settings. In *Somatization: physical symptoms and psychological illness* (ed. C. Bass) pp. 73-103. Blackwells, Oxford.

degruy, F., Columbia, L., and Dickinson, P. (1987). Somatization disorder in a family practice. *Journal of Family Practice*, **25**, 45-51.

Escobar, J.I., Burnham, A., Karno, M., Forsythe, A., and Golding, J.M. (1987). Somatization in the community. *Archives of General Psychiatry*, **44**, 713.

Ford, C.V. (1984). Somatizing disorders. In *Helping patients and their families cope with medical problems*, (ed. H.B. Roback), p. 39. Jossey-Bass Publishers, San Francisco.

Ford, C.V. and Long, K.D. (1977). Group psychotherapy of somatizing patients. *Psychotherapy and Psychosomatics*, **28**, 294-304.

Guze, S.B. (1970). The role of follow-up studies: their contribution to diagnostic classification as applied to hysteria. *Seminars in Psychiatry*, **2**, 392.

Kashner, T.M., Rost, K., Cohen, B., Anderson, M., and Smith, G.R. (1995). Enhancing the health of somatization disorder patients: the cost effectiveness of short term group therapy. *Psychosomatics*. In press.

Kashner, T.M., Rost, K., Smith, G.R., and Lewis, S. (1992). An analysis of panel data: the impact of a psychiatric consultation letter on the expenditures and outcomes of care for patients with somatization disorder. *Medical Care*, **30**, 811-21.

Kass, D.J., Silvers, F.M., and Abroms, G.M. (1972). Behavioral group treatment of hysteria. *Archives of General Psychiatry*, **26**, 42.

Katon, W., Kleinman, A., and Rosen, G. (1982). Depression and somatization: a review. *American Journal of Medicine*, **72**, 127.

Katon, W., Ries, R.K., and Kleinman, A. (1984*a*). The prevalence of somatization in primary care. *Comprehensive Psychiatry*, **25**, 208.

Katon, W., Ries, R.K., and Kleinman, A. (1984*b*). Part II: a prospective DSM-III study of 100 consecutive somatization patients. *Comprehensive Psychiatry*, **25**, 305.

Katon, W., Berg, A.O., Robins, A.J., and Risse, S. (1986). Depression: medical utilization and somatization. *Western Journal of Medicine*, **144**, 564.

Katon, W., Lin, E., Von Korff, M., Russo, J., Lipscomb, P., and Bush, T. (1991). Somatization: a spectrum of severity. *American Journal of Psychiatry*, **148**, 34.

Kessler, L.G., Cleary, P.D. and Burke, J.D., Jr (1985). Psychiatric disorders in primary care. *Archives of General Psychiatry*, **42**, 583.

Kimble, R., Williams, J.G., and Agras, S. (1975). A comparison of two methods of diagnosing hysteria. *American Journal of Psychiatry*, **132**, 1197.

Kirmayer, L.J. and Robbins, J.M. (1991). Three forms of somatization in primary care: prevalence, co-occurrence and sociodemographic characteristics. *Journal of Nervous and Mental Disorders*, **179**, 647.

Mally, M.A. and Ogston, W.D. (1964). Treatment of the 'untreatables'. *International Journal of Group Psychotherapy*, **14**, 369.

Melson, S.J., Rynearson, E.K., Dortzbach, J., Clark, R.D., and Snyder, A.L. (1982). Short-term intensive group psychotherapy for patients with functional complaints. *Psychosomatics*, **23**, 689.

Murphy, M. (1993). The psychological management of somatisation disorder. In *Psychological treatment in disease and illness*, (ed. M. Hodes and S. Moorey), pp. 65-87. Gaskell and The Society for Psychosomatic Research, London.

Purtell, J.J., Robins, E., and Cohen, M.E. (1951). Observations on clinical aspects of hysteria — a quantitative study of 50 hysteria patients and 156 control subjects. *Journal of the American Medical Association*, **146**, 902.

Robins, L.N., Helzer, J.E., Croughan, J. and Ratcliff, K.S. (1981). National Institute of Mental Health Diagnostic Interview Schedule: History, characteristics, and validity. *Arch. Gen. Psychiatry*, **38**, 381.

Rost, K., Kashner, T.M. and Smith, G.R., Jr (1994). Effectiveness of psychiatric intervention with somatization disorder patients: improved outcomes at reduced costs. *General Hospital Psychiatry* (in press).

Schoenberg, B. and Senescu, R. (1966). Group psychotherapy for patients with chronic multiple somatic complaints. *Journal of Chronic Diseases*, 19, 649.

Schreter, R.K. (1980). Treating the untreatables: a group experience with somaticizing borderline patients. *International Journal of Psychiatry and Medicine*, 10, 205.

Sharpe, M., Peveler, R., and Mayou, R.A. (1992). Treatment of functional somatic symptoms. *Journal of Psychosomatic Research*, 36, 515–29.

Smith, G.R., Jr, Monson, R.A., and Ray, D.C. (1986a). Psychiatric consultation in somatization disorder: a randomized, controlled study. *New England Journal of Medicine*, 314, 1407–13.

Smith, G.R., Kashner, T.M., and Rost, K. (1995). A trial of the effect of a standardized psychiatric consultation on health outcomes and costs in somatizing patients. *Archives of General Psychiatry*. In press.

Swartz, M., Landerman, R., George, L., Blazer, D., and Escobar, J. (1990). Somatization disorder. In *Psychiatric disorders in America*, (ed. L.N. Robins and D. Regier). Free Press, New York. pp. 220–55.

Shorter, E., Abbey, S.E., Gillies, L.A., Singh, M., and Lipowski, Z.J. (1992). Inpatient treatment of persistent somatization. *Psychosomatics*, 33, 295–301.

11 Psychiatric and psychological approaches to the treatment of chronic pain: concepts and individual treatments

Sidney Benjamin and Chris J. Main

In the first of two chapters, Dr Benjamin and Dr Main offer observations concerning the treatment of patients with chronic pain, which are relevant to the treatment of the other syndromes described in this book.

Patients with chronic pain (especially those attending pain clinics) may be regarded as having both physical and psychiatric disorder and successful treatment depends on understanding and treating both. Psychological treatment requires the identification of any specific and treatable mental disorder together with behavioural assessment of the ways in which pain and associated disability may be modified. The latter includes a full assessment of the role of care givers.

The authors review the principal forms of psychological treatment and conclude that there is no clear evidence for the superiority of any one type of intervention. It is also evident that many chronic pain patients are not able to benefit from psychological treatment, either because it is not available or because the patients are unsuitable or are unwilling to accept it. Since these patients are liable to be the most severely distressed and disabled and to make the greatest use of health services for their care, this failure of care constitutes a major clinical problem.

Introduction

This chapter reviews concepts underlying the psychological and psychiatric management of patients with chronic pain and discusses the clinical efficacy of recent developments in treatment. It is concerned with general principles underlying chronic pain management, rather than issues specific to particular regional pain syndromes. In the next chapter we examine the evidence for the value of the interdisciplinary management of chronic pain, consider issues of health care delivery and prevention, and make recommendations for the future directions of chronic pain management. The psychological aspects of treatment of acute pain and pain associated with specific organic disorders, such as malignant disease, are not covered.

Most of the chapters in this book focus on individual pain syndromes and their treatment. This reductionist approach has been an important step in the development of our knowledge of the causes and treatments of chronic pain and functional somatic syndromes but also has limitations.

We may lose sight of the extent to which different symptoms and syndromes occur in the same people at the same or different times (when their significance may be quite different from that of isolated syndromes), have shared causes, or respond to the same treatments (see Chapter 4). Furthermore, although specific types of treatment approaches are described, they are, in practice, not usually administered in isolation, even in research studies, making it difficult to evaluate their individual efficacy.

A further fundamental issue in the management of pain or other functional somatic symptoms is that they are commonly but inappropriately viewed as arising from *either* physical *or* mental causes. Whilst it is implicit in the definition of a 'functional' symptom that there was no adequate 'organic' explanation, the concept is often applied in an excessively simplistic manner (Kirmayer and Robbins 1991), ignoring the frequent co-occurrence of physical and psychosocial problems (Benjamin *et al.* 1988). Similarly, it is often assumed that treatments are *either* physical *or* psychosocial. In reality, a physical treatment may act on the mental state (for example an antidepressant may result in cognitive changes), whilst psychological approaches (for example, an operant behavioural programme or cognitive therapy) may have physical effects such as increased exercise or changes in autonomic function. Psychological strategies are often valuable regardless of whether there is a mental or physical illness (or both). This observation may help to make them acceptable to patients who are reluctant to acknowledge a diagnosis of mental illness.

The problem

The nature of pain mechanisms

Most medical approaches to treatment are based on ancient assumptions about the nature of pain (Bonica 1990). The early views of the Greek philosophers were not seriously challenged until the seventeenth century when Descartes (1664) and others proposed that nerves were tubes which connect the periphery of the body to the brain, a theory that has remained influential in perpetuating the belief in a close relationship between a peripheral noxious stimuli and the severity of the pain sensation. In recent years this simple model has been superseded by the Gate Control Theory (Melzack and Wall 1965, 1982) which incorporates evidence about physiological specialization, central summation, patterning, modulation of input, and the influence of psychological factors. Central to the theory is the concept of a 'gate' in the dorsal horn of the spinal cord where the effects of afferent nerve impulses can be modified by excitatory and inhibitory pathways descending from the brain stem. The gate theory is consistent with Beecher's (1959) observations that pain perception is only loosely related to underlying noxious sensory stimuli or physiological dysfunction.

More recent developments in theories of pain have included the concepts of dimensions of sensory input, motivation and emotion, conceptual evaluation, and the socio-cultural environment (Chapman 1977). Thus, peripheral and/or central nervous system disorder, if present, is likely to be only one of the factors contributing to the experience of pain and its consequences. This fact must be taken into account if treatment is to be successful. However, the current medical management as described in the next section clearly indicates that treatment is still steadfastly bound to an unsatisfactory seventeenth-century Cartesian model of pain.

Limitations of physical treatments

Pain is a symptom not a disease. Despite the wide range of investigations to which some patients are subjected, there is considerable difficulty in arriving at a diagnosis. The frustration caused by differing and often seemingly incompatible diagnoses and ineffective treatments only adds to the distress of inadequately relieved pain and associated disability. We discuss this problem further in the next chapter.

The traditional medical response to pain is to treat underlying organic pathology or to provide symptomatic relief or palliative care, using centrally or locally acting analgesia. Frequently the efficacy of this approach is limited, even when there is evidence of organic pathology. There is considerable doubt about the value of many of the physical procedures that are available. For example, facet joint injection and facet nerve block are fashionable and common procedures for the relief of back pain. A recent comparison of these two (Marks *et al.* 1992) demonstrated that two-thirds of patients experienced little or no improvement immediately after infiltration and only approximately one-fifth had any worthwhile improvement after 3 months. Although this study did not include a control procedure, the outcome is no better than that commonly resulting from placebos. There was little difference in the effects of the two treatments for these conditions.

The clinical problem is further illustrated by a survey of 181 UK consultants in neurology, anaesthetics, oncology, and surgical specialties who were all experienced in the treatment of 'chronic nerve-damage pain' (Davies *et al.* 1991). They were asked to rate the value of 16 different specific treatments (including surgery, nerve blocks, medication, and 'other treatments' — the latter including psychological approaches). Many consultants were unwilling to offer an opinion about the value of commonly used treatments, and, of those who did, the majority rated each treatment as having a 'poor' or 'limited' effect. The main finding was the gross divergence of views about the value of every treatment, even amongst consultants in the same specialty and this was not related to their levels of experience. Although there may be disagreement about the meanings of the results of these two studies, they do indicate serious limitations in the value of current physical treatments and services and in the confidence of those who provide them. It is unlikely that similar research on the opinions of psychiatrists and clinical psychologists would demonstrate a more consistent view of the efficacy of psychological treatments.

Not only may physical treatments be ineffective in some patients or some conditions, but they may also have unwanted effects. Psychological and physical dependence, particularly on analgesics and sedatives, are often a major secondary problem requiring treatment in their own right. This is particularly likely in 'chronic benign pain'. Patients expect to have their pain cured and pursue multiple ineffective referrals, physical assessments, and treatments which may be invasive and damaging. They are often disappointed and become angry with their doctors (Loeser *et al.* 1990). The latter feel they have to offer something and administer ineffectual physical treatments because they feel familiar with them. Management is expensive and may be of very little value.

General issues in treatment

Indications for psychological and psychiatric intervention

Psychiatrists and clinical psychologists have presented a profusion of models of chronic pain, often accompanied by related treatments and sometimes with extravagant claims backed by limited evidence of efficacy. It has been unhelpful to view chronic pain globally, primarily as a psychiatric disorder involving 'masked depression' (Blumer and Heilbronn 1982), or to apply DSM-III-derived psychiatric 'diagnoses' such as 'adjustment reaction' and 'psychological reaction to physical condition' (for example, Fishbain *et al.* 1986). Conversely, failure to diagnose and treat major depressive disorders that have been reported to occur in up to 45 per cent of chronic back pain patients and the assumption that distress is invariably the effect of pain, have sometimes been a serious impediment to effective treatment (Sullivan *et al.* 1992).

These problems have been enhanced by the narrow training and rigid agendas of the various health professions and specialties. There is no evidence that any simple model adequately accounts for the complexity of interactions found in many settings or leads to effective treatment for the majority of patients. The current range of models and treatments requires an empirical appraisal of their value, based on appropriate assessments of the characteristics of patients, disorders, treatments, and outcomes. Psychological approaches should be based on two separate but related issues.

1. Is there a mental illness associated with chronic pain? Mental illnesses should be diagnosed only on the basis of positive findings and not simply because organic pathology has not been identified. To what sort of treatment is the mental illness likely to respond and is the pain also likely to improve with that treatment?

2. Can the pain (or pain behaviours), whatever the cause, be modified using psychological techniques?

These two issues are often related but they are not equivalent. Most accounts of the treatment of chronic pain fail to offer a perspective in which these fundamental issues are either recognized or acknowledged. These approaches to treatment are summarized in Table 11.1.

Table 11.1 Summary of psychiatric and psychological treatments

---

Treatment for diagnosed mental disorders associated with pain

1. Depressive disorders
      Antidepressants
      Management of psychosocial problems
      Cognitive therapy
2. Somatoform disorders
      Containment, in general medical settings
      Behavioural, cognitive, or psychodynamic psychotherapy in specialist settings
3. Substance abuse
      Detoxification for alcohol and drug dependence
      Avoidance of inappropriate prescribing
      Time contingent analgesia

Psychological approaches to treatment of chronic pain

1. Psychodynamic psychotherapy
2. Behaviour therapy
3. Cognitive therapy
4. Psychophysiological treatments
5. Exercise
6. Multidisciplinary treatment programmes

The diagnosis and treatment of mental disorders in patients with chronic pain

Surveys of patients with chronic pain show that mental disorders occur in between 5 and 95 per cent, depending on setting, sample selection, and the range of diagnoses that are included. Frequently these disorders are not identified, not treated, or are treated inadequately (Benjamin and Barnes 1984; Sullivan *et al*. 1992; Benjamin and Bridges, 1994). One reason is that most doctors who specialize in treating chronic pain have little experience of diagnosing or treating psychiatric illness and most psychiatrists have no training in pain management. It is still relatively uncommon for psychiatrists to be directly involved in multi-specialty pain clinics, or to collaborate with physicians in joint clinics. A second reason is that patients and often their doctors assume that mood changes and mental disorders are invariably *caused* by the pain and therefore that only physical treatment of the pain will result in resolution of the pain and an improved mood. The chronicity of pain, despite multiple physical inter-ventions, demonstrates that this view is frequently unrealistic. Cartesian dualism leads to the belief that patients have either a physical or mental disorder, rarely both. In fact mental and physical disorders are particularly likely to be found *together* in the same chronic pain patients (Benjamin *et al*. 1988). Failure to recognize this fact is a further reason why these disorders tend to be unidentified and untreated by pain clinic staff. Psychiatric case identification can be improved using screening instru-ments for mental disorders generally (Benjamin *et al*. 1991*a*) or for mood disorders specifically (Turner and Romano, 1984). This simple and poten-tially cost-effective approach is not often used however, and its contribu-tion to pain management has not been adequately evaluated. The prevalence of specific psychiatric disorders varies considerably according to treatment settings (Benjamin *et al*. 1988; Benjamin 1989; Atkinson *et al*. 1991; Benjamin and Bridges 1994). The commonest diagnoses are affective disorders (depressive disorders are commoner than anxiety disorders in most studies of chronic pain), somatoform disorders, substance abuse, and personality disorders.

Depressive disorders In patients with pain, depressive disorders are diagnosed according to standard criteria, including consistently depressed mood, depressive cognitions and neuro-vegetative symptoms. Problems in diagnosis arise because depressed mood may be less evident than anger and irritability and because depressed mood and other symptoms (for example, sleep and appetite disturbance) may be attributed by patients and physi-cians to the pain or to the effect of (real or imaginary) underlying physical pathology. Thus, the diagnosis of depressive disorders in patients with chronic pain calls for special experience and skill (Sullivan *et al*. 1992).

Ideally, treatment should integrate psychosocial and biological appro-aches. Antidepressants are often effective but treatment adherence may be a problem, particularly because of unwanted effects which may create special difficulty in patients who are hypersensitive to somatic sensations. For some patients, acceptance of treatment may be difficult because of the potential gains derived from somatization. Although some patients will readily explore contributory psychosocial factors, others are more resistant (Bass and Benjamin 1993).

Sullivan *et al.* (1992) recently noted that the treatment of depression in patients with chronic low back pain has usually been aimed at pain rather than depression. The presence of depression may adversely affect the response to rehabilitation programmes and, as will be seen from recent research reports described below, this often leads to the exclusion of depressed patients from treatment programmes from which they might benefit. Where they are not excluded, they may be treated inappropriately: recent reports note that depressed chronic pain patients are more likely to be treated with narcotics than with antidepressants (Doan and Wadden 1989) and are less likely to receive antidepressants than chronic pain patients who are not depressed (Haythornthwaite *et al.* 1991). Those given antidepressants are likely to be given inadequate doses and therefore fail to benefit (Katon *et al.* 1985). However, there is some evidence that both antidepressant medication and cognitive therapy result in substantial improvement in depression and in pain, that these two treatments may be equally effective, and that they are as effective in depressed patients with pain as in depressed patients without pain (Onghena and van Houdenhove 1992; Sullivan *et al.* 1992).

Somatoform disorders   Chronic pain is often a presenting complaint in hypochondriasis and somatization disorder and is the central feature in somatoform pain disorder. Problems in diagnosis arise (see Chapter 3) because of the changing nomenclature and criteria used in different diagnostic systems (DSM-IIIR, DSM-IV, ICD-9, ICD-10) and also because of uncertainty regarding whether they are valid discrete disorders or part of a spectrum of inappropriate illness behaviour with somatic presentations. Further problems result from the failure to differentiate the *syndrome* diagnoses of somatoform disorder from the *process* of somatization (the latter can be found in association with any psychiatric diagnosis) (Bass and Benjamin 1993). Clinically, difficulties arise due to inappropriate diagnosis and treatment of non-existent depressive disorders, inappropriate focus on management of non-existent or trivial physical pathology (Bass and Benjamin 1993), and psychiatrists' limited experience of this group of disorders.

Somatoform disorders are generally regarded as having a poor prognosis. It is often difficult to engage the patient in treatment. There is little evidence that physical treatments are effective but there have been claims about the value of a range of psychological approaches (see Chapter 10). These usually include supportive containment in primary medical practice or behavioural or cognitive and, occasionally, dynamic psychotherapy in more specialized settings. Such strategies should not be assumed to have the same effect as when applied to other types of chronic pain patients included in the evaluations of treatment described below. The management of chronic somatization (Bass and Benjamin 1993; Benjamin and Bridges 1994) and somatization disorder (Smith 1991) are reviewed in Chapter 10.

Other mental disorders Alcohol dependence sometimes results from self-medication to reduce pain, although it has also been noted that alcohol abuse may pre-date pain onset by many years (Atkinson *et al.* 1991) and may contribute to it. Drug dependence, mainly with narcotics or ben-zodiazepines, results from self-medication or may be iatrogenic. Detox-ification will usually be a necessary early component of the treatment plan.

No psychiatric disorder Even when psychiatrists with a particular interest in pain and somatization find no evidence of a diagnosable mental illness, there may still be evidence that psychological factors have contributed to aetiology. Some patients have particular difficulty adjusting to a painful physical disorder, and sometimes the degree of disability is greater than would usually be expected. Such problems may be a major focus in the work of liaison psychiatrists; regardless of the use of psychiatric diagnoses, an understanding of the relevant psychosocial mechanisms and physiological processes, for example the effects of inactivity (Sharpe and Bass 1992), is an essential prerequisite for appropriate assessment and treatment.

The effects of care givers on pain and treatment

Family members and other care givers have been reported to have pro-found effects on both the origins of pain, its course, and the response to treatment (Turk *et al.* 1987; Roy 1988) but relevant research findings are few. There is a close relationship between pain, the patient's satisfaction with relationships, the severity of pain behaviour, and poor adherence and response to psychological treatment (Funch and Gale 1985; Flor *et al.* 1986; Gil *et al.* 1987). Findings tend to be consistent with an operant condi-tioning model whereby solicitous family members may reinforce patients' pain perceptions and behaviours. There is so far little evidence that family support facilitates improvement. Some pain treatment programmes have emphasized the importance of involving the care givers as therapists and, where necessary, training them to reinforce desirable rather than undesir-able behaviours. Others have claimed that chronic pain becomes a family problem which can best be resolved through family therapy based on a range of models including systems theory (Roy 1988).

Empirical research on the beliefs and behaviours of care givers is scanty.

To respond appropriately, family members require information about the nature and causes of pain, the extent to which physical treatments are likely to be effective, the potential for psychological approaches and their own contribution to them. In fact they are rarely provided with such information and it is therefore not surprising that they are either overwhelmed by uncertainty or have strongly held inappropriate beliefs (Rowat and Knafl 1985; Benjamin *et al.* 1991*b*). Care givers accompanying chronic pain patients to a pain clinic have been shown to cling to the belief that pain is caused by a disease which will be discovered by more investigations and will be cured by physical treatments, despite past failure to do so. Those care givers who have positive views about psychological contributions and rehabilitation have had no opportunity to influence management (Benjamin *et al.* 1991*b*).

The concept of 'tertiary gain' has been used to describe unconscious benefits that family members and others may derive through the role of care giver (Hughes *et al.* 1987). At times the reciprocal needs of patient and carer may cement an otherwise unviable relationship. Such mechanisms may contribute to the reluctance of some carers to allow pain patients to enter or remain in psychological treatment. When patients do improve, occasionally carers become seriously depressed and additional management may have to be directed to the carer's needs. These important interpersonal issues have received little systematic investigation.

Psychological treatments of chronic pain

Psychodynamic psychotherapy

Psychodynamic models have emphasized the use of pain as a *defence mechanism*, features of which may include somatization, dissociation, and introjection. Thus, pain can serve to protect the patient from conscious awareness of underlying conflicts (primary gain) as well as offering more direct benefit due to changes in the behaviours of others (secondary gain). Observations of severe depression following relief from chronic pain supports such views (Penman 1954). Engel (1959) particularly noted the contribution of experiences of loss, aggression, guilt, and atonement to the psychopathology of the 'pain prone patient' and recently these findings have received experimental support (Adler *et al.* 1989). Childhood experiences of deprivation, abuse, and unusual or excessive illness models are a precursor of inappropriate illness behaviour in later life (Benjamin and Eminson 1992). Suppressed reactions to such experiences can persist and find expression through the process of transference, a central focus of modern psychodynamic psychotherapy. Thus the overwhelming and seemingly inappropriate dependence on and hostility to doctors which characterize some chronic pain patients may be more than an understandable reaction to inept management. The continuing controversy concerning the extent to which such factors are relevant to the causation or persistence of chronic pain and to its treatment is partly due to differences in characteristics of patients seen in different settings, as well as the training and predilections of therapists.

The role of psychotherapy in chronic pain treatment has recently been reviewed (Tunks and Merskey 1990). There are remarkably few published studies on the effects of psychodynamic psychotherapy in the treatment of chronic pain. Whilst psychoanalytic experience may be helpful in understanding the process of pain development in some patients, there has been a widely held view that patients with chronic pain are unusually difficult to engage in treatment (Pilowsky 1986). Comparison of psychodynamic treatment with brief supportive treatment has shown that the former was not superior on any outcome measure apart from subjective reports of 'coping better' (Bassett and Pilowsky 1985). A more recent report (Pilowsky and Barrow 1990) compared brief psychotherapy with the effects of amitriptyline in patients with chronic intractable 'psychogenic' pain and found that the former resulted in increased pain intensity but improved productivity, whilst the latter was more effective in reducing pain and increasing activity. The increased pain following brief psychotherapy is consistent with psychodynamic theories described above. There is also recent evidence for more profound effects of brief, focused psychothcrapy in patients with abdominal pain arising from irritable bowel syndrome (Svedlund 1983; Chapter 8).

Behavioural approaches

As pain becomes more chronic, external factors are likely to exert an increasing influence. Behavioural medicine offers an alternate conceptualization to that of the disease model in which the report of pain is seen not only as evidence of an underlying disease or injury but as a problem worthy of assessment and management *in its own right*. The two principal processes suggested by learning theory are classical and operant conditioning (Fordyce *et al.* 1973).

According to the *classical conditioning model*, pain may arise as a conditioned response. For example, pain may be initiated by an injury (that is, as an unconditioned response) but is experienced in conjunction with a conditioned stimulus, such as anxiety, which was originally experienced at the time of the injury. Subsequently, pain is experienced in association with anxiety in other contexts. In *operant conditioning*, pain behaviours are understood in terms of their reinforcing consequences (or anticipated consequences). For example, powerful social consequences, such as the caring responses of a solicitous spouse, may become the key to understanding the persistence of a chronic maladaptive pain behaviour syndrome. In practice, both classical and operant conditioning seem to contribute. Fordyce (1985) recognized that pain perception and associated behaviours are often attenuated by environmental events which were regarded as positive or negative reinforcers, in accordance with operant conditioning principles. This applies regardless of whether or not any physical pathology or psychological factors have been identified as having initiated the pain. Thus, all pain can be divided into 'operant' or 'non-operant' pain and the former can be modified by a process of operant conditioning. Patients and their carers are often unaware of the fluctuations in pain, the circumstances in which these occur and the contribution made by carers (Rowat and Knafl 1985) but they may be identified by behavioural analysis. Pain diaries (Fordyce 1990) are now commonly used in the assessment of pain and associated environmental factors, although such self-report measures have a number of limitations (Chapman and Syrjala 1990). Behavioural techniques are usually incorporated to some extent into all pain programmes and are also used in work with individual patients. The treatment paradigm is similar to that of other applications of behaviour therapy. Following the behavioural assessment, specific goals for treatment will be agreed with the patient to help to develop or reintroduce desirable behaviours and diminish or eliminate undesirable ones. For example, goals might include increasing mobility (walking to the library or the shops daily) and social activities (visits to the social club twice weekly), using systematic stress control procedures, and decreasing unhelpful medication and the avoidance of further consultations. A phased programme involving a series of intermediate targets may be worked out and contingency management (Fordyce 1990) used. This may involve changing the way that family members respond to the patient or, in an in-patient environment, involve specially trained staff in selectively responding with positive (usually social) reinforcement of desirable behaviours and negative reinforcement (usually avoiding responses) of undesirable behaviours. The effects of behavioural treatment on acute back pain were demonstrated by the superiority of treatment (medication and exercise) given on a time-contingent basis compared with similar treatment which was dependent on the patient's pain ('pain contingent') (Fordyce *et al.* 1986). Linton (1986) has reviewed the efficacy of behavioural management and concluded that there is considerable evidence for the value of operant techniques in increasing activity levels and decreasing use of medication. Evidence for reduction in other inappropriate pain behaviours or actual pain levels is weaker. However, there is considerable difficulty in identifying the specific effects of behavioural techniques, even in behavioural programmes, because of the many other influences on outcome.

Early behavioural programmes (for example, Fordyce *et al.* 1973) placed particular emphasis on creating an environment, usually hospital based, which facilitated maximal behavioural change. Improvement was therefore highly dependent on the environment and frequently generalization to other non-hospital settings did not occur. Changing the home environment was more difficult to achieve and sustain, so that initial behavioural changes were followed by relapse and poor long-term outcome. Behavioural techniques are now commonly integrated into more comprehensive psychological programmes which include aspects of cognitive therapy.

Cognitive therapy

Cognitive therapy is directed specifically at conscious thoughts: beliefs about the ability to control symptoms, expectations about treatment, and the coping strategies used to try to reduce the impact of stressors. Measures of pain locus of control (Crisson and Keefe 1988; Toomey *et al.* 1988; C. Main, P.L.R. Wood, C.C. Spanswick *et al.*, in preparation) have been used to assess beliefs about pain control. Patients who rated their own ability to control and decrease pain as poor also viewed treatment outcome as determined by chance and were more likely to report depression, anxiety, and obsessive–compulsive symptoms (Toomey *et al.* 1988). Generally it seems that those with higher ratings for 'internal locus of control' have lower levels of physical and psychological symptoms and respond better to treatment than 'externals' but the mechanisms involved and the direction of possible causal relationships remain uncertain.

Cognitive distortions, such as overgeneralization, selective abstraction, and catastrophizing, are commonly found in pain patients and can be measured using the Cognitive Errors Questionnaire (Lefebvre 1981). It has been shown that such thoughts are associated with lower pain tolerance (Turk and Rudy 1986) and (independently of disease severity) with depression and disability (Smith *et al.* 1986; Smith and Peck 1988). Coping strategies can be broadly grouped into the use of imagery techniques, self-statements (as in stress-inoculation training), and attention-diversion techniques (Fernandez 1986). The Coping Strategies Questionnaire (Rosenstiel and Keefe 1983) is at present the most widely used assessment instrument. Different coping strategies (reinterpretation and distraction, with or without imagery) have been shown to have similar effects in controlling experimentally induced pain and are superior to expectation of pain relief or no intervention (Devine and Spanos 1990). Greater use of active coping and pain suppression strategies have been found to be related to greater functional impairment; catastrophizing and helplessness were related to anxiety and depression; and diverting attention and praying were associated with more severe pain and functional impairment (Rosenstiel and Keefe 1983). However, these findings may depend on the severity of pain, and other inconsistent findings have been reported (Turner and Clancy 1986). A recent study (Main and Waddell 1991) has also found cognitive factors to be related to disability, work loss, and depression.

Other recent research has examined the relationship between pain, coping strategies, and pain beliefs (Jensen *et al.* 1991). Patients who view pain as 'enduring and mysterious' are more likely to 'catastrophize', less likely to use coping strategies, and less likely to rate coping strategies as effective in controlling pain (Williams and Keefe 1991). Spinhoven and Linssen (1991) noted that, following treatment with 20 hours of instruction in cognitive strategies, including distraction and imaging, patients with chronic back pain had improved ratings for pain and 'perceived control' but not for 'active coping' or 'helplessness'. At 6-month follow-up, reduction in perceived pain was significantly related only to 'perceived control'.

If these findings are supported, it seems that beliefs about pain, including *belief in the ability to control it*, may be more salient for pain relief than either expectation of pain relief or the cognitive strategies actually used. Changing pain beliefs may be a key feature in effective treatment, but how this may best be achieved is open to question.

Clinical applications of cognitive therapy are based on the assumption that emotions and behaviours are strongly influenced by cognitions, emphasize the use of active structured techniques to modify cognitions, teach patients to use such methods on their own, and are usually time-limited (Turner and Romano 1990). They include an amalgam of psychological techniques, including identifying and changing maladaptive thoughts (cognitive restructuring), training in coping skills, various forms of relaxation training, and use of imagery, problem solving, and behavioural strategies to overcome disability. Early studies suggested that cognitive therapy was superior to placebo medication (Engstrom 1983) and to waiting list controls (Turner 1982; Moore and Chaney 1985).

The outcomes of recent treatment trials are inconsistent, however. They are difficult to compare because they use different sample selection criteria, different assessments and cognitive approaches, mix cognitive strategies with other psychological approaches, provide treatment of different duration and frequency, use different control groups, and have different attrition rates.

Philips (1987) reported that 83 per cent of her treatment group improved, compared with none of a waiting list control group, based on assessments of pain and pain behaviour, mood, and self-control of pain. At 12-month follow-up there were further improvements in the treatment group. Nicholas *et al.* (1992) compared back pain patients, treated with a rather brief 'cognitive package' plus physiotherapy, with an active control group which received physiotherapy plus discussion groups about pain problems, but not cognitive strategies or reinforcement. The treatment group showed more improvement than controls on disability as rated by others, use of medication, self-efficacy beliefs, and the use of active coping strategies, but there was little change in the ratings of pain, depression, self-rated disability, or pain beliefs. Increased active coping was not associated with reduced pain or change in pain beliefs. Benefits appear to have been less than those found by Philips (1987), but the latter excluded subjects with poorer prognoses and treatment was more prolonged. A further study (Spinhoven and Linssen 1991) found that more prolonged treatment (20 hours of cognitive strategies, including distraction and imagery) resulted in improvements in pain ratings but not in mood, use of medication, or 'uptime' (time spent out of bed).

A better indication of the effects of cognitive therapy delivered in relatively 'pure' form comes from the treatment of chronic non-cardiac chest pain (Klimes *et al.* 1990) in which education, reinterpretation of symptoms, and training in coping skills were compared with a waiting list control (see Chapter 18). The treatment group showed an overall improvement in measures of pain frequency, mood, and self-assessment of activity. Diagnosed mental disorders were reduced from 62 per cent to 28 per cent. Changes persisted at 6 month follow-up. There was no change in the control group but, when switched to active treatment, they too showed similar improvement. Unfortunately changes in pain beliefs and cognitive strategies were not assessed, so this study does not provide us with insight into the processes involved.

Psychophysiologically based treatments

Psychophysiological approaches to treatment may include progressive muscle relaxation, autogenic training (Davis *et al.* 1982), breathing control, biofeedback, hypnosis and meditation but to some extent they overlap with cognitive strategies. Muscle relaxation (Turner and Romano 1984) is the technique which has been used most widely in pain management. In general it has been demonstrated to have a profound peripheral effect on psychophysiological arousal. Breathing control is commonly used in association with relaxation and may have particular value in the control of hyperventilation (Glynn *et al.* 1981; Parker and Main 1990). Relaxation with breathing control may have particular value in pain syndromes in which guarding and bracing are used to protect against pain but actually enhance it. Clinical experience suggests that hypnosis may have a profound effect in controlling pain but there is poor agreement about the mechanisms concerned and well-controlled research is lacking, particularly on long-term effects (Turk and Flor 1984). Biofeedback has mainly involved electromyogram (EMG) feedback and can best be regarded as a form of relaxation. It has been used, in combination with autogenic training, with some success in the treatment of tension headache

(Blanchard and Ahles 1990) and in the treatment of low back pain (Keefe *et al*. 1981*a*,*b*; Flor and Turk 1989). Recent developments, including the use of surface electromyography, are discussed in the next chapter. Whilst all these techniques have been used extensively, usually as an adjunct to other psychological approaches and are regarded as helpful, there have been relatively few trials demonstrating their specific effects. Whilst relaxation training is possibly beneficial to almost anyone with a chronic pain problem, the role of psychophysiological variables in the development, maintenance, and response to the treatment of pain requires clarification.

Exercise

Exercise has been a central feature of many psychological treatments for chronic pain (Fordyce *et al*. 1973) and may in itself result in pain reduction (Fordyce *et al*. 1981). A recent review of 16 studies comparing exercise administered by physiotherapists with other conservative physical treatments (such as heat, bed-rest, or manipulation) found that most studies were of insufficient quality to reach any conclusions (Koes *et al*. 1991). One recent report indicates the potential effect of psychological intervention on exercise. Systematic contingent reinforcement (with a points system and functional reward) of exercise (walking) in patients with low back pain resulted in increments in walking rate and reduction in pain ratings, whilst no reinforcement and non-contingent reinforcement had no systematic effect (Geiger *et al*. 1992).

Even though psychological intervention can increase the amount of exercise, it is not clear to what extent either or both are necessary components of successful pain management. As in other aspects of psychological treatment of pain, recent reports are disappointingly inconsistent. Cognitive and behavioural treatments have been found to be more effective than exercise in some studies (Turner *et al*. 1990; Nicholas *et al*. 1991). By contrast, Altmaier *et al*. (1992) compared a 3-week in-patient programme of physiotherapy, exercise, and education with similar treatment plus operant conditioning, cognitive approaches, biofeedback, and relaxation. Both treatment packages resulted in marked improvement in pain and function, which was sustained at 6 month follow-up, but there was no difference between the groups at any stage. Overall, 57 per cent returned to work, with no significant difference between the groups.

Comparison of treatments

There have been very few investigations comparing clearly identified specific psychological treatments with each other or with non-psychological treatments. However, there has been some evidence that both operant-based behavioural and cognitive treatments may result in some sustained improvement (Turner and Clancy 1988); operant treatment may be more effective in changing behaviour whilst cognitive therapies may have more effect on pain (Linton and Götestam 1984).

A meta-analysis of 109 studies of non-medical treatments of chronic pain (Malone and Strube 1988) suggested substantial improvements for most treatments as well as for no-treatment and placebo-pill groups. At this stage there is no clear evidence for the long-term superiority of any one psychological intervention, either alone or in combination with exercise, over exercise alone, when applied to the sort of subjects included in these studies. It is important to note that many studies exclude patients with any marked psychopathology. These are the very patients who might be expected to have the worst prognosis and have the greatest need for psychological intervention.

Multidisciplinary treatment programmes

Multidisciplinary pain clinics have developed since the 1960s. The management employed is eclectic and is usually provided by multiple medical specialties as well as by clinical psychologists, nurses, physiotherapists, occupational therapists, social workers and others (Hallett and Pilowsky 1982; Aronoff *et al.* 1983). Treatment usually incorporates a number of the psychological approaches described above, with considerable variation between centres in the type, duration, and amount of treatment and in the disorders treated. The emphasis has usually been on reducing disability rather than 'curing' pain. Behavioural principles have been prominent, with specified goals, structured hierarchies of activities, 'pacing' to prevent inappropriate excessive or erratic exercise, and positive reinforcement (usually social) of achievements, whilst avoiding reinforcement of 'pain behaviours'. Further details are presented in the next chapter.

Originally, it was usual to offer an in-patient treatment programme of 3–4 weeks' duration. More recently, out-patient treatment programmes have been used but reports usually fail to indicate whether they provide treatment for patients with severely restricted mobility or serious physical or mental disorders. There have been claims for the superiority of 'field' (that is, domiciliary) management over out-patient treatment (Cott *et al.* 1990), which are not yet supported by adequate data. A recent meta-analysis of 65 reports of multimodal treatment of chronic back pain (Flor *et al.* 1992) found that, overall, treatment groups improved 30 per cent more than control groups in the short-term (less than 6 months post-treatment) and 38 per cent more in the longer term (over 6 months, mean 2 years). Multimodal treatment was superior to all types of control procedures, including no-treatment, placebo, waiting list, physical therapy, or medical treatment alone. Outcome for treatment groups was superior on a wide range of both subjective and objective assessments, including pain behaviour, activity, use of medication and health services, and they were twice as likely to return to work. The authors of this meta-analysis argue that their findings support the superiority of multimodal treatments and that their benefits are sustained. Unfortunately many individual studies, including some of the most recent, have serious limitations in both the assessments and design used (described below). In particular, some studies have failed to use appropriate randomization procedures and have even allocated patients who lack adequate health insurance to no-treatment control groups, where social disadvantage may contribute to their worse outcome.

Cost-effectiveness

There have been few studies directly comparing the costs of in-patient with out-patient treatment. Recently, Peters *et al.* (1992) found that both in- and out-patient groups receiving multimodal treatment improved post-treatment and at 9–18 months follow-up, with regard to measures of pain, activity, return to work, and appropriate use of medication. The in-patient group was functioning better at follow-up than the out-patients, whilst a no-treatment control group had deteriorated. Treatment for in-patients cost seven times more per patient than for out-patients. Costs were compared with savings in accident compensation and sickness benefits (but excluding additional savings in health service costs) for those who had returned to work. Calculated over 1 year, the out-patient programme showed a gain, the in-patient programme a small deficit; calculated over 5 years, assuming that the benefits of treatment will be sustained, both programmes would result in substantial savings, the in-patient programme saving twice as much as the out-patient treatment. Unfortunately, pre-treatment assessments showed that the groups were not comparable, the in-patient group being more severely disabled. Failure in randomization may have been determined by selective drop-outs, with the most disordered out-patients and controls seeking alternative treatments. It is likely that out-patient treatment is less acceptable and successful, particularly if offered to more disabled patients. The best clinical and financial arrangement may be to assign patients to in-patient or out-patient treatment depending on severity and psychopathology.

The evaluation of treatment outcome

The assessment of chronic pain and the efficacy of its treatment have recently been reviewed (Turk and Melzack 1992). Appraisal of the efficacy of the different treatment approaches described above requires careful

Table 11.2 Requirements for research design

Assessments

    Wide range required
    Subjective and objective
    Physical pathology
    Mental disorders — diagnose severity
    Related to type of treatment and goals
    Cross-modal
    Cost-savings

Other design requirements

    Identify psychological procedures used
    Identify proportions not entering or completing treatment
    Identify disorders/syndromes treated
    Randomization—after initial assessment
    Control groups—waiting list inadequate
    Duration of follow-up to steady state
    Treatment effects on multiple symptoms
    Effects of multiple symptoms on outcome

scrutiny of the outcome measures and other aspects of research design. These are summarized in Table 11.2.

Assessments

Within the last few years, most researchers have recognized the importance of including a range of assessment measures, including measures of pain and pain behaviour, mood, social dysfunction, and sometimes use of medication and health services. However, the use of objective assessments is still comparatively rare. The common practice of follow-up assessments by telephone is inadequate. Evidence of return to work and reduction in disability payments have become increasingly important. Detailed cost-savings analyses of short- and long-term benefits will need to be included in all future investigations.

Few reports of chronic pain treatment adequately assess the presence and severity of mental disorders or the effects of psychological treatments on them. The assessment of physical pathology is also frequently omitted, apart from the exclusion of patients with malignant disorders, but may be equally important in influencing outcome in reported studies. Investigations of 'chronic benign pain' may include both patients with physiologically determined symptoms due to stress and others with chronic, progressive physical disorders such as osteoarthritis. It is unlikely that the treatment responses of these conditions will be similar, yet this issue is rarely considered.

Investigations of specific types of treatment, for example behavioural or cognitive, should obviously include assessments of what they purport to change. Thus, assessments of beliefs and cognitive strategies should be mandatory for research into the effects of cognitive therapy, as should objective assessments of behavioural changes for the effects of operant-based treatments. However, it is also important to use cross-modal assessments, for example to determine the extent to which cognitions are changed by behavioural treatments or cognitive treatment leads to improved mobility. These will lead to better understanding of the mechanisms involved in the therapeutic process. They will also help to determine whether different treatments have different effects and, if so, whether they are all necessary, whether they have similar cumulative effects, or whether some are clearly superior for different groups of patients.

Other problems in research design

The review of psychological treatments suggests that there is a broad range of approaches which may have rather similar beneficial effects. However, studies of apparently similar treatments indicate inconsistencies both in the effects of treatment and in the modalities that change. In addition to the limitations in assessments described above, a number of other problems in research design are likely to contribute to these disparate findings:

(1) results have been confounded by failure to limit treatment procedures to those being investigated;

(2) it is often difficult to identify the specific psychological procedures that are being used;

(3) failure to report the proportion of patients who do not complete treatment;

(4) failure to randomize subjects after initial assessment and to use appropriate control groups;

(5) waiting list control groups can be subject to excessive attrition, thus disrupting randomization;

(6) failure to control for non-specific treatment effects;

(7) some experimental work provides very brief intervention which would not usually be expected to be effective in the clinical management of severe chronic disorders.

These are likely to account for at least some of the considerable differences that have emerged between different studies, although there is also general agreement about improvement in the majority of patients who persist with treatment.

The duration of treatment and the persistence of its effects also requires further consideration. Most investigations are designed to demonstrate the effects of relatively brief intensive treatment and there has been little attention to the possible benefits of longer-term interventions aimed at maintaining and building on initial improvements.

Most research now includes some follow-up to determine whether changes persist, but this is usually quite brief, rarely more than 1 year, and longer periods are essential. Whilst some reports suggest that treatment effects persist or even increase, others show regression. Some studies with longer follow-up periods, up to 3 years, indicate an increasing relapse rate for at least the first 2 years, suggesting that this should be the minimum follow-up period.

To what extent do treatment outcomes based on one syndrome apply to others? Surprisingly, there has been little research comparing the effects of the same treatment on different pain syndromes, such as headache, back pain, irritable bowel syndrome, or atypical facial pain and we know little about the extent to which findings can be generalized.

In addition, there is evidence that some patients collect multiple symptoms and the diagnosis or pain syndrome to which they are allocated at any time will depend mainly on which symptom happens to predominate when they are seen and on the interests of their latest therapist. Research on chronic pain rarely includes longitudinal assessment of multiple symptoms. We therefore know little about the extent to which subjects included in treatment studies have single or multiple symptoms or the effect that this may have on outcome.

Conclusions

The diagnosis and treatment of associated mental disorders is an effective approach for some patients with chronic pain but requires special skills. Psychological treatments can probably make a valuable contribution to treatment for many patients and may be most useful when used in combination. However, despite considerable advances in our knowledge of the efficacy of psychological and psychiatric treatment it is still not clear what is the best treatment for patients with chronic pain. There is also substantial evidence that many chronic pain patients are not able to benefit from psychological treatments. Specialist therapy may not be available, patients are regarded as unsuitable, or patients may be unwilling to accept or persist with treatment. These patients are liable to be the most severely disordered, distressed, and dependent and those who impose the greatest financial burden on health and social services. The available data indicate that this group is large and may even constitute the majority in some settings.

There is a risk that the successful use of relatively brief, cheap out-patient programmes for ambulant patients will be regarded as an indication to close more costly in-patient programmes. However, there is already some indication that the latter are necessary for the treatment of more severe disorders and may actually be more cost-effective in the longer term. It is unlikely that out-patient services will ever satisfy the needs of chair-bound or bed-bound patients. There is therefore a good case for treatment to be planned on the basis of *disability* rather than on *symptoms*. The implications for health care delivery are addressed in the next chapter.

At present there is little evidence for the long-term superiority of any one psychological procedure over others or even that they are much better than education and exercise. It is tempting to draw on the paradigm of research into the treatment of phobias and to speculate that psychological treatments are effective only when they result in behavioural change, particularly exercise and that different treatments will be effective for different patients, depending on the causes and effects of their chronic pain.

References

Adler, R.H., Zlot, S., and Hurny, C. (1989). Engel's 'Psychogenic pain and the pain-prone patient': a retrospective, controlled clinical study. *Psychosomatic Medicine*, **51**, 87–101.

Altmaier, E.M., Lechmann, T.R., Russell, D.W., Weinstein, J.N., and Kao, C.F. (1992). The effectiveness of psychological interventions for the rehabilitation of low back pain: a randomized controlled trial evaluation. *Pain*, **49**, 329–35.

American Psychiatric Association (1987). *Diagnostic and statistical manual*, (3rd edn), (revised). American Psychiatric Association, Washington, DC.

Aronoff, G.M., Evans, W.O., and Enders, P.L. (1983). A review of follow-up studies of multidisciplinary pain units. *Pain*, **16**, 1–11.

Atkinson, J.H., Slater, M.A., Patterson, T.L. Grant, I., and Garfin, S.R. *et al.* (1991). Prevalence, onset, and risk of psychiatric disorders in men with chronic low back pain: a controlled study. *Pain*, **45**, 111–21.

Bass, C. and Benjamin, S. (1993). The management of chronic somatization. *British Journal of Psychiatry*, **162**, 472–80.

Bassett, D.L. and Pilowsky, I. (1985). A study of brief psychotherapy for chronic pain. *Journal of Psychosomatic Research*, **29**, 259–64.

Beecher, H.K. (1959). *Measurement of subjective responses*. Oxford University Press, New York.

Benjamin, S., (1989). Psychological treatment of chronic pain: a selective review. *Journal of Psychosomatic Research*, 33, 121-31.

Benjamin, S. and Barnes, D. (1984). Can anaesthetists detect depression in pain patients? *Pain*, Suppl. 2, s365.

Benjamin, S. and Bridges, K. (1994). The need for specialist services for chronic somatization. In *Liaison psychiatry: defining needs and planning services*, (ed. S. Benjamin, A. House, and P. Jenkins). Gaskell, London.

Benjamin, S. and Eminson, D.M. (1992). Abnormal illness behaviour: childhood experiences and long-term consequences. *International Review of Psychiatry*, 4, 55-70.

Benjamin, S., Barnes, D., Berger, S., Clarke, I., and Jeacock, J. (1988). The relationship of chronic pain, mental illness and organic disorders. *Pain*, 32, 185-95.

Benjamin, S., Lennon, S., and Gardner, G. (1991a). The validity of the general health questionnaire for first stage screening for mental illness in pain clinic patients. *Pain*, 47, 197-202.

Benjamin, S., Mawer, J., and Lennon, S. (1991b). The knowledge and beliefs of family care givers about chronic pain patients. *Journal of Psychosomatic Research*, 36, 211-17.

Blanchard, E.B. and Ahles, T.A. (1990). Biofeedback therapies. In *The management of pain*, (2nd edn), (ed J.J. Bonica), pp. 1722-32. Lea and Febiger, Philadelphia.

Blumer, D. and Heilbronn, M. (1982). Chronic pain as a variant of depressive disease. The pain prone disorder. *Journal of Nerve and Mental Disorders*, 170, 381-406.

Bonica, J.J. (1990). *The management of pain*, (2nd edn). Lea and Febiger, Philadelphia.

Chapman, C.R. (1977). Psychological aspects of pain patient treatment. *Archives of Surgery*, 112, 767-72.

Chapman, C.R. and Syrjala, K. (1990). The measurement of pain. In *The management of pain*, (2nd edn), (ed. J.J. Bonica), pp. 580-4. Lea and Febiger, Philadelphia.

Cott, A., Anchel, H., Goldberg, W.M., Fabich, M. and Parkinson, W. (1990). Non-institutional treatment of chronic pain by field-management: an outcome study with comparison group. *Pain*, 40, 183-94.

Crisson, J.E. and Keefe, F.J. (1988). The relationship of locus of control to pain coping strategies and psychological distress in chronic pain patients. *Pain*, 35, 147-54.

Davies, H.T.O., Crombie, I.K., Lonsdale, M. and Macrae, W.A. (1991). Consensus and contention in the treatment of chronic nerve-damage pain. *Pain*, 47, 191-6.

Davis, M., Eshelman, E.F., and McKay, M. (1982). *The relaxation and stress reduction workbook*. New Harbinger Publications, Oakland.

Descartes, R. (1664). L'Homme. Reported in Bonica J.J. (1990). History of pain concepts and therapies. In *The management of pain*, (2nd edn), (ed. J.J. Bonica), pp. 2-17. Lea and Febiger, Philadelphia.

Devine, D.P. and Spanos, N.P. (1990). Effectiveness of maximally different cognitive strategies and expectancy in attenuation of reported pain. *Journal of Personality and Social Psychology*, 58, 672-8.

Doan, B.D. and Wadden, N.P. (1989). Relationship between depressive symptoms and descriptions of chronic pain. *Pain*, **36**, 75–84.

Engel, G. (1959). 'Psychogenic' pain and the pain prone patient. *American Journal of Medicine*, **26**, 899–918.

Engstrom, D.E. (1983). Cognitive behavioural therapy methods in chronic pain treatment. In *Advances in pain research and therapy*, Vol. 5, (ed. J.J. Bonica, U. Lindblom, A. Iggo, L.E. Jones, and C. Benedetti), pp. 829–38. Raven Press, New York.

Fernandez, E. (1986). A classification system of cognitive coping strategies of pain. *Pain*, **26**, 141–51.

Fishbain, D.A., Goldberg, M., Meagher, B.R., Steele, R., and Rosomoff, H. (1986). Male and female chronic pain patients categorized by DSM-III psychiatric diagnostic criteria. *Pain*, **26**, 181–97.

Flor, H. and Turk, D.C. (1989). Psychophysiology of chronic pain: do chronic pain patients exhibit symptom-specific psychophysiological responses? *Psychological Bulletin*, **105**, 205–59.

Flor, H., Turk, D.C., and Scholz, O.B. (1986). Impact of chronic pain on the spouse: marital, emotional and physical consequences. *Journal of Psychosomatic Research*, **31**, 63–71.

Flor, H., Fydrich, T., and Turk, D.C. (1992). Efficacy of multidisciplinary pain treatment centers: a meta-analytic review. *Pain*, **49**, 221–30.

Fordyce, W.E. (1985). The behavioural management of chronic pain: a response to critics. *Pain*, **22**, 113–25.

Fordyce, W.E. (1990). Contingency management. In *the management of pain*, (2nd edn), (ed. J.J. Bonica), pp. 1702–10. Lea and Febiger, Philadelphia.

Fordyce, W.E., Fowler, R.S., Lehmann, J.F. Delateur, B.J., Saud, P.L., and Treischmann, R. (1973). Operant conditioning in the treatment of chronic pain. *Archives of Physical and Medical Rehabilitation*, **54**, 399–408.

Fordyce, W., McMahon, R., and Rainwater, G. (1981). Pain complaint–exercise performance relationship in chronic pain. *Pain*, **10**, 311–21.

Fordyce, W.E., Brockway, J., Bergman, J.A., and Spengler, D. (1986). Acute back pain: a control group comparison of behavioural versus traditional management methods. *Journal of Behavioural Medicine*, **9**, 127–40.

Funch, D.P. and Gale, E.N. (1985). Predicting treatment completion in a behavioural therapy programme for chronic temporomandibular pain. *Journal of Psychosomatic Research*, **30**, 57–62.

Geiger, G., Todd, D.D., Clark, H.B., Miller, R.P., and Kori, S.H. (1992). The effects of feedback and contingent reinforcement on the exercise behaviour of chronic pain patients. *Pain*, **49**, 179–85.

Gil, K.M., Keefe, F.J., Crisson, J.E., and Van Dalfson, P.J. (1987). Social support and pain behaviour. *Pain*, **29**, 209–17.

Glynn, C.J., Lloyd, J.W., and Folkhard, S. (1981). Ventilatory responses to chronic pain. *Pain*, **11**, 201–12.

Hallett, E.C. and Pilowsky, I. (1982). The response to treatment in a multidisciplinary pain clinic. *Pain*, **12**, 365–74.

Haythornthwaite, J.A., Sieber, W.J., and Kerns, R.D. (1991). Depression and the chronic pain experience. *Pain*, **46**, 177–84.

Hughes, A.M., Medley, I., Turner, G.N., and Bond, M.R. (1987). Psychogenic pain: a study of marital adjustment. *Acta Psychiatrica Scandinavica*, **75**, 166-70.

Jensen, M.P., Turner, J.A., Romano, J.M., and Karoly, P. (1991). Coping with chronic pain: a critical review of the literature. *Pain*, **47**, 249-83.

Katon, W., Egan, K., and Miller, D. (1985). Chronic pain: lifetime psychiatric diagnosis and family history. *American Journal of Psychiatry*, **142**, 1156-60.

Keefe, F.J., Block, A.R., Williams, R.B., and Surwit, R.S. (1981a). Behavioural treatment of chronic low back pain: clinical outcome and individual differences in pain relief. *Pain*, **11**, 221-31.

Keefe, F.J., Shapira, B., Brown, C., Williams, R.B., and Surwit, R.S. (1981b). EMG-assisted relaxation training in the management of chronic low back pain. *American Journal of Clinical Biofeedback*, **4**, 93-103.

Kirmayer, L.J. and Robbins, J.M. (1991). Functional somatic symptoms. In *Current concepts of somatization*, (ed. L.J. Kirmayer and J.M. Robbins). American Psychiatric Press, Washington, DC.

Klimes, I., Mayou, R.A., Pearce, M.J., and Coles, L. (1990). Psychological treatment for atypical non-cardiac chest pain: a controlled evaluation. *Psychological Medicine*, **20**, 605-11.

Koes, B.W., Bouter, L.M., Beckerman, H., van der Heijden, and Knipschild, P.G. (1991). Physiotherapy exercises and back pain: a blinded review. *British Medical Journal*, **302**, 1572-6.

Lefebvre, M.F. (1981). Cognitive distortion and cognitive errors in depressed psychiatric and low back pain patients. *Journal of Consulting and Clinical Psychology*, **49**, 517-25.

Linton, S.J. (1986). Behavioural remediation of chronic pain: a status report. *Pain*, **24**, 125-41.

Linton, S.J. and Gotestam, K.G. (1984). A controlled study of the effects of applied relaxation and applied relaxation plus operant procedures in the regulation of chronic pain. *British Journal of Clinical Psychology*, **23**, 291-9.

Loeser, J.D., Seres, J.L., and Newman, R.I. (1990). Interdisciplinary, multimodal management of chronic pain. In *The management of pain*, (2nd edn), (ed. J.J. Bonica), pp. 2107-20. Lea and Febiger, Philadelphia.

Main, C. and Waddell, G. (1991). A comparison of cognitive measures in low back pain: statistical structure and clinical validity at initial assessment. *Pain*, **46**, 287-98.

Malone, M.D. and Strube, M.J. (1988). Meta-analysis of non-medical treatments for chronic pain. *Pain*, **34**, 231-44.

Marks, R.C., Houston, T., and Thulbourne, T. (1992). Facet joint injection and facet nerve block: a randomised comparison in 86 patients with chronic low back pain. *Pain*, **49**, 325-28.

Melzack, R. and Wall, P.D. (1965). Pain mechanisms: a new theory. *Science*, **150**, 971-9.

Melzack, R. and Wall, P.D. (1982). *The challenge of pain*. Basic Books, New York.

Moore, J.E. and Chaney, E.F. (1985). Outpatient group treatment of chronic pain: effects of spouse involvement. *Journal of Consulting and Clinical Psychology*, **53**, 326–34.

Nicholas, M.K., Wilson, P.H., and Goyen, J. (1991). Operant-behavioural and cognitive-behavioural treatment for chronic low back pain. *Behaviour Research and Therapy*, **29**, 225–38.

Nicholas, M.K., Wilson, P.H., and Goyen, J. (1992). Comparison of cognitive-behavioural group treatment and an alternative non-psychological treatment for chronic low back pain. *Pain*, **48**, 339–47.

Onghena, P. and Van Houdenhove, B. (1992). Antidepressant-induced analgesia in chronic non-malignant pain: a meta-analysis of 39 placebo-controlled studies. *Pain*, **49**, 205–19.

Parker, H. and Main, C.J. (1990). *Living with back pain*. Manchester University Press, Manchester.

Penman, J. (1954). Pain as an old friend. *The Lancet*, **1**, 633–9.

Peters, J., Large, R.G., and Elkind, G. (1992). Follow-up results trom a randomised controlled trial evaluating in- and outpatient pain management programmes. *Pain*, **50**, 41–50.

Philips, H.C. (1987). The effects of behavioural treatment on chronic pain. *Behavioural Research and Therapy*, **25**, 365–77.

Pilowsky, I. (1986). Psychodynamic aspects of pain. In *The psychology of pain* (2nd edn), (ed. R.A. Sternbach). Raven, New York.

Pilowsky, I. and Barrow, C.G. (1990). A controlled study of psychotherapy and amitriptyline used individually and in combination in the treatment of chronic, intractable. 'psychogenic' pain. *Pain*, **40**, 3–19.

Rosenstiel, A.K. and Keefe, F.J. (1983). The use of coping strategies in chronic low back pain patients: relationship to patient characteristics and current adjustments. *Pain*, **17**, 33–4.

Rowat, K.M. and Knafl, K.A. (1985). Living with chronic pain: the spouse's perspective. *Pain*, **23**, 259–71.

Roy, R. (1988). Impact of chronic pain on marital partners: systems perspective. In *Proceedings of the Vth World Congress on Pain*, (ed. R. Dubner, G.F. Gebhart, and M.R. Bond), pp. 287–97. Elsevier, Amsterdam.

Sharpe, M. and Bass, C. (1992). Pathophysiological mechanisms in somatization. *International Review of Psychiatry*, **4**, 81–97.

Smith, R. (1991). *Somatization disorder in the medical setting*. American Psychiatric Press, Washington, DC.

Smith, T.W. and Peck, J.R. (1988). Cognitive distortion in rheumatoid arthritis: relation to depression and disability. *Journal of Consulting and Clinical Psychology*, **3**, 312–16.

Smith, T.W., Aberger, E.W., Follick, M.J., and Ahern, D.K. (1986). Cognitive distortion and psychological distress in chronic low back pain. *Journal of Consulting and Clinical Psychology*, **54**, 573–5.

Spinhoven, P. and Linssen, A.C.G. (1991). Behavioral treatment of chronic low back pain. I. Relation of coping strategy use to outcome. *Pain*, **45**, 29–34.

Sullivan, M.J.L., Reesor, K., Mikail, S. and Fisher, R. (1992). The treatment of depression in chronic low back pain: review and recommendations. *Pain*, **50**, 5–13.

Svedlund, J. (1983). Psychotherapy in irritable bowel syndrome: a controlled outcome study. *Acta Psychiatrica Scandinavica*, **67** (Suppl. 306), 1-86.

Toomey, T.C., Finneran J., and Scarborough, W.B. (1988). Clinical features of health locus of control beliefs in chronic facial pain patients. *Clinical Journal of Pain*, **3**, 213-18.

Tunks, E.R. and Merskey, H. (1990). Psychotherapy in the management of chronic pain. In *The management of pain*, (2nd edn), (ed. J.J. Bonica), pp. 1751-6. Lea and Febiger, Philadelphia.

Turk, D.C. and Flor, H. (1984). Etiological theories and treatments for chronic back pain: II psychological models and interventions. *Pain*, **19**, 209-33.

Turk, D.C. and Melzack, R. (1992). *Handbook of pain assessment*. Guilford, New York.

Turk, D.C. and Rudy, T.E. (1986). Assessment of cognitive factors in chronic pain: a worthwhile enterprise? *Journal of Consulting and Clinical Psychology*, **54**, 760-8.

Turk, D.C., Flor, H., and Rudy, T.E. (1987). Pain and families I. Etiology, maintenance and psychosocial impact. *Pain*, **30**, 3-27.

Turner, J.A. (1982). Comparison of group progressive-relaxation training and cognitive-behavioural group therapy for chronic low back pain. *Journal of Consulting and Clinical Psychology*, **50**, 757-65.

Turner, J.A. and Clancy, S. (1986). Strategies for coping with chronic low back pain: relationships to pain and disability. *Pain*, **24**, 355-64.

Turner, J.A. and Clancy, S. (1988). Comparison of operant behavioural and cognitive-behavioural group treatment for chronic low back pain. *Journal of Consulting and Clinical Psychology*, **56**, 261-6.

Turner, J.A. and Romano, J.M. (1984). Self report screening measures for depression in chronic pain patients. *Journal of Clinical Psychology*, **40**, 909-13.

Turner, J.A. and Romano, J.M. (1990). Cognitive-behavioural therapy. In *The management of pain*, (2nd edn), (ed. J.J. Bonica), pp. 1711-21. Lea and Febiger, Philadelphia.

Turner, J.A., Clancy, S., McQuade, K.J., and Cardenas, D.D. (1990). Effectiveness of behavioral therapy for chronic low back pain: a component analysis. *Journal of Consulting and Clinical Psychology*, **58**, 537-79.

Williams, D.A. and Keefe, F.J. (1991). Pain beliefs and the use of cognitive-behavioral coping strategies. *Pain*, **46**, 185-90.

12 Psychological treatment and the health care system: the chaotic case of back pain. Is there a need for a paradigm shift?

Chris J. Main and Sidney Benjamin

In the second of their two chapters, Dr Main and Dr Benjamin examine the social context of treatment. They begin by discussing the ways in which occupational, financial, and other social factors contribute to the aetiology and influence the prognosis of chronic pain and then consider the various types of pain management programmes. The section on treatment guidelines is concerned particularly with specialist programmes. The final section makes recommendations for service development in terms of community education, improved health care delivery, and changes in health care policy. The issues discussed in this chapter are relevant to the provision of care for all the functional somatic syndromes discussed in this book. They are considered further in Chapters 21 and 22.

Introduction

The previous chapter gave an overview of the value of individualized psychological approaches to the treatment and management of the patient with pain. Here we argue that in order to understand chronic disability and pain-related dysfunction and to provide cost-effective treatment, we must also consider the wider socio-economic and occupational context in which treatment is delivered. Consideration of the place of psychological treatment for pain in general invites further consideration of the data concerning back pain in particular, since of all pain problems it has been perhaps the most extensively researched and has generated the widest range of treatment approaches.

The problem

Back pain and sciatica affect approximately 80 per cent of the population at some time in their life and 5 per cent of the adult population consult their doctor each year with back trouble. Although 80–90 per cent of attacks of pain recover within 6 weeks, a significant number of patients remain incapacitated. Low back disability has increased dramatically in Western societies since the 1950s. In the UK, work loss due to back pain has doubled during the last 5 years and back-related incapacities now account for one-seventh of all sickness and invalidity benefit (Waddell 1993). The increasing sophistication of high-technology medicine has singularly failed to halt this increase (Waddell 1993). More alarming for the future, it is increasing faster than any other form of incapacity. The chronic back pain patient may see several specialists and be given a range of diagnoses, sometimes accompanied by inconsistent and even conflicting advice. Investigation of the influence of psychological factors on response to treatment has therefore to be set against a background of treatment failure and a plethora of new 'miracle cures' ranging from the crassly inept to the fanciful. Failed treatment is associated with a higher prevalence of inappropriate symptoms (Waddell *et al.* 1986). Patients attending pain clinics have much longer present episodes and show higher levels of distress than routine referrals to departments of orthopaedic surgery (Main *et al.* 1992).

Aetiology

Although the Gate Control Theory (Melzack and Wall 1965) has been extremely influential in current conceptualizations of pain (Bonica 1990), many patients implicitly hold a view much more akin to the simpler Cartesian model (see Chapter 11). More sophisticated aetiological formulations have incorporated new developments in the understanding of the nervous system. Of particular importance has been the recognition that *chronic pain* differs in important respects from post-operative pain and from other kinds of *acute pain*. Specific pharmacological control of post-operative pain has been one of the success stories of this century (Ready and Edwards 1992). If pain persists beyond the acute phase, however, patients begin to change both physically and psychologically. Furthermore, persistent pain and limitation in activities of daily living, as with any other life stress, will eventually have a psychological impact on the patient. Once the pain and disability has progressed beyond the acute phase, the chronic pain patient is likely to become progressively demoralized and distressed (Sternbach 1974). It is against such a complex background that psychological management and treatment must be considered. The complex interplay between physical, psychological, and socio-economic factors can be addressed in the biopsychosocial model of low back pain (Waddell 1992; see Chapter 11).

New understandings of the neuroplasticity of the nervous system may also lead to clarification of the roles of both the central and peripheral nervous systems in the aetiology of pain (Woolf 1991). In addition, more complex multidimensional pain models involving physiological, behavioural, cognitive, and socio-biological components have been promulgated in the last decade. Flor *et al.* (1990) offer an excellent

Table 12.1 Specific psychological influences in industrial and occupational settings (adapted from Bigos *et al.* 1990)

Effects on claims:	Risks of chronicity:
Severity of symptoms	History of low back pain
Perceptions of safety	Distress
Perceptions of impact	Low job satisfaction

overview of these. A summary of psychological influences on chronic pain in occupational settings is shown in Table 12.1.

Compensation   Since the increase in injuries at the time of the building of railways in the nineteenth century, the importance of psychological factors has been (implicitly) recognized in the evaluation of compensation after back injury (Allen and Waddell, 1989) and there have been repeated attempts to 'disentangle' physical from psychological components. Litigation made it seem important to identify malingerers and indeed this is still a concern of the modern medico-legal process. Concepts such as 'real' and 'imaginary' pain entered the professional lexicon and, following psychiatric fashion in the early part of the century, terms such as 'conversion hysteria' were frequently used to describe symptomatology for which no adequate organic basis could be found. As a consequence much effort has been directed at an inappropriate diagnostic classification which divides symptoms into 'functional' and 'organic'. Clinically, interest in the nature of back pain has been maintained by differences in disability in response to apparently similar levels of incapacity and by difficulties in predicting response to physical methods of treatment.

Occupational factors   In a comprehensive review of industrial back pain, Bigos *et al.* (1990) consider risk factors in relation to back pain disability. They highlight the 'unfounded tendency to label normally occurring back symptoms as industrial injuries' and describe how psychosocial factors influence recovery from symptoms and return to work. While acknowledging the methodological limitations of many of the studies which they review, they present a strong case for the importance of psychological factors in determining compensation claims for back pain, the perception of symptom severity, and the associated disability. They conclude 'Once an individual is off work, perceptions about symptoms, about the safety of returning to work, and about the impact of returning to work on one's personal life can affect recovery even in the most well-meaning worker (Bigos *et al.* 1990, p. 854).

It is time to acknowledge the importance of an occupational perspective for clinical evaluation. Recently a new generation of tests specifically validated for back pain sufferers has been developed. The first of these, the Fear–Avoidance Beliefs Questionnaire or FABQ (Waddell *et al.* 1993), derived from a study of more than 200 back pain patients, comprises two factors:

(1) fear–avoidance beliefs about work;

(2) fear–avoidance beliefs about physical activity.

Specific beliefs about work accounted for more than 20 per cent of the variance in activities of daily living and more than 25 per cent of the variance in the amount of work loss, even after controlling for the reported severity of pain.

The development of psychological treatment

During the last two decades the role of psychological factors in the genesis and maintenance of pain problems has been increasingly recognized. Unfortunately, much treatment has also been construed and delivered as *either* physical *or* psychological. In the previous chapter the importance of the recognition and treatment of primary psychiatric disorder has been discussed. However, in the majority of pain patients a primary psychiatric diagnosis is inappropriate and the psychological significance of chronic pain and associated dysfunction has to be assessed from cognitive, behavioural and psychophysiological perspectives as well as its affective impact (see Chapter 11).

Research into the factors contributing to the incapacity associated with back pain have led not only towards a broader view of aetiology (Waddell 1992), but also to a wider range of approaches to treatment. Thus, the specific psychological treatments reviewed in the previous chapter and elsewhere (Main 1992), are (with the exception of clearly identifiable psychiatric disorders such as depressive illnesses), frequently incorporated within interdisciplinary pain management programmes (PMP).

The behavioural perspective

Historically, the behavioural approach (Fordyce 1976) to the treatment and management of pain problems has been the most influential. Early pain management programmes (PMPs) were explicitly behavioural in nature to the extent that other psychological mechanisms were deemed irrelevant to understanding the process of treatment and its delivery. The importance of the shift in attention from the physical origin of pain to the circumstances in which pain occurs and is reported can hardly be over-emphasized. The behavioural approach often offers a way of re-establishing more normal functioning in a patient who has become a chronic invalid by establishing a systematic graded approach to rehabilitation. Whilst it is tempting to caricature the behavioural approach to pain as an environmental management system in which the individual plays little part, self-learning and self-help are fundamental to the modern PMP and active involvement is a prerequisite to a successful outcome.

Physiologically based stress reduction

Many of the self-control methods originally developed for the treatment of anxiety and depression have been adapted for the treatment of pain patients. Of the physiologically based approaches, the most widely known technique is Jacobsonian muscle relaxation (Jacobsen 1962), although biofeedback is also widely used. The original simple techniques have now been developed into much more sophisticated treatments using computerized myography from specific muscle groups in which abnormal electrical activity has been identified (Cram 1990).

Psychologically based stress reduction

Psychological approaches to the management of pain and its effects have been of equal importance. Traditional psychoanalytic psychotherapy has not been shown to be effective with pain patients, but cognitive therapy has been widely used (Turk *et al.* 1983). Early studies identified a series of cognitive abnormalities or distortions similar to those found in depressed patients and enabled the development of a range of therapies aimed at improving coping strategies. Therapy aims to help patients to regain some control over their pain and to boost their confidence. Cognitive therapy, whether offered to patients individually or as part of a group, is frequently combined with behavioural approaches to produce an amalgam known as cognitive behavioural therapy (CBT). A comprehensive review of cognitive behavioural therapy is offered by Turner and Romano (1990) (see also Chapter 7).

Pain programmes

Psychological approaches to the treatment and management of pain are frequently embedded within more broadly based programmes incorporating a variety of ingredients. With the progressive shift from the *disease* model of pain to the *illness* model of pain (see Chapter 1), there has been increasing recognition that successful rehabilitation of pain patients may require a wide range of professional skills. The range and importance of the psychological components varies between programmes. A brief overview of the general medical approach (GMA), back schools (BS), functional restoration programmes (FRP) and pain management programmes (PMP) will now be presented. The key features are presented in Tables 12.2–12.4.

Table 12.2 Comparison of general medical approach, back schools, functional restoration (work hardening) programmes, and pain management programmes

	General medical approach	Back schools	Functional restoration programmes	Pain management programmes
Stage in illness	Acute/chronic	Pre-acute Subacute	Chronic	Chronic
General aim	Treatment	Prevention	Rehabilitation	Rehabilitation
Occupational influence	Minor	Moderate	Major	Minor/major
Professional contact	Individual/ multidisciplinary	Multidisciplinary/ group	Multidisciplinary/ individual	Interdisciplinary/ group

Table 12.3 Therapeutic content. Comparison of general medical approach, back schools, functional restoration (work hardening) programmes, and pain management programmes

	General medical approach	Back schools	Functional restoration programmes	Pain management programmes
Pain reduction	Major	Minor	Minor	Minor
Increase mobility	Minor	Moderate	Major	Major
Increase power and strength	Minor	Minor	Major	Minor
Reduce distress	None	Minor	None/minor	Major
Reduce invalidism	None	Minor	Minor	Minor
Give coping skills	None	Moderate	Minor	Major

Table 12.4 Philosophy of care. Comparison of general medical approach, back schools, functional restoration (work hardening) programmes, and pain management programmes

	General medical approach	Back schools	Functional restoration programmes	Pain management programmes
Education	None	Major	Moderate/major	Major
Patient involvement				
Treatment	None	Major	Major	Major
Decision making	None	Minor	Minor	Major
Emphasis on self-help	None	Major	Major	Major
Emphasis on return to work	Minor	Minor	Major	Minor

The general medical approach   This is usually delivered on an individual basis. The focus of treatment is on pain reduction with the assumption that if pain is successfully reduced, normal functioning will automatically be restored. Little need is seen for education or for self-help. While such a straightforward approach may be successful for acute pain, such as postoperative pain, chronic pain presents a much more complex problem.

Back schools   Back schools were established initially in Sweden as educational back care programmes designed to prevent back pain in occupational settings (Zachrisson-Forssett 1980). A number of clinical variants have emerged. The Canadian back school (Hall and Iceton 1983) contains more psychological content than the Swedish back school, but is still run essentially on an educational model, with a class of 15–20 patients receiving four weekly lectures on various aspects of back pain. It is claimed to be more appropriate for chronic back sufferers, but there is little evidence for the efficacy of the simpler back school approach for chronic back pain (Linton and Kamwendo 1987; Nordin *et al*. 1992). The Californian back school (Matmiller 1980) differs in the inclusion of an obstacle course. There is a specific emphasis on improving physical function which can be seen as the forerunner of the work-hardening approach which typifies functional restoration programmes, but there is little specific psychological content.

Functional restoration programmes These are vigorous treatments focused almost entirely on return to work (Mayer and Gatchel 1988) and designed to 'normalize' back function. They combine a sports medicine approach with ergonomic assessment and an individualized computer-assisted programme designed to increase muscle power (particularly back strength) and range of movement. Psychological factors are addressed primarily in the context of obstacles to the achievement of progressively more demanding exercise targets. Impressive results are claimed for this approach (Mayer *et al*. 1987; Hazard *et al*. 1989). These may however reflect the financial implications for the North American patient if failure to achieve satisfactory progress is admitted, since the results have not been so impressive in other health care settings.

Pain management programmes These are characterized by their high psychological content and emphasis on self-help. Many of the early North American programmes were run as 3- or 4-week in-patient programmes within which a wide range of education and therapy was offered (Loeser *et al*. 1990). Restoration of fitness and increase in tolerance for exercise, however, has always been a fundamental component in such programmes. Modern pain management programmes are often run on an out-patient basis. A group of 10–12 patients will attend once or twice per week and be required to carry out a range of homework assignments (Main and Parker 1989). The psychological effect of being part of a group on the reduction of distress and on general confidence should not be underestimated. Traditionally such programmes have been offered to chronically incapacitated patients. Some pain management programmes have been geared almost exclusively towards return to work, while others have taken a broader view of rehabilitation. It is normally only in functional restoration programmes that specific attention is directed towards the role of spouses and families in maintaining pain behaviour (Romano *et al*. 1991). Such multidisciplinary treatments are superior to other forms of treatment for chronic pain (Nicholas *et al.* 1992), but maintenance of treatment gains is particularly important and needs to be specifically addressed during the programme itself (Turk and Rudy 1991).

In general pain management programmes are now established as an important approach to chronic back pain. Unfortunately, many published research studies are methodologically flawed (Flor *et al.* 1992). Future studies need to determine which patients are likely to benefit from a vigorous exercise programme (Manniche *et al.* 1991) and which require a programme including a higher proportion of psychological techniques.

Advances in psychological assessment have identified an increasingly wide range of potential therapeutic targets for psychological intervention. While it is acknowledged that there will always be a need for individual psychological therapy, it is becoming increasingly evident that training of the whole treatment team in psychological treatment skills needs to be included. In attempting to overcome patients' fears and anxieties about increasing function, it is important that the patients receive clear and consistent advice from all members of staff. All staff should be familiar with the general principles of pain management and skilled in 'reorienting' the patient successfully towards a more self-directed approach.

Treatment is however delivered in a socio-economic context. The health care system needs reappraisal if rehabilitation is to be facilitated rather than hindered by government policy regarding benefits and allowances.

The relationships between assessment and treatment: a reappraisal

Recent research and literature reviews have highlighted the importance of psychological factors in the development of low back pain. The importance of early mobilization and return to work has been recognized (Waddell 1992) and an equally 'aggressive' approach for the identification of individuals at risk of developing chronic back pain or failing to respond to rehabilitation is required. While it may be comforting to construe socio-economic factors as extrinsic to the treatment process, they clearly have a major influence on outcome and in the case of many of the North American pain management programmes have become a specific objective in terms of return to work.

A number of recommendations for psychological assessment and intervention are outlined in Table 12.5. Clearly at the stage of *primary prevention*, psychological treatment as such is not appropriate, but evaluation of the occupational environment may indicate the need for an appraisal of the psychological risk factors (Bigos *et al.* 1990). Although psychological influences on pain may be addressed within the overall teaching of some of the back schools, such themes are not normally given more than limited attention (Zachrisson Forssell 1980).

Table 12.5 Recommendations for the psychological assessment and prevention of low back pain

Primary prevention
  Assess the psychological stress in work environments
  Educational approach towards back care and stress reduction

Secondary prevention
  Identify risks of low back pain recurrence
  Multidimensional assessment of individuals 'at risk'
  'Preventative pain management programme'

Occupational rehabilitation
  Socio-economic evaluation of low back pain
  First stage psychological screening (distress and fear–avoidance beliefs)
  Second stage psychological evaluation (coping strategies and psychophysiology)
  Individualized or group rehabilitation

Secondary prevention programmes are aimed at patients with acute or subacute back pain. While the traditional back school approach has not been found to be particularly effective (Nordin *et al.* 1992) this may in part be a function of problems with the selection of patients and their compliance with treatment (Schlapbach and Gerber 1991). While such back schools may be more effective in achieving return to work when incorporated within more extensive rehabilitation programmes (Choler *et al.* 1985; Lindstrom *et al.* 1992), use of health care resources by symptomatic acute back pain patients is significantly reduced if psychological principles are incorporated into the management plan (Fordyce *et al.* 1986). In clearly symptomatic patients adequate physical and psychosocial appraisal is fundamental to any decisions regarding treatment and treatment failure is frequently a direct consequence of inadequate decision making based on an oversimplistic model of pain (Waddell 1987). The same observations may be made in the context of occupational rehabilitation. An approach to clinically oriented psychological assessment and intervention is shown at the foot of Table 12.5.

Guidelines for treatment

1. Far too much emphasis in planning treatment programmes has been placed on the *self-report* of pain. It is also necessary to consider physical, psychological, and socio-economic factors in the assessment of the low back pain patient and in the selection of treatment (Waddell 1992).

2. The use of simple *screening questionnaires* does not constitute adequate psychological assessment. In addition to screening for treatable mental illness, psychological assessment should contain an appraisal of the patients' pain, disability, distress, beliefs about treatment, and coping strategies (Main and Spanswick 1991). Most of these can be assessed by means of existing scales, but it is important that the assessor has a thorough understanding of their use. A *behavioural assessment* (Keefe and Hill 1985) is of considerable value and may be essential in planning treatment. Clinical assessments of illness behaviour during physical examination or videotaped assessment may be useful, but should only be carried out by adequately trained observers and as no more than a screening procedure (Waddell and Richardson 1991). Determination of suitability for psychological treatment will require a clinical interview designed to assess disproportionate disability, response to previous treatment, the psychosocial concomitants of the pain behaviour, and to elicit objectives for pain management (Main and Spanswick 1991). When possible, *psychophysiological assessment* should also be undertaken (Flor *et al.* 1990). This is of importance not only in deciding whether to offer a specific psychophysiological programme, but also in educating the patient about the nature of chronic pain. New assessment techniques are being continually developed. It is important however that any new test is evaluated carefully in clinical practice before it is uncritically accepted.

3. The role of benefits (such as disability awards, invalidity awards, and mobility allowances) and medico-legal issues have to be considered, together with an evaluation of occupational factors (Bigos *et al.* 1990). Although some pain programmes will not accept any patients currently involved in compensation claims (statistically, such patients respond less well), they are often significantly distressed and alleviation of distress may outweigh the extra financial costs (Loeser *et al.* 1990).

4. Selection for psychological treatment must be on the basis of identified distress or disproportionate disability, together with a willingness to consider a self-help approach once this has been carefully explained (Main 1992). Selection must never be made on the basis of tests alone. A robust 'no nonsense' approach has already been tried with many of these patients in an effort to get them to improve their mobility. The topic of assuming more responsibility for increasing their mobility must be handled with sensitivity.

5. As early as the first contact a potential treatment contract has been established. Much of the distress evident in patients with chronic back

pain is a consequence of bad medical management in the form of poor doctor–patient communication, unnecessary assessment, and ineffectual treatment which does not match promises patients have been given (Main and Parker 1989). Psychological management should not be conceptualized as an alternative to pharmacological treatment. Rather it represents a radically different way of understanding back pain and the back pain patient. It need not just be a desperate attempt to 'salvage' the patient when everything else has failed, but a perspective which needs to be considered from the early stages of consultation. Psychological treatment is no more a 'miracle cure' than anything else; it has a place as part of an interdisciplinary treatment approach which offers sensible physical treatment when indicated, good doctor–patient communication, and considers the *person* who has the low back problem and not just their back.

Specific attention must also be directed towards the successful integration of psychological methods with other treatments, such as physiotherapy and pharmacology. A wider perspective on the role of psychological influences needs to be taken since psychological factors are important not only in the outcome of psychological interventions but also conservative treatment, both at the chronic (Main *et al.* 1992) and the acute stage (A. Roberts, submitted). Intensive psychological interventions are sometimes necessary even in rehabilitation programmes with a strong exercise component (Mayer and Gatchel 1988).

Recommendations for service development

In the UK, the Department of Health, in recognition of the need to address the increase in low back disability, has established a Clinical Services Advisory Group with the remit of reappraising future priorities for back pain research. It is likely that this will lead to a major re-examination of the way in which services for back pain are delivered. The following recommendations (which are the personal views of the authors) are offered for consideration.

Community education

Most bouts of low back pain do not even require a consultation with a general practitioner. The general public need to know when consultation is appropriate and this means they must be offered an alternative to a narrow medical model in which low back pain can be demythologized and demedicalized.

With more serious back trouble, appropriate investigation and acute treatment should lead to a management plan in which the responsibility is shared by the doctor and patient. The promotion of *self-help* will require a prolonged and active media campaign, directed not only at the general public but also at health care professionals.

Improved health care delivery

The range and quality of educational material (both verbal and visual) about back pain must be improved, on the premise that access to sensible and accurate information will enhance the likelihood of optimal health care delivery. Materials should be made available to the general public, patients in treatment, general medical practitioners, undergraduate and postgraduate students, and also to hospital specialists involved in the treatment and management of back pain. It should be anticipated that although a general perspective may be offered, specific educational modules are likely to be needed for each of the groups mentioned.

As part of this process, it is to be hoped that communication between patients and professionals and also between professionals will be improved. Unfortunately this problem is not always sufficiently recognized by the professional staff themselves. A wider range of video-based training materials should be developed for this purpose.

Much greater emphasis must be placed on earlier intervention and prevention. The distinctions between primary, secondary, and tertiary prevention (Weiser and Cadraschi 1992) must be borne in mind, since the level of professional input required is dependent on the stage of chronicity. Services of varying levels of sophistication in assessment and treatment should be established. These could range from simple clinics using only simple screening procedures to larger much more comprehensive interdisciplinary treatment programmes (see Chapter 4).

Assessment of risk

Recent studies reviewed by Halpern (1992) have identified basic ergonomic factors important in prevention. Psychosocial factors are also of importance (Weiser and Cedraschi 1992) and research into the development of chronic incapacity has demonstrated the major role of psychological factors in the prediction of outcome (Main *et al.* 1992). Similar 'risk' factors have been identified for patients with acute back pain (A. Roberts, submitted) and suggest a role for psychological intervention much earlier in the treatment process.

With back problems lasting longer than approximately 6 weeks a psychosocial assessment should be undertaken and a management strategy developed which includes both medical treatment and psychosocial rehabilitation. A plan to maximize the maintenance of treatment gains should be part of the overall strategy.

Changes in health care policy

The essence of psychological treatment is to develop the individual's personal responsibility for their back pain and to maximize their capacity to control and manage it. The limitations of the traditional disease model of back pain and the restricting role of the benefit system (and assessment for benefits) need to be recognized and reorganized if optimal psychological management is to be achieved. It is important to recognize that low back pain treatment and management take place within the confines of the health care policy of a particular country. In the UK, the benefit system mitigates against successful rehabilitation: attempts to return to part-time work, as a sensible stage in returning to full-time work, can endanger invalidity benefits. It is time to consider a benefit system which reinforces progress in rehabilitation, promotes learning of appropriate self-care procedures, and encourages people to return to work. A number of other countries have a much better integration between medical and occupational rehabilitation. Unfortunately, at a time of high unemployment, it is parficularly difficult for patients with back problems to return successfully to the workplace.

Recommendations for design and delivery of health care for back problems

This review of the nature and efficacy of psychological methods of management has illustrated not only the value of psychological methods of management of low back pain, but also has highlighted a number of major limitations in the disease model. As far as psychological management is concerned, a number of objectives would seem to be appropriate.

1. Establishment of adequate biopsychosocial assessment in clinical and occupational settings.

2. Identification of patients at risk of chronic incapacity or in need of psychological treatment.

3. Prevention of iatrogenic disability and distress by avoiding unnecessary investigations and speculative or inadequate medical or psychological treatment.

4. Development of psychological techniques designed to enhance patients' responses to rehabilitation.

5. An increase in the sophistication of current psychological therapy both for individuals and in groups.

Conclusions

A review of the wide-ranging influence of psychological factors in the development of chronic back pain and response to treatment makes the case for a biopsychosocial approach (Waddell 1992). Although this chapter has concentrated on the specific problem of back pain, the arguments have wider implications for understanding chronic incapacity in general. There are considerable similarities to the problems of patients with other illnesses, such as chronic fatigue syndrome, fibromyalgia, irritable bowel syndrome, and non-specific chest pain (see Chapters 16, 14 and 18). We believe that not only is a biopsychosocial perspective relevant to all these disorders, but that many of the principles of psychological intervention and management described for back pain (and in the previous chapter) have a more general relevance to the understanding, prevention, and management of chronic disability.

Acknowledgements

To Professor S. Bigos for permission to precis, in the form of text and two tables, some of the key features from his 1990 article.

References

Allen, D.B. and Waddell, G. (1989). An historical perspective on low back disability. *Acta Orthopaedica Scandinavica.* **60**, (Suppl. 234) 1–23.

Bigos, S.J., Battie, M.C., Nordin, M., Spengler, D.M., and Guy, D.P. (1990). Industrial low back pain. In *The lumbar spine*, (ed. J.N. Weinstein and J.W. Wiesel), pp. 846–59. W.B. Saunders, Philadelphia.

Bonica, J.J. (1990). History of pain concepts and therapies. In *The management of pain*, (2nd edn), (ed. J.J. Bonica), pp. 2–17. Lea and Febiger, Philadelphia.

Choler, U., Larsson, R., Nachemson, A. *et al.* (1985). 'Back pain: attempt at a structural treatment program for patients with low back pain. Unpublished report. Cited in Nordin *et al.* (1992).

Cram, J.R. (1990). *Clinical EMG for surface recordings*, Vol 2. Clinical Resources, Nevada City.

Flor, H., Birbaumer, N., and Turk, D.C. (1990). The psychobiology of chronic pain. *Advances in Behaviour Research and Therapy*, **12**, 47–84.

Flor, H., Fydrich, T., and Turk, D.C. (1992). Efficacy of multidisciplinary pain treatment centers: a meta-analytic review. *Pain*, **49**, 221–30.

Fordyce, W.E. (1976). *Behavioral methods in chronic pain and illness*. C.V. Mosby, St Louis.

Fordyce, W.E., Brockway, J., Bergman, J.A, and Spengler, D. (1986). Acute back pain: a control group comparison of behavioral versus traditional management methods. *Journal of Behavioral Medicine*, **9**, 127–40.

Hall, H. and Iceton, J.A. (1983). Back school. An overview with specific reference to the Canadian back education units. *Clinical Orthopaedics*, **179**, 10–17.

Halpern, M. (1992). In *Baillière's clinical rheumatology 6 (3) Prevention of low back pain: basic ergonomics in the workplace and clinic*, (ed. M. Nordin and T.L. Vischer), pp. 705–30. Baillière Tindall, London.

Hazard, R.G., Fenwick, J.W., Kalisch, S.M., Redmond, J., Reeves, V., Reid S. *et al.* (1989). Functional restoration with behavioural support: a one year prospective study of patients with chronic low back pain. *Spine*, **14**, 157–61.

Jacobsen, E. (1962). *You must relax.* (4th edn). McGraw-Hill, New York.

Keefe, F.J. and Hill, R.W. (1985). An objective approach to quantifying pain behavior and gait patterns in low back pain patients. *Pain*, **21**, 153–61.

Lindstrom, I., Ohlund, C., Eek, C., Wallin, L., Peterson, L.E., and Nachemson, A. (1992). Mobility, strength and figures after a graded activity program for patients with subacute low back pain. A randomized prospective clinical study with a behavioural therapy approach. *Spine*, **17**, 641–52.

Linton, S.J. and Kamwendo, K. (1987). Low back schools: a critical review. *Physical Therapy*, **67**, 1375–83.

Loeser, J.D., Seres, J.L., and Newman, R.I. Jr (1990). Interdisciplinary, multimodal management of chronic pain. In *The management of pain*, (2nd edn), (ed. J.J. Bonica), pp. 2107–20. Lea and Febiger, Philadelphia.

Main, C.J. (1992). Psychological treatment. In *The lumbar spine and back pain*, (4th edn), (ed. M.I.V. Jayson), pp. 487–505. Churchill Livingstone, Edinburgh.

Main, C.J. and Parker, H. (1989). The evaluation and outcome of pain management programmes for chronic low back pain. In *Back pain: new approaches to rehabilitation and education*, (ed. M. Roland and J.J. Jenner), pp. 129–56. Manchester University Press, Manchester.

Main, C.J. and Spanswick, C.C. (1991). Pain: psychological and psychiatric factors. In *Pain mechanisms and management*, (ed. J.C.D. Wells and C.J. Woolf). *British Medical Bulletin*, **47**, 732–42.

Main, C.J., Wood, P.L.R., Hollis, S., Spanswick, C.C., and Waddell, G. (1992). The distress and risk assessment method: a simple patient classification to identify distress and evaluate the risk of poor outcome. *Spine*, **17**, 42–52.

Manniche, C., Lundberg, E., Christensen, I., Bentzen, L., and Hesselsoe, G. (1991). Intensive dynamic back exercises for chronic low back pain: a clinical trial. *Pain*, **47**, 53–63.

Mattmiller, A.W. (1980). The California back school. *Physiotherapy*, **66**, 118–22.

Mayer, T.G. and Gatchel, R. (1988). *Functional restoration for spinal disorders: the sports medicine approach.* Lea and Febiger, Philadelphia.

Mayer, T.G., Gatchel, R.J., Mayer, H., Kishino, N., Keeley, J., and Mooney, V. (1987). A prospective two-year study of functional restoration in industrial low back injury. *Journal of the American Medical Association*, **258**, 1763–7.

Melzack, R. and Wall, P.D. (1965). Pain mechanisms: a new theory. *Science*, **150**, 3699–709.

Nicholas, M.K., Wilson, P.H., and Goyen, J. (1992). Comparison of cognitive-behavioral group treatment and an alternative non-psychological treatment for chronic low back pain. *Pain*, **48**, 339–47.

Nordin, M., Cedraschi, C., Balague, F., and Roux, E.B. (1992). Back schools in the prevention of chronicity. In *Baillière's clinical rheumatology 6 (3) common low back pain: prevention and chronicity*, (ed. M. Nordin and T.L. Vischer), pp. 685–703. Bailliere Tindall, London.

Ready, L.B. and Edwards, W.T. (1992). *Management of acute pain: a practical guide (IASP task force on acute pain)*. IASP Publications, Seattle.

Romano, J.M., Turner, J.A., Friedman, L.S., Bulcroft, R.A., Jensen, M.P., and Hops, H. (1991). Observational assessment of chronic pain patient–spouse behavioral interactions. *Behavioural Therapy*, **22**, 549–67.

Schlapbach, P. and Gerber, N.S. (1991). Back school. *Rheumatology*, **14**, 25–33.

Sternbach, R.A. (1974). *Pain patients: traits and treatment*. Academic Press, New York.

Turk, D.C., and Rudy, T.E. (1991). Neglected topics in the treatment of chronic pain patients: relapse, non-compliance and adherence enhancement. *Pain*, **44**, 5–28.

Turk, D.C., Meichenbaum, D.H., and Genest, M. (1983). *Pain and behavioral medicine: a cognitive-behavioral perspective*. Guilford Press, New York.

Turner, J.A. and Romano, J.M. (1990). Cognitive-behavioural therapy. In *The management of pain*, (2nd edn), (ed. J.J. Bonica), pp. 1711–21. Lea and Febiger, Philadelphia.

Waddell, G. (1987). A new clinical model for the treatment of low back pain. *Spine*, **12**, 632–44.

Waddell, G. (1992). Biopsychosocial analysis of low back pain. In *Baillière's clinical rheumatology 6 (3) common low back pain: prevention and chronicity*, (ed. M. Nordin and T.I.L. Vischer), pp. 523–57. Baillière Tindall, London.

Waddell G. (1993). Simple low back pain: rest or active exercise? *Annals of Rheumatic Diseases*, **52**.

Waddell, G. and Richardson, J. (1991). Clinical assessment of overt pain behaviour by physicians during routine clinical examination. *Journal of Psychosomatic Research*, **136**, 77–87.

Waddell, G., Morris, E.W., DiPaola, M.P., Bircher, M., and Finlayson, D. (1986). A concept illness tested as an improved basis for surgical decisions in low back disorders. *Spine*, **11**, 712–19.

Waddell, G., Somerville, D., Henderson, I., Newton, M., and Main, C.J. (1993). A fear–avoidance beliefs questionnaire (FABQ) and the role of fear–avoidance beliefs in chronic low back pain and disability. *Pain*, **52**, 157–68.

Weiser, S. and Cadraschi, C. (1992). Psychosocial issues in prevention of low back pain. In *Baillière's clinical rheumatology 6 (3) common low back pain: prevention and chronicity*, (ed. M. Nordin and T.L. Vischer), pp. 657–84. Baillière Tindall, London.

Woolf, C.J. (1991). Central mechanisms of acute pain. In *Proceedings of the VIth World Congress on Pain*, (ed. M.R. Bond, J.E. Charlton, and C.J. Woolf), pp. 25–34. Elsevier, Amsterdam.

Zachrisson-Forssell, M. (1980). The back school. *Spine*, **6**, 104–6.

13 Dysmorphophobia in plastic surgery and its treatment

Tim E.E. Goodacre and Richard Mayou

Dr Goodacre and Dr Mayou suggest that the aetiology of dysmorphophobia and the general approach to management has much in common with other functional somatic symptoms. Since Goodacre is a plastic surgeon, their chapter is largely written from a surgical perspective. However, the general principles of management also apply to dysmorphophobia in other settings.

The authors begin by reviewing the psychology of normal appearance and the role of aesthetic surgery in general. It is apparent that many patients, whose appearance is not regarded as abnormal by others, obtain great psychological benefit from surgery. In contrast, a small proportion of patients have a very poor outcome and it is this subgroup who attracted the interest of psychiatrists. Published clinical descriptions of dysmorphophobia are generally unsatisfactory and reflect the substantial biases in the sample studies. However, the authors conclude that those who have major mental illness and those who have notably vague and unrealistic expectations of the ways in which surgery might change their lives are least likely to benefit from surgery.

The authors believe that surgery is often an effective treatment for those who are preoccupied with their appearance, but that in those cases where the surgeon is doubtful about the indications, joint surgical and psychiatric assessment and management is important. There is a role for psychiatric treatment as an alternative to surgery and this may include the treatment of major psychoses and depression, as well as cognitive behavioural therapy. Whatever the proposed treatment, sympathetic assessment and discussion of management with patients and families is essential.

Introduction

A normal appearance is considered by most people to be an important determinant of social acceptance. Surgery to change appearance has been sought for centuries for a variety of reasons, including the intention of removing a source of mental distress and of enhancing well-being. Most patients requesting plastic surgery have an obvious abnormality of appearance, but a minority of those who seek help have an apparently inappropriate and excessive subjective concern about perceived deformity, which in objective terms may be minimal or even non-existent. These patients often consume considerable medical resources and yet remain dissatisfied and distressed. As a result, plastic surgeons are especially likely to suffer persecution and litigation by disappointed patients.

This chapter aims to describe this group of patients, review what is known of the effectiveness of treatment, and outline a strategy for their management. In order to do so, however, we begin by setting their condition within the context of the psychology of appearance and of the range of aesthetic ('cosmetic') surgery. We suggest that the principles of management of 'misinterpretation' of appearance are similar to those described in other chapters for misinterpretation of physical symptoms.

Understanding the patient's beliefs and anxieties may lead to successful treatment, whereas failure to accept and to deal with the reality of the patient's complaint and underlying beliefs may lead to increased distress, disability, and dissatisfaction. The relevant psychiatric literature is sparse and is based on highly selected and extreme cases. Case series of body image problems reported by plastic surgeons suggest generally good results, but usually give disappointingly little information about those who have poor outcome.

The problem

Psychology of normal and abnormal appearance

A large anthropological literature describes the very considerable cultural influences which shape beliefs and behaviour concerning physical appearance and dress. Dissatisfaction with appearance is very common in the general population, especially in women and in certain subgroups such as athletes and ballet dancers (Thompson 1991). In a survey of 258 college students, 70 per cent agreed with one of three questions based on the three principle DSM-IIIR criteria for body dysmorphic disorder and 28 per cent agreed with all three (Fitts *et al.* 1989). Psychological research has largely been concerned with obesity and other eating disorders, but other worries about body shape and individual features are also frequent (Slade 1994). It has been consistently found that there is little relationship between self-rated physical attractiveness and ratings by others, whilst there are associations between such self-ratings and self-esteem, confidence, and social skills (Feingold 1992).

Awareness of congenital disfiguring defects becomes apparent in early childhood, whereas worry about developmental disproportion is likely to be become prominent only in early adolescence. It seems that reactions to acquired disfigurement are most severe when this occurs in adolescence or later. Overall, reactions to disfigurement are not closely related to the objective severity of the abnormality. There appears to be no correlation between the objective defect and the extent of any psychopathology

(Harris 1982; Hill-Beuf and Porter 1984; Wengle 1986). Characteristic behavioural responses have been described and include defensive behaviours, such as camouflage, restriction of activities, avoidance, and difficulties with personal relationships (Harris 1982). The onset of worries is often attributed to the critical remarks and behaviour of others. There is no doubt that those who are disfigured have to suffer frequent and hurtful comments as well as intrusive scrutiny from other people, especially in childhood (Harris 1989). For example, in his large study of 750 patients seeking cosmetic surgery, Reich (1969) identified the desire 'to eliminate a feature causing self-consciousness, unwelcome attention, or adverse comment' as the principle motivating factor in 59 per cent of the group, although he also pointed to a number of possible subconscious factors. Since teasing about some element or other of body appearance is almost uniformly experienced by all members of society at some time or other, it would appear to be an inadequate explanation for why certain people subsequently become acutely sensitive.

Personality vulnerability is clearly important and has often been described in psychodynamic terms. Harris (1982) hypothesized that '. . . the factors which determine whether or not a subject becomes self-conscious of an abnormality of appearance are circumstantial and constitutional' and that 'the constitutional factor could be the subject's aestheticality — his innate sensitivity of aesthetic perception'. Others have suggested that extreme narcissism was the most significant factor separating cosmetic rhinoplasty patients from other control groups. Whatever the role of such psychosocial variables it would seem that although teasing may be one precipitant of the request for surgery it is a less important aetiological factor than has been generally acknowledged. We prefer the more comprehensive approach to predisposing, precipitating, and maintaining factors as described throughout this book for all types of functional somatic symptoms.

Aesthetic surgery

This branch of plastic surgery has been defined as being devoted to the normalization of abnormal appearance for the relief of psychological distress which stems from self-consciousness of the abnormality (Harris 1989). We can identify four broadly defined groups of abnormality (Table 13.1). Those in the first group (congenital conditions) are frequently referred for treatment before maturity by concerned parents and it is helpful to consider the factors that drive patients to request a change in appearance separately. Several categories can be defined.

Appearance outside social norms A significant proportion of patients seeking surgery (at least 50 per cent in the first author's experience) request

Table 13.1 Types of abnormal appearance presenting for aesthetic surgery

	Group	Examples	Usual age of presentation
1.	Congenital malformations	Bat ears Skin blemishes Cleft lip/palate	Childhood and adolescence
2.	Developmental disproportion	Large/small breasts Large nose 'Jodhpur' hip fat	Late teens and young adults
		Gynaecomastia Buck teeth	(Usually childhood)
3.	Ageing processes	Sagging cheeks Baggy eyelids Drooping breasts Post-partum abdomen Skin laxity/striae	Age 40 years onwards
4.	Consequences of injury and disease	Scars, tattoos Acne Surgical loss (breast, nose, ear, etc.) Facial palsy	All ages

it for the correction of a bodily feature which is outside the normal distribution of size or shape for their social group. This is usually a rational and understandable request, with a predictably good outcome. Examples would be the woman with little or no breast tissue, who wishes to look 'normal' in a society in which breasts have an association with femininity or the person with prominent teeth which results in others not taking him/her seriously. Some conditions cannot be surgically corrected (such as dwarfism). Some patients try to change their condition without resort to surgery, for example by gluing back bat ears or dieting excessively to lose breast tissue. Occasionally this may lead to a secondary psychological disorder, such as bulimia or anorexia, but this does not contraindicate surgery and is not an indicator of dysmorphophobia. The secondary condition frequently disappears when the primary physical abnormality is dealt with and sometimes in a most spectacular way in cases where psychological treatment has failed.

Perceived adverse social response   In this related group the main factor driving the patient to surgery is an adverse external response to one or other of their features (Table 13.2). Within this group, doctors need to

Table 13.2 Areas of preoccupation with appearance

Facial flaws	Minor scars, deep wrinkles, mild acne
Minor asymmetries	Nasal tip bulges, wide or narrow nasal base, upper eyelid fullness, slightly asymmetric cheeks (normal in all people)
Facial prominences	Chubby cheeks, minor nasal lumps, receding chin on full set of teeth, etc.
Facial shape	Too wide, too narrow, too long, too short, 'an ugly shape', etc.
Size or shape of other body parts	Breasts, buttocks, genitals, abdomen, hands and feet
Minor skin blemishes or scars anywhere on the body	

be aware of the very considerable cultural variations in what is regarded as normal appearance, for example the considerable social implications which loss or damage to a bodily part creates in some societies. Compared with the preceding category, the bodily 'feature' may be within the normal distribution of society, but be seen by the patient as the stimulus for adverse comment and therefore actively disliked. These patients may already have taken considerable steps to minimize their psychological distress, such as avoiding certain forms of social contact or undressing in front of anyone else.

Although in many ways similar to the first group, motivation for surgery is much more complex and the potential for post-surgical disappointment far greater. Since their well-being depends upon removing the source of adverse comments and anxiety, their response to surgery will to some extent be governed by how they feel others have changed their attitudes to them as well as to their own perceptions of the change.

This diverse group of patients includes those who perceive that society has 'dumped them on the scrap-heap' because they look old or feel that they are stigmatized as a member of one or other racial group because they possess a characteristic nose, lips, or facial structure. Some of those within this group will have very minimal deformities, but still be entirely rational in their approach, and be satisfied with surgery. An example might be the television actor whose features, albeit 'normal', look unfavourable from certain camera and lighting angles.

It is within this group that the patients who are the subject of this chapter also fall. They may have a minor feature which they consider to be 'abnormal', or even no abnormality at all other than a self-perception of being ugly, which they might attribute to one or other (usually facial)

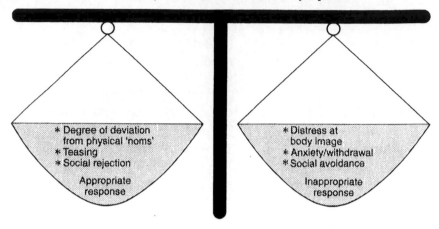

Fig. 13.1   Response to concern about appearance

feature. Their response to this perceived body image is excessive, and may manifest itself in anxiety states, paranoid symptoms (ideas of reference), delusions of being laughed at, and as the reason behind unemployment. These factors will be enlarged upon later, but the difficulty in separating this group from those with an appropriate response can be illustrated by the concept of a balance (Fig. 13.1). The greater the actual deformity (as perceived by 'normal' outside assessors with experience of the whole variety of patients seeking body image correction, rather than by the patients, friends, and relatives who may carry all of society's prejudices and double-standards about 'cosmetic surgery'), the greater the 'allowable' patient response before the balance swings to the side of inappropriateness. There is, of course, a spectrum of appearance which constitutes the left side of this balance, from those with a clearly abnormal appearance, through those with minor abnormalities, to those generally regarded as of normal appearance. There is, equally, a wide range of response which constitutes the right side of the balance. Some of those with undoubtedly abnormal appearance are phlegmatic, while others are self-conscious and become socially limited. The definition of minimal deformity is obviously arbitrary, and is determined by cultural and social factors. There is a large 'grey area' of patients with some sort of minor abnormality whose response to their deformity varies from the mild to the strong. However, there are clearly a group at the far extreme whose response is pathologically excessive and can be classsified as dysmorphophobic.

Although a large number of patients (perhaps 30–40 per cent of the total seeking cosmetic surgery) fall within this second category, only a minority have such an inappropriate response as to require immediate referral to a psychiatrist. Reich (1969) suggested 1–2 per cent. Similarly Fukuda (1977) suggests in a review of Japanese patients that 2 per cent of all patients in a plastic surgery out-patient department could be regarded as having severe psychiatric symptoms. Of 179 patients in this category, 22 had delusions and 26 were 'polysurgical addicts'. However, in an ideal setting with no restriction upon resources, a far larger proportion might benefit from formal psychiatric and/or clinical psychological assessment. Although there are few psychiatrists and psychologists working primarily with these patients, there is some evidence to suggest that easy access to a clinical psychologist can reduce the frequency of inappropriate operations (E. Bradbury, personal communication).

Beautification   A third group of patients seek aesthetic surgery for beautification rather than for the correction of any perceived 'deformity'. This relatively small group (perhaps 5 per cent of the total seeking cosmetic surgery in the UK at present) is slowly becoming more conspicuous and is likely to continue to do so as the social acceptability of such surgery increases. There has, of course, always been a tendency for the 'beautiful people', especially women, to rise in social standing. However, the rise of mass media, including the dramatic increase in visual exposure of successful figures via television has lead to a stronger association between success and beauty.

These patients are usually highly informed and motivated and include a subgroup of those seeking changes of appearance for fashion (the 'Madonna lips', 'Michael Jackson nose', etc.). Such people, who perhaps should not be called 'patients' at all, are important in creating the predominant image of 'plastic surgery' in the minds of those whose need to change appearance relates to definite physical pathology. This distorted image lead to a sense of shame and sometimes disgust in the subject and only increases the dilemma facing many needy patients.

Suppressed desire for surgery   It is widely believed that there are many other people who do not seek surgery but would like to have some alteration to one or other aspect of their body image, despite having a reasonably appropriate view of their appearance and fully accepting that others see them as being within normal limits. Evidence to support or refute this suggestion is virtually non-existent, but it is likely that such people are swayed sufficiently by the comments of their peers and relatives and by the unpalatable practical and financial difficulties and other aspects of undergoing surgery, to tolerate aspects of their appearance which they would ideally like to change. In recent years increased public acceptance of cosmetic surgery has been accompanied by increasing demand from people who would formerly have not considered the possibility.

The outcome of surgery   The efficacy of plastic surgery in satisfying the desires of patients for a changed appearance is well documented. However, the difficulty in subdividing patients with differing degrees of deformity (such as nasal humps) has meant that there have been no studies comparing social outcome in those with an appearance slightly outside the average with those with an entirely average appearance. Anecdotal teaching in plastic surgery traditionally suggests that the latter group are far less likely to be satisfied with surgery and, indeed, can become a 'millstone around the neck' of any surgeon who has the misfortune (or poor judgement) to operate upon them. In a study comparing purely 'cosmetic' rhinoplasty patients with post-traumatic deformity rhinoplasty patients, Slator and Harris (1992) challenged this traditional teaching and introduced the concept of 'aestheticality' to describe the heightened response of some patients to a minimal deformity by the norms of most of society. They went on to suggest that, whilst cosmetic rhinoplasty patients will usually be pleased with their surgery, they remain sensitive to and self-conscious of their appearance. They also have high expectations and are aware of and are troubled by minor imperfections. Reich's (1969) comment in his 1970 paper still remains true: 'While it is generally agreed that the incidence of psychiatric disorders is high amongst the group who are concerned with purely marginal deformities, opinions vary as to the place of plastic surgery in dealing with these cases. This variation appears to depend not only on whether the author is a plastic surgeon or a psychiatrist, but also on the existence of a personal bias, based on his own psychological make-up as well as on his professional experience.' There seems to have been little advance in this dilemma since the statement was made 23 years ago.

Apart from Reich's (1969) series of 750 applicants for cosmetic surgery there have been numerous reports of case series for particular procedures, including augmentation mammoplasty, rhinoplasty, face lift, and recontouring for deformities in the width of the face. Results must be interpreted with considerable caution (Wengle 1986), since little is known about the measures used. Furthermore, there has been a dramatic increase in the number of cosmetic operations and selection criteria have changed. It is apparent that many of the patients who request cosmetic surgery appear normal both clinically and as assessed by psychological tests. It is also evident that there is no simple relationship between the degree of psychopathology and the motivation for surgery. Severe psychopathology is rare and the outcome from surgery is usually excellent. These accounts of surgical series are consistent with plastic surgeons' clinical experience that many patients with apparently minimal deformity have an excellent outcome, with improvement in mood, confidence, and social lives.

Overall, cosmetic surgery results not only in improved satisfaction but also benefits in self-assessments of attractiveness, confidence, quality of relationship, sexuality and ability to cope with stress. Positive changes in psychometric testing have also been demonstrated. However, since reports of surgical series have generally concentrated on good outcome for the majority, we know little about those who have a poor outcome. The characteristics of those patients may well be rather different from the arbitrarily selected group of severe psychiatric series with dysmorphophobia.

The dysmorphophobic patient

The history of the term dysmorphophobia and of its classification both as a primary disorder and as a secondary feature of other psychiatric disorders has been well reviewed (Hay 1970; Phillips 1991; Hollander *et al.* 1992*a*). The term dysmorphophobia was introduced in 1891 by Morselli. It has was widely used within European psychiatry, but is rarely mentioned in the USA. It is usually classifiable as an over-valued idea, but may occasionally be delusional. Hay (1970) reintroduced it into modern British literature in 1970 with a review based on 17 cases and on a study of 45 patients requesting surgery because they were dissatisfied with their noses. Independently, but several years later, Andreasen and Bardach (1977) described six patients in a paper published in the USA. Most case series have been small and it is unclear how subjects were selected. Comparison with consecutive surgical series suggests they represent an arbitrary extreme of a spectrum of concern about appearance.

Although Hay (1970) considered dysmorphophobia to be a symptom and Andreasen and Bardach (1977) entitled their paper "Dysmorphophobia: symptom or disease?" the term has recently been used as a diagnostic category. It was referred to as a form of atypical somatoform disorder in DSM-III (Phillips 1991) and *body dysmorphic* disorder was introduced as a separate primary category within DSM-IIIR. This condition was differentiated from as *delusional disorder, somatic type*, and other conditions detailed in Table 17.1 (Hollander *et al.* 1992*b*). DSM-IV allows a co-morbid diagnosis of *Delusional Disorders: Somatic Type*. ICD-10 includes body dysmorphic disorder and dysmorphophobia (non-delusional) in a list of subgroups within *hypochondriacal disorder*. There remain serious difficulties in those definitions which make the arbitrary distinctions on a spectrum between, on the one hand concern and dissatisfaction with appearance common in the general population and, on the other, a severe psychiatric disorder. This has led to arguments about the nature of the association with depression and obsessive–compulsive disorder. We believe that it is more appropriate to consider dysmorphophobia as a common functional syndrome, similar to the many others considered in this book, which is frequently, but not universally, associated with several types of psychiatric disorder (Table 13.3). Psychiatrists see a small proportion of such patients, particularly those with severe handicaps and major management problems; plastic surgeons see a much wider population, but still a self-selected subgroup.

This chapter is concerned with dysmorphophobia as a symptom among those seeking plastic surgery. Dysmorphophobia also presents to dermatologists: complaints of facial skin roughness and redness, excessive sweating, hair baldness and hair loss, and excessive bodily hair have all been recorded.

Table 13.3 Body image disorders

1. Dysmorphophobia
Body dysmorphic disorder
Secondary to major psychiatric disorder
2. Social phobia
3. Eating disorders
4. Obsessive-compulsive disorder
5. Transsexualism

Clinical features

The clinical features of dysmorphophobia as described in case reports and series and reviews (Hay 1970; Andreasen and Bardach 1977; Frank 1985; Phillips 1991; Hollander *et al.* 1992*a*; Nreziroglu and Yaryura-Tobias 1993) are summarized in Table 13.4. There is a wide range of individual variation in the severity and pattern of symptoms. Subjects may be extremely secretive and avoid all mention of their worry or may go out of their way to mention their supposed defect and to seek reassurance. Some can describe clear dissatisfaction with a particular body feature and of the change that they desire; others are more vague. Some see surgery as offering a prospect of improving their own body image and self-esteem and thereby enabling them to achieve confidence in changing their own lives, whereas others believe that surgery will achieve magical changes in their circumstances and in the behaviour of others. Many patients attribute problems at work and even unemployment to their body image.

Presentation to the surgeon

Unlike most patients seeking plastic surgery, the dysmorphophobic patient often presents him or herself directly to the plastic surgeon for treatment. The majority of truly dysmorphophobic patients will present in their late

Table 13.4 Clinical features of dysmorphophobia

Onset
 History of low self-esteem
 Usually in adolescence
 Precipitation by teasing, distressing incidents

Symptoms
 Often ill defined
 Unrealistic expectations of benefits
 History of previous worries about appearance and failed surgery.

Preoccupation with appearance
 Rumination
 Preoccupation with reactions of others
 Concern that appearance results in misjudgments about character, ethnic origins
 Self-examination (looking in mirrors, examining photographs, etc.)

Defensive behaviour
 Secrecy (occasionally insistent on mentioning in conversation)
 Avoidance of public situation (especially changing rooms, swimming, etc.)

Social relationships
 Low self-esteem
 Difficulty in friendships
 Social problems
 Avoidance

Mood
 Depression
 Social anxiety

Consultation
 Often initial difficulty in admitting concern
 Repeated consultation
 Dissatisfied with medical care

teens and early twenties and this has been reflected in the DSM-IV estimate of onset being most common from adolescence through to the third decade. There has almost always been a considerable delay between onset of the complaint and presentation to the specialist. If there is any detectable blemish or physical abnormality (however insignificant), it is likely that the passage of the patient from the primary practitioner to the specialist (usually either plastic surgeon or dermatologist, rarely psychiatrist) will have been relatively rapid. In the more severe cases with no perceptible deformity, the patient will frequently have demanded second opinions, 'shopped around' for sympathetic doctors, or self-referred to private practitioners. After initial rebuttal at early consultations, the patient frequently attends with a sympathetic relative or friend for support. This person may well support the cause of the patient well beyond what he or she deems realistic because of experience of the patient's distress.

Although there may be a wide variety of psychological symptoms, there is always an overwhelming concern about some aspect or other of the physical appearance. It is common for the patient to complain of one or other of these symptoms in a strange and poorly defined way, which often alerts the physician to the predominantly psychological nature of the disorder. Occasionally the patient will present a catalogue of very minor facial features which culminate in the overall impression of ugliness and extreme lack of self-esteem. However, there is not an overall disturbance of the body image as with patients suffering from eating disorders or transsexualism.

In addition to the presenting anomaly, the patient often forcefully expresses the dramatic impact of the perceived deformity on their social lives. Social contact may progressively be avoided and the patient's occupation affected by the presumption of being talked about or laughed at. There may be an almost morbid preoccupation with not being observed from certain angles and, in particular, of being photographed.

Co-morbid psychiatric disorder

Most authorities would agree that dysmorphophobia has a complex aetiology which is unrelated to one specific cause or underlying condition. Certain personality traits have been associated with the syndrome, with obsessive–compulsive, schizoid, and narcissistic being predominant. Other factors identified are perfectionism, self-criticism, insecurity, sensitivity, and reservedness. However, several of these factors are also associated with those whose request for cosmetic plastic surgery is deemed entirely 'appropriate', and in whom such surgery produces a successful outcome.

The co-morbid psychological disorder most often reported is depression, but this may be secondary to the dysmorphophobia. Schizophrenia and other psychotic symptoms have been reported to occur in some psychiatric case series. Although eating disorders reflect a 'total' body image problem, it is not uncommon for patients seeking cosmetic plastic surgery to starve themselves (or become bulimic) in attempts to change the bodily 'defect' which disturbs them so much. However, these patients usually do not exhibit the features of dysmorphophobia and in the first author's experience often sustain spectacular and lasting 'cures' of the eating disorder when the surgery is undertaken.

Comparison with other functional symptoms

Although the aetiology of dysmorphophobia is disputed, the suggested aetiological factors indicate clear parallels with other conditions described in this book. The problems are those of individual interpretation or misinterpretation, of minor or perceived abnormalities affected by presenting events, previous experience, and the reaction of others, including doctors. There is some evidence that unsympathetic medical care may substantially worsen problems.

Treatment

Reports of the outcome for patients diagnosed as suffering from dysmorphophobia are generally poor (Hay 1970; Phillips 1991; Hollander *et al.* 1992*a*). This is not surprising since failed surgery and other treatment has often been an inclusion criterion for the diagnosis. On the other hand, there is little guidance available on the selection of patients for aesthetic surgical procedures, since plastic surgery case series give a generally optimistic view but provide scant detail about the characteristics or outcome of patients who present with little objective abnormality.

Role of surgery

There is considerable divergence of opinion among plastic surgeons about the benefit (or otherwise) of operating on such patients (Reich 1975; Harris 1989). Consensus is strongest concerning the cases in whom there is no perceived deformity at all. Few surgeons would agree to change a normal appearance to satisfy a patient's misperception. However, the larger group consists of those with minor deformities and here the accepted teaching is, again, that the surgeon should decline to operate under any circumstances whatsoever. It is almost impossible to define 'normal' in such circumstances, but an example might be a patient claiming to have a lump on the bridge of a nose which is objectively entirely straight. In such cases, opinion on management amongst surgeons would range from a vigorous confrontational approach with associated refusal to discuss surgery, to a sympathetic hearing which might entertain the possibility of surgical modification of the part in order to satisfy the patient's desires regardless of the surgeon's own perception. The majority of plastic surgeons would steer a middle course between these two extremes of management, often relying upon the clarity with which the patient can express their discontent at whichever feature troubles them to decide whether a surgical solution is conceivable.

Andreasen and Bardach (1977) suggested that because the imagined defect is emotional rather than physical, the patient will rarely be satisfied with the result of surgery and will often find another 'defect' postoperatively for which further surgery is demanded. This view was vigorously challenged by Reich (1969, 1975) in the previously mentioned study of 750 consecutive patients requesting surgery to change appearance.

Of 518 reviewed post-surgery, there were no cases of acute psychological breakdown or of attempted or actual suicide. These he contrasted with four cases who exhibited a deterioration of mental health, two of whom attempted suicide, following the refusal of a psychiatrist to allow an operation for the improvement in appearance of a feature which constituted significant objective deformity (in the opinion of the surgeon). These findings were in general agreement with other authors (Edgerton *et al.* 1993) who challenged the belief that neurotic or psychotic patients were a poor risk in respect of cosmetic operations.

The paucity of the literature dealing specifically with the dysmorphophobic group of patients and their response to treatment (other than largely anecdotal case reports) leaves little to guide the surgeon faced with a patient with an excessive response to a minor deformity. The authors cautiously recommend combined management with a psychiatrist, only embarking upon surgery with considerable pre- and post-operative psychological support for the patient.

Table 13.5 Indicators of poor outcome

Vague ill-defined dissatisfaction
Unrealistic expectation that surgery will lead to change in the behaviour of others
Previous failed surgery
Paranoid beliefs
Major psychiatric disorder
Pressure for surgery from others

Factors which are believed to be associated with a poor outcome from surgery are summarized in Table 13.5. We believe that caution about surgery is indicated when the abnormality is barely detectable (if at all). The presentation in such cases is often forceful, associated with anxiety that the doctor is going to reject the plea as unnecessary, and an inability to be rational about the anomaly. The social effect of the supposed anomaly is often stressed at length (for example, the inability to hold down a job, to make friends, etc.) The patient almost always relates examples of being talked about or laughed at because of the supposed anomaly at some time or other. This may relate back to a single episode or comment in the distant past, which appears to have been magnified out of all proportion. Newspaper clippings or other examples of people reported to be suffering in a similar way may be produced as evidence of the 'genuineness' of the request.

During the consultation the patient will often avoid revealing the affected part to the doctor and may do so only under some duress or with extreme embarrassment. Such patients are often unwilling to be seen by medical students or clinic nurses. In these circumstances the doctor almost always feels uncomfortable about the request for surgery and, indeed, the prospect of operating on the patient. This sense of unease should lead to further assessment rather than to either an abrupt refusal or to agreement to the patient's demand for surgery.

Non-surgical treatment

The minority of patients with major depression, delusional disorders, or other major psychiatric disorders require specific psychiatric treatment. The role of psychiatric and psychological treatments in the majority of patients who do not have such disorder is less certain. In the absence of adequate treatment trials, clinical experience and the findings of a number of small uncontrolled surveys suggest that such treatments can be effective (Phillips 1991; Phillips *et al.* 1993). Psychological treatments may also be an important adjunct to surgery, since the patient with low self-esteem and social problems may well require psychological treatment to make the most of any improvement in self-confidence.

Antipsychotic drugs   A proportion of patients with dysmorphophobia either have or later develop schizophrenia or other delusional disorders. Standard antipsychotic medication is appropriate in such cases (Phillips 1991). However, such drugs are generally unhelpful for patients with dysmorphophobia which is not clearly of delusional intensity.

Antidepressants   Case reports have reported the successful treatment of dysmorphophobia with antidepressant drugs (Phillips *et al.* 1993). The drugs used include clomipramine, fluoxetine, and other tricyclics. Lithium, benzodiazepines, and electroconvulsive therapy (ECT) have also been reported as unsuccessful treatments. Overall, antidepressants appear mostly likely to have an important role when there are clear symptoms of major depression and the newer selective serotonin reuptake inhibitors (SSRI) drugs may be more effective than tricyclic agents (Phillips *et al.* 1993).

Psychological treatments   The complex nature of this condition and the lack of understanding of its cause, have led to a diverse range of psychological treatments being proposed (Phillips 1991). These include psychoanalytical psychotherapy, behavioural treatment with systematic desensitization (Munjack 1978), and a cognitive behavioural approach (Marks 1987). In a review of treatment for body image disturbance, Thompson (1991) states 'At the top of the list (i.e. of treatment for body dysmorphic disorder), I would place the cognitive techniques, followed by some of the behavioural exposure techniques'. Case reports are encouraging. For example, Marks and Mishan (1988) have described good results from exposure therapy in five chronically disabled dysmorphophobic patients. Improvement in avoidance and anxiety were associated with reduction in concern about appearance.

Practical guidelines

The majority of patients present initially to their general practitioner. They may be referred to the plastic surgeon or, occasionally, if the psychological response to the deformity is thought to be inappropriate, to the psychiatrist. It is important at these early stages to detect any major psychiatric disorder, since the consequences of surgery in these patients can be catastrophic and has been implicated in the violent deaths of plastic surgeons.

When considering surgery, the balance of appropriateness of response has to be determined by the surgeon, who assesses the patient's attitude and expectations alongside the ease (or otherwise) of correcting the supposed deformity. In the minimal but distinct lesion (perhaps a minimal nasal hump or small blemish) it may be that the ease of surgery makes a simple procedure justifiable, even in the presence of an exaggerated response by the patient. Such decisions should not be taken by junior members of the surgical team and the patient should be made fully aware of the experienced surgeon's views and the probability of the success of the procedure.

If the deformity seems minimal and the surgeon suspects dysmorphophobia, surgery should not be discussed further until a formal psychiatric assessment has been completed. If surgery is even tentatively held out as a possibility, further psychiatric management can be prejudiced and the situation may never be satisfactorily resolved. Once the patient has been seen by a psychiatrist, surgery can still proceed if it is felt to be of likely benefit. The support of the psychiatric team is desirable to provide back-up if post-surgical complications occur. Fukuda (1977) has advocated a decisive refusal of operations for patients who refuse psychiatric assessment.

Patients with objectively normal appearance or with concerns about appearance that fall within the normal range of aging or development require further assessment. The fundamental requirement of the management of such cases is sympathetic listening and discussion of the patient's beliefs and wishes. Just as with the symptoms described in other chapters, understanding the patient's beliefs and taking them seriously can produce a useful consultation with a positive outcome. Refusal of referral to a specialist or a dismissive reaction from a specialist are likely to worsen the problem. Significant distress and disability and realistic expectations of the benefits of surgery are indications for intervention. The doctor's personal view of what is normal should not be allowed to prevent a surgical procedure that may transform a young person's life. As stated above, the

Table 13.6 Management of patients with 'excessive' worries about their appearance

1. Full and sympathetic assessment and discussion

2. Identify and treat major psychiatric disorder

3. Consider surgery

4. Consider psychological treatment
    Psychotropic medication
    Cognitive behavioural therapy
    Psychotherapy

symptoms are often ill-defined, but the belief should clearly not be of delusional intensity.

A plan for consistent management is outlined in Table 13.6. It is important to stress both the need for a sympathetic hearing for a group of patients who have often had to struggle for some time to reach a wise opinion and the need for consistency in advice, particularly when general practitioners, plastic surgeons, and psychiatrists may all be involved at different times. Given that there is some debate within almost all health care systems on the funding and accessibility of services to correct body image, it would seem to be a basic right for all with such concerns to have at least a consultation on the value of surgery or psychiatric treatment.

Combined approach to consultation

Ideally, every patient presenting to a plastic surgeon with a complaint about an aspect of their body image would be seen initially by a clinical psychologist or psychiatrist with an interest in body image disorders. The aim would be to screen out cases for whom surgery would be inappropriate and to advise the surgeon on the management of the remaining cases. In the UK, this model has only been employed in private practice, where cost constraints are less severe than in the NHS. Pruzinsky (1988) has written about a collaborative approach in the USA, stressing the need for specialization and integration of the psychotherapist, whilst Bradbury, E.T. (personal communication) has reported the value of a similar system in the UK. It may well be that such procedures are highly cost-effective ways of ensuring the best use of resources and improving the quality of life. In more usual circumstances, the surgeon can choose to insist upon a pre-consultation psychiatric assessment whenever any of the criteria for dysmorphophobia are mentioned in the referring letter. An insistence upon a formal and full GP referral letter before agreeing to consultation is one means by which surgeons prevent the arrival of inappropriate patients into the consulting room. Although no data is available on the subject, it is the authors' impression that a far higher proportion of 'self-referrals' fall into the dysmorphophobic category than those who have followed the normal channel of referral.

Once the surgeon has encountered a patient with possible dysmorphophobia, the consultation should be steered firmly in the direction of a team review in order to determine the best management. It is helpful if the surgeon can introduce the fact that they work together with a specialist in the area of body image problems early on in the interview; the more natural and frequent this can be made to seem, the less the patient will feel branded 'mad' or feel that they are not being taken seriously. The surgeon would ideally introduce the patient to the psychologist or psychiatrist personally in a combined clinic setting. This rarely occurs outside private practice and care should then be taken to ensure that any cross-referral process occurs smoothly. In referring the patient, it is helpful if the surgeon gives some indication of their assessment of the value of surgery, as well as advice on whether they feel that further surgical assessment is really indicated. In the more severely dysmorphophobic cases, the prospect of a further visit to the plastic surgeon is sufficient to mar the value of any psychological treatment. Likewise, it is important that the psychiatrist indicates clearly to their surgical colleague whether they feel that psychological or other non-surgical treatment would be of value and, if so, where it fits within the overall treatment strategy.

A good working relationship between the surgeon and psychiatrist or psychologist is essential for this form of combined management. This will often take time to develop, as the 'barriers' of specialty and terminology must be overcome. The special importance of clear and comprehensive referral letters must be stressed particularly if patients with complex psychological conditions are being referred to surgeons.

Surgical outcome

Assessing the outcome of surgical intervention is difficult in plastic surgery and there is little published data. Since the goal of treatment is a satisfied patient with an acceptable perception of their appearance, there has to be something of the 'salesman's approach' in the pre- and post-operative surgical consultations. These need not be in any way deceptive; rather they should emphasize the positive yet realistic outlook of the mutually agreed treatment protocol. In particular, the post-operative consultation should avoid asking questions (such as 'do you think that you look better now?) and concentrate rather on positive affirmation that the problem has now been resolved. A post-operative visit to the psychiatrist should be arranged before the procedure is undertaken to ensure that the surgery is seen as only part of the overall management of the problem.

The dissatisfied patient

When dealing with a patient with an imagined or minimal disorder, the potential risk of dissatisfaction with treatment is high. Despite careful pre-operative counselling and preparation, the mystique surrounding surgery can reinforce unrealistic expectations. A critical period for determining the patient's acceptance or otherwise of the changes wrought by surgery is in the first 2 weeks following dressing removal. Constant positive reinforcement is required from the surgeon and associated medical and nursing staff if the new 'normal' state of the patient's appearance is to be fully accepted. If the patient exhibits early dissatisfaction, it is important to spend as much time as necessary to hear their point of view.

If the surgeon feels that a technical error has occurred in the surgery, then an open yet positive approach is recommended, usually leading to further surgery. The more common situation of dissatisfaction with an acceptable surgical result should be managed initially by a sympathetic but firmly confident attitude. Ideally, immediate post-operative counselling or therapy will have been arranged, so that the patient is carefully 'managed' through the critical early days following surgery. In practice this ideal is difficult to follow and there may be some delay in the patient undergoing review by the psychologist or psychiatrist who undertook the pre-operative assessment. The temptation for the surgeon to refuse to see the patient again should be resisted and instead the opposite approach of reviewing more frequently than normal adopted. This concept of support of the disgruntled patient ensures that they do not feel rejected by the surgeon and enables them to express all their anxieties and concerns. It is particularly in such cases that the mutual support of a close surgeon-psychiatrist liaison is invaluable in sharing the load.

The most difficult aspect of management concerns the patient who continues to demand surgical intervention. Without prior psychiatric involvement, such requests can be pathologically persistent and disquieting to the surgeon. The surgeon frequently feels bereft of colleagues in such instances, since professional friendships rarely stretch to taking on another's problem cases. However, it is vital that the patient feels that their problems are being taken seriously and case conferences with the opportunity for the patient to hear several opinions are valuable management strategies. Ultimately, however, the non-surgical treatment options outlined above will be the only lasting hopes for obtaining patient satisfaction and the goal of all consultations and case conferences should be directed to persuading the patient to accept this line of management. The subject of managing the dissatisfied plastic surgery patient has been well discussed by Goldwyn (1984).

Conclusion

Review of published evidence supports the clinical experience of plastic surgeons that the outcome of surgery is excellent for many people who are dissatisfied with their appearance and who seek surgery for well formulated reasons. At the same time, it is apparent that a small minority of those who consult not only have no clear objective disfigurement, but describe a severity of disability and a degree of expectations which arouse concern about their mental health. Even among these patients the outcome of surgery can be highly beneficial. Psychiatric and psychological treatment are an alternative especially for those unsuitable for surgery. It is unfortunate that reports of psychotropic drug treatment and psychological management are largely based on small series of severely disabled subjects as those methods may be especially useful for patients with less extreme problems.

The authors recommend collaborative surgical and psychiatric assessment which considers not only surgery, but also the use of antidepressant drugs and the cognitive techniques that have been used successfully to treat other groups of patients with functional somatic symptoms (such as chest pain and backache). However, further evaluation of the treatment of dysmorphophobic patients is clearly indicated and, in particular, attempts to define the condition more precisely and delineate the indications for surgery and psychiatric treatment more clearly.

References

Andreasen, N.C. and Bardach, J. (1977). Dysmorphophobia: Symptom or disease? *American Journal of Psychiatry*, **134:6**, 673–6.

Edgerton, M.T., Langman, M.W., and Pruzinsky, T. (1993). Patients seeking symmetrical recontouring for "perceived" deformaties in the width of the face and skull. *Aesthetic Plastic Surgery*, **14**, 59–73.

Feingold, A. (1992). Good-looking people are not what we think. *Psychological Bulletin*, **111:2**, 304–41.

Frank, O.S. (1985). Dysmorphophobia. In *Current themes in psychiatry*, (ed. R.N. Gaind, and F.I. Fawzy). Spectrum, London.

Fukuda, O. (1977). Statistical analysis of dysmorphophobia in an out-patient clinic. *Japanese Journal of Plastic and Reconstructive Surgery*, **20**, 569–77.

Goldwyn, R.M. (1984). The dissatisfied patient. In *The unfavourable result in plastic surgery: avoidance and treatment*, (ed. R.M. Goldwyn). Little, Brown, and Co, Boston.

Harris, D. (1982). The symptomatology of abnormal appearance an anecdotal survey. *British Journal of Plastic Surgery*, **35**, 312–23.

Harris, D.L. (1989). Cosmetic surgery. *Annals of the Royal College of Surgeons of England*, **71**, 195–9.

Hay, G.G. (1970). Dysmorphophobia. *British Journal of Psychiatry*, **116**, 399–406.

Hill-Beuf, A. and Porter, J.D.R. (1984). Children coping with impaired apperance:social and psychologic influences. *General Hospital Psychiatry*, **6**, 294–301.

Hollander, E., Neville, D., Frenkel, M., Josephson, S., and Liebowitz, M.R. (1992). *Psychosomatics*, **33**, 156–165.

Hollander, E., Neville, D., Frenkel, M., Josephson, S., and Liebowitz, M.R. (1992.) Body dysmorphic disorder. Diagnostic issues and related disorders. *Psychosomatics*, **33**, 156–165.

Marks, I.M. (1987). *Fears, phobias, and rituals*. Oxford University Press, Oxford.

Marks, I.M. and Mishan, J. (1988). Dysmorphophic avoidance with disturbed bodily perception. *British Journal of Psychiatry*, **152**, 674–8.

Munjack, D.J. (1978). The behavioural treatment of dysmorphophobia. *Journal of Behavioural Therapy and Experimental Psychiatry*, **9**, 53–6.

Nreziroglu, F.A. and Yaryura-Tobias, J.A. (1993). Body dysmorphic disorder: phenomenology and case descriptions. *Behavioural Psychotherapy*, **21**, 27–36.

Phillips, K.A. (1991). Body dysmorphic disorder: the distress of imagined ugliness. *American Journal of Psychiatry*, **148:9**, 1138–49.

Phillips, K.A., McElroy, S.L., Keck, P.E., Pope, H.G. and Hudson, J.1. (1993). Body dysmorphic disorder: 30 cases of imagined ugliness. *American Journal of Psychiatry*, **150**: No 2, (Abstract)

Pruzinsky, T. (1988). Collaboration of plastic surgeon and medical psychotherapist: elective cosmetic surgery. *Medical Psychotherapy*. **1**, 1–13.

Reich, J. (1969). The surgery of appearance: psychological and related aspects. *Medical Journal of Australia*, **2**, 5–13.

Reich, J. (1975). Factors influencing patient satisfaction with the results of esthetic plastic surgery. *Esthetic Surgery*, **55**, 5–13.

Slade, P.D. (1994). What is body image? *Behaviour Research and Therapy*, **32**, 497–502.

Slator, R. and Harris, D.L. (1992). Are rhinoplasty patients potentially mad? *British Journal of Plastic Surgery*, **45**, 307–310.

Thompson, J.K. (1991). *Body image disturbance, assessment and treatment*, Pergamon Press, New York.

Wengle, H.P. (1986). The psychology of cosmetic surgery: a critical overview of the literature 1960-1980-Part 1. *Annals of Plastic Surgery*, **16**, 435–443.

PART 4 SPECIFIC SYMPTOMS

14 Psychological treatment of irritable bowel syndrome and abdominal pain

Francis Creed

Professor Creed describes the high prevalence of functional gastrointestinal complaints — as high as 22 per cent in some community studies — as well as the considerable health care costs incurred by this group of patients. He also points out that patients attending a gastrointestinal clinic with irritable bowel syndrome differ from those in the community and that these critical differences have to be addressed in treatment. An overview of the physical and psychological treatment of patients with functional bowel disorders is presented and the importance of selection criteria and concurrent psychiatric illness emphasized. Professor Creed describes those factors that predict a favourable outcome with psychological treatment and concludes with practical guidelines for treatment.

Introduction

There are a number of important practical points to consider in the treatment of patients with irritable bowel syndrome and functional abdominal pain. First, these disorders are probably the most common functional syndromes in clinical practice, second, it is important to decide the most appropriate psychological intervention for a particular patient — a decision that is usually based on the duration of symptoms, third, engaging a patient in treatment is a critical process, and, fourth, it is important to be aware of the possibility of underlying organic disease such as Crohn's disease.

The latter two issues are dealt with in Chapters 5 and 8 and will not be addressed in detail here.

The prevalence of functional abdominal symptoms

It is well known that many patients attending a gastroenterology unit do not have organic disease. For example, in two district general hospital gastroenterology out-patient clinics in the UK 25 to 45 per cent of attenders were found to have functional complaints, including functional dyspepsia, irritable bowel syndrome, diarrhoea or constipation, or nonspecific abdominal pain (Harvey *et al.* 1983; Holmes *et al.* 1987).

The problem is less frequent and has been less well studied among medical in-patients. Nevertheless, the diagnosis of 'non-specific abdominal pain' (ICD code 785.5) is often made; it leads to observation in hospital and may result in laparotomy. Raheja *et al.* (1990) estimated that hospital admissions given this diagnosis cost the NHS £16.5 million per year (1980 figures). This group of patients clearly merit further study.

The diagnosis 'non-specific abdominal pain' includes patients who have an appendicectomy but in whom the appendix is found not to be inflamed (Donnan and Lambert 1976). It was this group of patients that, many years ago, led Oxford epidemiologists to link abdominal pain with psychiatric disorder. Rang *et al.* (1970) identified a group of young females admitted for appendicectomy but discharged with a diagnosis of 'undiagnosed abdominal pain', whose admission rate to a psychiatric unit over the 2 year study period was 13 times greater than expected. There have been no psychological treatment studies of these surgical in-patients but there is evidence that

(1) they have increased anxiety and abnormal illness behaviour (Joyce *et al.* 1986);

(2) a proportion of such patients are later diagnosed as having irritable bowel syndrome (Chaudhury and Truelove 1962; Lane 1973; Keeling and Fielding 1975).

There are no satisfactory studies of psychological aspects of abdominal complaints in general practice. The most common diagnosis in general practice in the digestive disease category is 'functional disorders of the stomach', reflecting the high rate of bowel symptoms in the community (Johnsen *et al.* 1986). Community studies, mostly performed in the USA, have demonstrated that up to 20 per cent of the population report bowel symptoms, the majority of whom have not consulted a doctor (Creed 1990). In the UK there is a similar high prevalence of individuals in the population who have experienced specific symptoms which fulfil 'Manning' criteria for irritable bowel syndrome (Whitehead *et al.* 1988; Jones and Lydeard 1992).

These studies confirm that bowel symptoms, including abdominal pain, are very common in the general population. Clinical assessment must address not only the patient's somatic symptoms, but also the reasons for

(1) attending the family doctor for treatment;

(2) referral to hospital.

The range of illness severity

In this overview patients with irritable bowel syndrome and abdominal pain will be considered at different stages along a pathway of severity. There may be patients in the community who develop bowel symptoms but do not seek medical help. It is not known whether these patients directly seek psychological treatment independent of medical consultations, although Blanchard *et al.* (1990) described a sample that included patients '(directly) seeking psychological treatment for their bowel symptoms'.

The next group of patients are those attending a general practitioner (GP); such patients experience more severe pain and more anxiety about serious illness than those in the general population who do not seek medical treatment. Two reports indicate that excessive anxiety about physical illness underlies consultation with the general practitioner for dyspepsia and irritable bowel syndrome (Lydeard and Jones 1989; Kettell *et al.* 1992). Some of these patients attending the general practitioner are referred to the hospital clinic; such patients are likely to have the most severe bowel symptoms, co-existing psychiatric symptoms, and the most severe illness worries.

Two groups of patients can be identified in clinical settings: those who respond to initial treatment and those who do not. Harvey *et al.* (1987) estimated that 85 per cent of irritable bowel syndrome patients respond to clinic treatment but 15 per cent do not. Psychological treatment therefore needs to be considered separately for each of the following groups:

(1)   GP attenders;

(2)   first time attenders at the hospital clinic who respond to treatment;

(3)   the non-responders or 'refractory' irritable bowel syndrome patients.

The available evidence concerns only the latter two groups.

The relative importance of physical and psychological symptoms

Having delineated three groups of patients, the next stage is to consider the relative importance of bowel symptoms and psychological problems in these groups. Treatment studies will then be considered in detail.

The severity of bowel symptoms   Two studies indicate that the bowel symptoms are more severe in those patients who consult doctors. Kettell *et al.* (1992) demonstrated that patients consulting a general practitioner had experienced more abdominal distention and more severe pain than

Table 14.1 Results of anxiety and depression scores on the Hospital Anxiety and Depression Scale (HADS) (Heaton *et al.* 1991)

	Anxiety	Depression
Clinic patients	11	6
Non-complainers	9	3
Controls	5	3

The table shows median scores for patients with irritable bowel syndrome attending a gastroenterology clinic, those in the community who have irritable bowel syndrome symptoms but do not seek medical treatment, and healthy controls in the community.

those persons in the community who reported symptoms of irritable bowel syndrome but who did not consult a doctor. The second study (Heaton *et al.* 1991) measured the severity of bowel symptoms using an 'intestinal suffering score'. The median 'intestinal suffering score' for patients attending a clinic was 88, compared with 27 for community sufferers who did not seek medical treatment and 17 in healthy controls. The latter reported mild bowel symptoms which were insufficient to merit the diagnosis of irritable bowel syndrome. Another study revealed that chronic attenders at a gastroenterology clinic report more severe pain than first time attenders (Guthrie *et al.* 1992).

The severity of the emotional disorder   The Heaton *et al.* (1991) study also included administration of the Hospital Anxiety and Depression Scale and the corresponding scores for anxiety and depression are shown in Table 14.1.

Clinic patients therefore have not only more severe bowel symptoms but also report more anxiety and depressive symptoms than healthy controls. These issues need to be addressed in treatment. There is, however, a third dimension to be considered: abnormal illness behaviour.

Abnormal illness behaviour and beliefs   Two papers have documented the increased scores on the Illness Behaviour Questionnaire (IBQ) among clinic attenders with functional bowel complaints (Colgan *et al.* 1988; Drossman *et al.* 1988). The suggestion that the increased IBQ scores might simply reflect more severe bowel symptoms was not supported by Drossman *et al.* (1988), who controlled for bowel symptom severity but still found significantly higher scores on the illness worry and disruption subscales of the IBQ in those subjects attending the clinic.

One further recent study is of interest. Gomborone *et al.* (1992) compared the Attitude to Illness Questionnaire scores of irritable bowel syndrome patients with depressed in-patients in a psychiatric unit. The former scored *higher* than both the depressed patients and other controls with organic gastrointestinal disease on the scales of *hypochondriacal beliefs*, *disease phobia*, and *bodily preoccupation*. This indicates the need to address these concerns as part of the psychological treatment.

The skills required in psychological treatment Psychological treatment should begin with those skills used by all doctors, not just those employed by psychologists and psychiatrists (Creed and Guthrie 1989). Such skills should be used by both general practitioners and gastroenterologists, but to date there has been little systematic study of their use. A survey of gastroenterologists in the USA showed that half of those in academic practice used 'personal psychological support' as the main treatment of patients with irritable bowel syndrome. The figure was less in gastroenterologists in private practice and in trainees. No further details of this study were published, but it suggests that difficult irritable bowel syndrome patients referred to academic gastroenterologists require considerable time in consultation.

In a recent audit of our own gastroenterology clinic, letters to the GP were screened for psychological aspects of treatment (Hamilton, personal communication). Only in a very small proportion were specific instructions for psychological treatment given. The largest proportion replied simply that no organic disease was found, suggesting possibly a 'technician's' role for the physician who has access to specialized investigations. In only 1 per cent was referral to the psychiatrist made.

Overview of evaluative research

Studies of patients presenting to the gastroenterology clinic

Randomized clinical trials of treatment for irritable bowel syndrome have been firmly criticized in an interesting article by Klein (1989). He outlined stringent criteria for an acceptable treatment trial and concluded that no satisfactory study had demonstrated unequivocal superiority of any active treatment over placebo. Klein's (1989) stringent criteria are necessary because of not only a pronounced placebo response but also the variable nature and severity of the symptoms seen in patients attending a gastroenterology clinic with this diagnosis. Klein (1989) advocates

(1) the recruitment of adequate numbers of patients, with a clear description of how they are selected;

(2) true random allocation;

(3) the use of sound measures of severity of symptoms to accurately detect change.

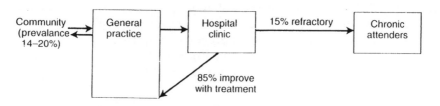

Fig. 14.1   Figure to illustrate the selection of patients reaching primary and secondary care with irritable bowel syndrome and the derivation of 'consecutive attenders' and 'refractory' groups, which have been entered into treatment trials

His paper was primarily concerned with the various drug treatments of irritable bowel syndrome, but the framework is also helpful in selecting the most satisfactory studies evaluating psychological treatments. In this section a number of studies will be discussed, all of which used ratings of both psychological and gastroenterological symptoms.

'Consecutive' versus refractory patients   There are six studies of psychological treatment of irritable bowel syndrome which have used both large numbers of patients and paid close attention to measures of symptom severity. Two have used cognitive behavioural treatment (Corney *et al*. 1991; E.B. Blanchard, unpublished), one stress management (Rumsey *et al*. 1989), a further two have used psychotherapy (Svedlund 1983; Guthrie *et al*. 1991), and one has used hypnosis (Whorwell 1984).

Four of the studies concluded that psychological treatment was significantly superior to a control condition in relieving bowel symptoms (Svedlund 1983; Whorwell 1984; Rumsey *et al*. 1989; Guthrie *et al*. 1991). On the other hand, two studies produced a negative result (Corney *et al*. 1991; E.B. Blanchard, unpublished). It is important to understand the reasons for this. Three of the successful studies were performed exclusively on patients with 'refractory' irritable bowel syndrome (Svedlund 1983; Whorwell 1984; Guthrie *et al*. 1991), whereas the fourth and the two unsuccessful studies (Rumsey *et al*. 1989; Corney *et al*. 1991; E.B. Blanchard, unpublished) were performed on a more general group of patients, most of whom had probably reported a more recent onset of symptoms (Fig. 14.1).

Selection criteria   The first three studies selected patients as follows. Corney *et al*. (1991) included patients who 'had symptoms for at least six months and were prepared to accept a trial which involved either psychological treatment or drug treatment'. No other data were provided regarding selection. Rumsey *et al*. (1989) included consecutive irritable bowel syndrome clinic patients, who were compared with those treated with medication alone. The description suggests that they were able to involve *consecutive* patients at a district general hospital gastroenterology clinic. E.B. Blanchard (unpublished) included patients 'seeking non-drug treatment for the IBS'.

For the refractory patients Svedlund (1983) indicated that 76 per cent had 'no improvement after previous treatment'. Whorwell (1984) also only included patients whose symptoms were refractory to conventional treatment. Guthrie *et al*. (1991) included patients who had symptoms for 1 year or more in the present episode and had been attending the clinic for at least 6 months without response to usual medical treatment.

Measure of symptoms – psychological scores   Two of the consecutive patient studies used the Hospital Anxiety of Depression Scale (HADS) and their scores can be compared with those of Heaton *et al*.'s (1991) study. The results were very similar: anxiety was more common than depression and the levels were very similar in the treatment studies of Rumsey *et al*. (1989) and E.B. Blanchard (unpublished) to those in the clinic population studied by Heaton *et al*. 1991.

Only one of the studies which included refractory patients used a psychiatric measure which is comparable to other studies. Guthrie *et al*. (1992) found that cases of depression were more common than cases of anxiety in their cohort entering the treatment study – this pattern is similar to chronic clinic attenders rather than recent attenders.

Measures of symptoms – gastrointestinal symptoms   Unfortunately no two studies have used the same measure of gastrointestinal symptoms, so a systematic comparison between studies is very difficult.

Psychological treatment   Behavioural therapy has been used in three studies of 'consecutive' patients attending a clinic. The 'refractory' patients have been treated by hypnotherapy and psychotherapy. Table 14.2 demonstrates that there are numerous differences between the groups of patients included in the two types of study. Thus, behavioural therapy has been used in patients with milder symptoms (both bowel and psychological symptoms) because the patients recruited have had less severe irritable bowel syndrome (consecutive attenders). Only one of the three studies has been successful, possibly because the 'less severe' group of patients showed a more marked placebo response, making it more difficult to demonstrate the effectiveness of behavioural therapy.

Table 14.2 An overview of psychological treatment trials (see text for details)

	Behaviour therapy	Hypnotherapy/ dynamic psychotherapy
Reduction in bowel symptoms	One out of three	Three out of three
Patient recruitment	Consecutive	'Refractory'
Psychological symptoms	Mild/anxiety	Severe/depression
Reduction in psychological symptoms	Significant in one only	psychotherapy + + hypnotherapy = ?
Poor prognostic indicators indicators	Trait anxiety	Hypnotherapy: anxiety or depression Psychotherapy: constant pain, absence of anxiety or depression

Reduction in psychological symptom scores   Table 14.3 demonstrates the differences between the five studies which reported psychiatric symptom scores before and after treatment for both treatment and control groups. In the study by E.B. Blanchard (unpublished), which used the Beck Depression Inventory, the control group experienced a *greater* reduction in symptom scores than the treatment group — hence the negative score in the right-hand column. The next study by Corney *et al.* (1991) used the Clinical Interview Schedule. The treatment group showed a greater reduction in psychiatric symptom score (21.3 per cent) compared with the control group (11.7 per cent), but the difference (9.5) was slight.

By contrast, the study by Rumsey *et al.* (1989) (which used the HADS) and by Svedlund (1983) (which used a unique scale of mental symptoms) showed a much greater reduction in psychiatric score in the treatment group than in the control group. The figures for the Guthrie *et al.* (1991) study are given both for the Psychiatric Assessment Schedule and the Beck Depression Inventory. Both indicate an enormous difference between treatment and control group, which may well underline the success of the treatment in reducing bowel symptoms. Guthrie has explained in Chapter 8 that the reduction of bowel symptom scores was highly correlated with reduction in psychiatric scores.

Predictors of outcome   Factors related to outcome in the treatment group during the first 3 months of the Guthrie *et al.* (1991) study included

(1)   current anxiety/depression (predicting a good response);

(2)   constant, as opposed to intermittent, pain (poor prognosis);

Table 14.3 Reduction in psychological symptom scores recorded in psychological treatment trials of irritable bowel syndrome

| | Percentage reduction of score | | |
	Treatment group (%)	Control group (%)	Difference
'Consecutive' patient studies			
Blanchard (1992) (BDI)	31.5	53	− 21.5
Corney *et al.* (1991) (CIS)	21.3	11.7	9.5
Rumsey *et al.* (1989) (HADS)	38.2	11	27.7
'Refractory patient studies			
Svedlund (1983) (mental symptoms)	35	7.7	27.3
Guthrie *et al.* (1991) (PAS)	76	8	68
(BDI)	68.7	23	45

BDI, Beck Depression Inventory.
CIS, Clinical Interview Schedule.
HADS, Hospital Anxiety and Depression Scale.

(3) irritable bowel syndrome symptoms clearly exacerbated by stress (good prognosis);

(4) the duration of weeks off work (poor prognosis in those with symptoms of longer duration).

Discriminant function analysis indicated that at 3 months after treatment a number of factors correctly classified 79 per cent of patients. These included intermittent versus constant pain, short duration of the present episode, presence of anxiety/depression, and number of sites of abdominal pain. However, at 1 year, the single factor 'intermittent versus constant pain' correctly classified outcome in 86 per cent of patients, that is, those with constant pain had a poor outcome.

Turning to other studies, E.B. Blanchard (unpublished) and Whorwell (1984) both examined outcome in terms of previous psychiatric status. They both found that anxiety or psychiatric symptoms at the beginning of the study predicted a *poor* response. In our own study, however, they predicted a good response (Guthrie *et al.* 1991). This suggests that psychotherapy may work in a different way from hypnosis or cognitive behavioural therapy.

Patients' opinions about psychological treatment   What do patients say helped them most? Svedlund (1983) found that the psychotherapy group rated 'increased understanding providing possibilities to change' three times more often than controls. Rumsey *et al.* (1989) reported a number of factors which patients found helpful: these included the beneficial effect of relaxation, the increase in feelings of control over the condition, increased understanding of how to deal with stress, and an increase in self-confidence. The Corney *et al.* (1991) study was less conclusive: 11 (50 per cent) of the 22 in the experimental group mentioned that their stomach pain had been helped compared with five (25 per cent) out of 20 in the control group. Six of the experimental group reported that their anxiety had been helped.

Chronic abdominal pain

The more severe forms of irritable bowel syndrome merge into a clinical picture of chronic abdominal pain which cannot be simply attributed to bowel dysfunction. This pain does not vary with defecation and the group can be delineated clinically as a separate subgroup of patients with functional bowel disorder (Thompson *et al.* 1992). In their descriptive paper, Drossman and Thompson (1992) indicated that these patients should be managed in a similar way to patients with chronic pain (see Chapter 11).

Practical management

It is clear from the above that three factors have to be considered in the management of patients with irritable bowel syndrome/chronic abdominal pain: the bowel symptoms, concurrent emotional distress, and abnormal illness beliefs and behaviour. These will be considered in turn.

Bowel symptoms − explanation and reassurance

Many patients referred to a psychologist or psychiatrist begin the consultation with a question about why the referral took place. The session must therefore commence with an explanation of the aetiology of irritable bowel syndrome/abdominal pain and how psychological factors make a contribution (see Chapter 5).

The therapist must have an explanatory model which is reasonably accurate and understandable by the patient. Explaining that emotions can affect the gut is important and providing examples of certain activities such as a visit to the dentist, sitting an exam, or a driving test causing 'butterflies in the stomach' is a good way of facilitating such an explanation. It is wise to establish that the patient fully understands this model before proceeding further.

The next point to make is that a subgroup of the population, perhaps one in five, are prone to develop abdominal pain with diarrhoea when under stress. A hallmark of the pain is its modification by defecation or passing flatus.

Next comes a *positive diagnosis* of irritable bowel syndrome. Typical features, which are much more common in irritable bowel syndrome than organic disease, are relief by defecation, passage of slime or mucus with the stools, bloating, varying sites of the pain, including dyspeptic symptoms, absence of weight loss, and passage of blood. At this point the patient may initiate a discussion about fear of cancer or other serious disease. These fears should be explored when they are mentioned. Many patients worry about serious physical illness, and this concern is usually increased by knowledge of a relative or friend whose symptoms, although similar to those of irritable bowel syndrome, were subsequently found to be caused by cancer, ulcer, or inflammation. It is necessary to explore each patient's worries about his/her own bowel symptoms. Sooner or later the therapist establishes that the patient has been reasonably reassured by the negative investigations, but there is still a nagging doubt. There are usually protestations at this stage that the pain is causing much suffering and 'something must be done'.

One then has to speculate about the actual cause of pain. It is best to be honest and say that the mechanism is not fully understood. There are, however, a number of research studies upon which an explanation can be based. These have found that the pain of irritable bowel syndrome can be reproduced when a balloon inserted into the colon is inflated (Swarbrick *et al.* 1980) and that patients with irritable bowel syndrome are particularly sensitive to this pain, developing it at a lower volume of distention than those who do not have irritable bowel syndrome. The observation that pain may be relieved by passing flatus or defecating lends further support to the notion that it is distension of the bowel that causes the pain. Having established that pain results from a distended bowel and that activity of the bowel may be related to stress, the next step is to proceed to possible lines of treatment.

Three forms of treatment can be offered. The first is aimed at altering the contents of the bowel. Bulking agents, such as Fybogel, are intended to soften the contents of the gut and prevent solid masses forming thereby leading to smooth propulsion of the contents along its length. The second line of treatment is to influence bowel function using a drug which affects the smooth muscles in the gut wall. These antispasmodic agents may be successful in relieving the pain in a proportion of people.

When neither of these simple treatments work a third more psychological type of treatment approach may be considered. It is well known that the gut has a rich nerve supply (this is why emotional reactions lead to butterflies in the stomach). If someone is severely stressed, this may result in abnormal gut contraction with pockets of high pressure and/or painful contractions. Therefore, any way of relaxing the person may lead to fewer of those signals reaching the gut which cause abnormal contractions. Some patients may have noticed that their symptoms improve at times when they are relaxed, for example on holiday. For example, one patient claimed that diet was the cause of his symptoms. He reached this conclusion because his regular trips to France, his wife's country of origin, were always associated with improved symptoms. He attributed this to a change in diet. It became clear in conversation, however, that he was also much more relaxed when he went on holiday to France. In particular, he was away from stressful situations at work which caused him concern.

The aims of these discussions with the patient are three-fold. First, one is hoping to help the patient to understand his/her condition more fully. Second, a positive explanation along these lines may help more than any amount of negative investigations in reassuring the patient that pain does not signify serious tissue damage. Third, it greatly improves the rapport between the patient and therapist if such a quasi-physiological discussion can take place; it can also help to prevent the patient from dismissing psychological treatment as irrelevant.

Emotional distress — psychological treatment

The first task is to detect and appropriately treat any anxiety state or phobic or depressive illness. It is reasonable to explain that treatment of the anxiety or depressive symptoms alone may lead to some improvement of the bowel symptoms or it might just make the person feel generally better in themselves. The treatment of these syndromes is the same as in any other setting. Psychological approaches are effective but antidepressant drugs may also be used (see Chapter 6).

In linking bowel symptoms and psychological factors, the use of a *bowel chart* is enormously helpful. The patient is asked to keep a daily record of the severity of the pain and bloating together with the number of bowel movements and the nature of the stools. For pre-menopausal women it is advisable to have a column for menstruation. A final column can be used to record whether the person has any noticeable stresses or disruptions in their life.

It should be explained clearly to the patient that the bowel chart is extremely important in monitoring symptoms and must be recorded diligently and accurately if the information is to be useful. At all subsequent visits to the clinic the bowel chart is reviewed. This monitoring is likely to reveal variations in bowel symptoms over time. This observation should be discussed with the patient with the aim of identifying patterns. It may then become clear that exacerbations are related to external events, in which case links between life stress and bodily symptoms can be made.

Some patients are resistant to the suggestion that bowel complaints are related in any way to stress. Such patients may avoid psychological treatment, but can be coerced into this approach if either of the following two conditions pertain. First, the patient may accept that they are tense and require help with this but will not acknowledge that the bowel symptoms are linked to the tension. Alternatively, the patient may be persuaded that all other treatments have been tried and a trial of relaxation or anti-depressants may be worthwhile simply 'to leave no stone unturned'. If the bowel chart is used the patient can be engaged in further discussions about the nature and variability of the symptoms and any possible precipitant. The advantage of this approach is that it will permit further consultations during which rapport and trust between patient and therapist may develop to the point where the patient feels able to discuss personal problems more freely. For this reason it is unwise to try and establish a contract of a number of sessions at the outset. It is sometimes better to adopt an empirical approach, encouraging the patient 'to wait and see' whether two or three further sessions help. The specific psychotherapy used may be either dynamic psychotherapy as described Chapter 8, or cognitive behavioural therapy as described in Chapter 7.

Abnormal illness attitudes and behaviours — overcoming resistance to psychological therapy

These aspects of irritable bowel syndrome are the most difficult to treat because they usually reflect an underlying resistance to a psychological approach. The patient may display abnormal illness behaviour during the consultation, for example exaggerated non-verbal complaints of pain, requesting a relative to re-enforce the description of extremely disabling pain (for example, 'I couldn't get out of bed yesterday because the pain was so bad, could I?'), denial of any psychological problem (even though the pain commenced at a time of bereavement or divorce), or an insistence that the pain dominates the person's life to the extent that they cannot leave the house except to visit the hospital.

It is worth addressing these attitudes and behaviours as they emerge. Care must be taken however to avoid making the patient feel threatened and gentle exploration is usually preferable to a direct challenge. The patient may emphasize the physical nature of their problem. This is an opening for the therapist to explain that all pain has both psychological and physical aspects, rather than just one or the other. Alternatively, the patient may describe in detail his or her extreme disability. This presents an opportunity for the therapist to ask what the patient's life would be like if he/she did not have the pain, and then to an examination of the difference between the patient's life before the symptoms began and the current situation. In this way the extent of the disability and other changes in life circumstance can be elicited.

It is also important to seek, often overcoming resistance in the process, a description of the important psychological events which have occurred in the patient's life over recent years and, in particular, those which preceded the onset of the symptoms. This discussion may reveal important life events which the patient is reluctant to disclose.

At this stage in the interview, it is worth repeating that the pain and/or bowel disturbance is severe and distressing. It is also worth pointing out that numerous promises of new treatments have failed to bring relief, and the patient was reluctant to have a psychological assessment for fear of the symptoms being dismissed as 'all in the mind'. This leads to a discussion of the importance of both physical and psychological factors in somatic complaints and the proposal of a plan to attempt to reduce disability, even though the symptoms may remain unchanged. These strategies are discussed more fully in Chapters 8 and 11.

Progress of treatment

At the first interview it often becomes clear that the patient is totally resistant to any form of psychological intervention. In these cases it is best to use the approach outlined for chronic pain or fatigue (see Chapters 11 and 16). For many other patients, however simply making the link between the symptoms and life stresses can result in significant improvement in their symptoms. Such improvements have been documented in the controlled trial by Guthrie *et al.* (1991) and is described in more detail in Chapter 8.

Conclusion

The essential components of psychological treatment that have been used in severe functional bowel disorder are also applicable to those patients with milder forms of the disorder seen in general practice or in gastro-enterology clinics. These components include establishing rapport with the patient, providing a positive diagnosis and a comprehensible explanation for the symptoms, and using negative investigations as secondary evidence. The patient's fears of disease must be addressed and abnormal illness behaviours (if present) sympathetically pointed out and explained. A positive approach of this nature should prevent the milder forms of functional bowel disorder from developing into more chronic forms, for which numerous investigations are often performed with little benefit to the patient.

References

Blanchard, E.B., Scharff, L., Schwarz, S.P., Suls; J.M., and Barlow, D.H. (1990). The role of anxiety and depression in the irritable bowel syndrome. *Behaviour Research and Therapy*, **28**, 401–5.

Chaudhury, N.A. and Truelove, S.C. (1962). Irritable colon syndrome. A study of the clinical features, predisposing causes, and prognosis in 130 cases. *Quarterly Journal of Medicine*, **31**, 307–22.

Colgan, S., Creed, F.H., and Klass, S.H. (1988). Psychiatric disorder and abnormal illness behaviour in patients with upper abdominal pain. *Psychological Medicine*, **18**, 887–92.

Corney, R.H., Stanton, R., Newell, R., Clare, A., and Fairclough, P. (1991). Behavioural psychotherapy in the treatment of irritable bowel syndrome. *Journal of Psychosomatic Research*, **35**, 46–9.

Creed, F.H. (1990). Functional abdominal pain. In *Somatization: physical symptoms and psychological illness*, (ed. C. Bass). pp. 141–70, Blackwell, Oxford.

Creed, F.H. and Guthrie, E. (1989). Psychological treatment of the irritable bowel syndrome: a review. *Gut*, **30**, 1601–9.

Donnan, S.P.B. and Lambert, P.M. (1976). Appendicitis: incidence and mortality. *Population Trends*, **5**, 26–8.

Drossman, D.A. and Thompson, W.E. (1992). The irritable bowel syndrome and a graduated multicomponent treatment approach. *Annals of Internal Medicine*, **116**, 1008–16.

Drossman, D.A., McKee, D.C., Sandler, R.S., Mitchell, C.M., Lowman, B.C., *et al.* (1988). Psychosocial factors in irritable bowel syndrome. A multi-variate study of patients and non-patients with IBS. *Gastroenterology*, **95**, 701–8.

Gomborone, J.E., Dewsnap, P.A., Libby, G.W., and Farthing, M.J.G. (1992). A specific illness-related schema in irritable bowel syndrome (IBS). *Abstract British Society of Gastroenterolgy*, S23.

Guthrie, E., Creed, F.H., Dawson, D., and Tomenson, B. (1991). A controlled trial of psychological treatment for the irritable bowel syndrome. *Gastroenterology*, **100**, 450–7.

Guthrie, E., Creed, F.H., and Whorwell, P.K. (1992). Outpatients with irritable bowel syndrome: a comparison of first time and chronic attenders. *Gut*, **33**, 361–3.

Harvey, R.F., Salih, S.Y., and Read, E.A. (1983). Organic and functional disorders in 2000 gastroenterology outpatients. *Lancet*, **i**, 632–4.

Harvey, R.F., Mauad, E.C., and Brown, A.M. (1987). Prognosis in the irritable bowel syndrome: a 5-year prospective study. *Lancet*, **i**, 963–5.

Heaton, K.W., Ghosh, S., and Braddon, F.E.M. (1991). How bad are the symptoms and bowel dysfunction of patients with irritable bowel syndrome. A prospective, controlled study with special reference to stool form. *Gut*, **32**, 73–9.

Holmes, K.M., Salter, R.H., Cole, T.P., and Girdwood, T.G. (1987). A profile of district gastroenterology. *Journal of the Royal College of Physicians*, **21**, 111–14.

Johnsen, R., Jacobsen, B.K., and Forde, O.H. (1986). Association between symptoms of irritable colon and psychological and social conditions and lifestyle. *British Medical Journal*, **292**, 1633–5.

Jones, R. and Lydeard, S. (1992). Irritable bowel syndrome in the general population. *British Medical Journal*, **304**, 87–90.

Joyce, P.R., Bushnell, J.A., Walsh, J.B.W., and Morton, J.B. (1986). Abnormal illness behaviour and anxiety in acute non-organic abdominal pain. *British Journal of Psychiatry*, **149**, 57–62.

Keeling, P.W.N. and Fielding, J.F. (1975). The irritable bowel syndrome: a review of 50 consecutive cases. *Journal of Irish College of Physicians and Surgeons*, **4**, 91–4.

Kettell, J., Jones, R., and Lydeard, S. (1992). Reasons for consultation in irritable bowel syndrome: symptoms and patient characteristics. *British Journal of General Practice*, **42**, 459–61.

Klein, K.B. (1989). Controlled treatment trials in the irritable bowel syndrome: a critique. *Gastroenterology*, **95**, 232–41.

Lane, D. (1973). The irritable colon and right iliac fossa pain. *Medical Journal of Australia*, **1**, 66–7.

Lydeard, S. and Jones, R. (1989). Factors affecting the decision to consult with dyspepsia: comparison of consulters and non-consulters. *Journal of the Royal College of General Practitioners*, **39**, 495–8.

Raheja, S.K., McDonald, P.J., and Taylor, I. (1990). Non-specific abdominal pain – an expensive mystery. *Journal of the Royal Society of Medicine*, **83**, 10–11.

Rang, E.H., Fairbairn, A.S., and Acheson, E.D. (1970). An enquiry into the incidence and prognosis of undiagnosed abdominal pain treated in hospital. *British Journal of Preventative and Social Medicine*, **24**, 47–51.

Rumsey, N., Wilkinson, S., and Walker, R. (1989). *A comparison of group stress management programmes with conventional pharmacological treatment in the treatment of the irritable bowel syndrome.* South Western Gastroenterology Group, Thurlstone.

Svedlund, J. (1983). Psychotherapy in irritable bowel syndrome: a controlled outcome study. *Acta Psychiatrica Scandinavica*, **67** (Suppl. 306), 1–86.

Swarbrick, E.T., Hegarty, J.E., Bat, L., Williams, C.B., and Dawson, A.M. (1980). Site of pain from the irritable bowel. *Lancet*, **11**, 443–6.

Thompson, W.G., Creed, F., Drossman, D.A., Heaton, K.W., and Mazzacca, (1992). Functional bowel disease and functional abdominal pain. Working Team Report. *Gastroenterology International*, **5**, 75–91.

Whitehead, W.E., Bosmajian, L., Zonderman, A., Costa, P., and Schuster, M.M. (1988). Symptoms of psychological distress associated with irritable bowel syndrome: comparison of community and clinic samples. *Gastroenterology*, **92**, 709–14.

Whorwell, P.J., Prior, A., and Faragher, E.B. (1984). Controlled trial of hypnotherapy in the treatment of severe refractory irritable bowel syndrome. *Lancet*, **ii**, 1232–4.

15 Psychological aspects of premenstrual syndrome: developing a cognitive approach

Fiona Blake, Dennis Gath, and Paul Salkovskis

Many symptoms have been reported to be associated with the changes of the menstrual cycle. The premenstrual syndrome has been difficult to define but refers to symptoms which are clearly premenstrual, recurrent and distressing. Whilst many aetiological mechanisms have been proposed, there is substantial evidence that psychological factors are of particular importance in the determinance of the severity of symptoms and associated disability. Dr Blake and her colleagues describe a pilot study which focuses on the cognitions of people with premenstrual syndrome and of a new cognitive behavioural treatment. Their findings suggest that this approach can be effective and that it has practical implications for the provision of both primary and specialist care.

Introduction

The term 'premenstrual tension' was introduced by Frank (1931). Interest in this condition was greatly increased by publications by Dalton (1964, 1984) who identified a specific disorder, premenstrual syndrome, characterized by disturbances of mood and behaviour during the luteal phase of the menstrual cycle. Whilst premenstrual syndrome has received considerable attention from clinicians and others, there has been little agreement about its defining characteristics, aetiology, and management (Gath and Iles 1989).

This chapter considers the relevance of cognitive factors to premenstrual syndrome and the implications of those factors for treatment.

Definition and diagnosis

Up to 150 symptoms have been reported as associated with changes in the menstrual cycle (Moos 1968b). These symptoms are physical, cognitive, emotional, and behavioural. Women often describe these symptoms in general terms such as 'feeling out of control', or 'not my usual self', but these terms are too broad to define the syndrome. Amongst lay people, the term 'premenstrual syndrome' is often applied to any fluctuating disturbance of a woman's feeling of well-being during the reproductive years. These lay views have been influenced from time to time by arguments about the role and behaviour of women in society.

Since there are no biological markers of premenstrual syndrome, medical definitions put most emphasis on the timing of the symptoms. Thus, the symptoms should be prominent in the luteal phase of the cycle, relieved by menstruation, and minimal or absent in the follicular phase. Apart from the timing, operational definitions rely largely on women's subjective accounts of their symptoms. These accounts can be difficult to interpret because symptom severity often varies from month to month. Moreover, it has been show that women rate their symptoms more severely in retrospective accounts than they do in concurrent daily diaries (Clare 1983; Slade 1984). Hence, the standard practice now is to ask women to keep daily ratings for at least two cycles.

With this approach, it is possible to distinguish a subgroup of women whose symptoms are mostly premenstrual and also recurrent and distressing. Women with this symptom pattern can be said to have premenstrual syndrome; such women can be distinguished from a much larger number of women who have symptoms that are not strictly premenstrual in their timing, are less severe, and less specific (see below). There is controversy as to whether premenstrual syndrome should be a separate category in psychiatric classifications. Of the two main systems of classification, ICD-10 does not include premenstrual syndrome but DSM-IIIR includes *Late Luteal Phase Dysphoric Disorder* in an appendix as a condition requiring 'further investigation' (American Psychiatric Association 1987). DSM-IV lists *Premenstrual Dysphasic Disorder* as a syndrome 'provided for further study'. In research and in clinical practice the diagnosis of premenstrual syndrome must be distinguished from premenstrual exacerbation of an underlying emotional disorder (for example, a depressive disorder) and from emotional problems that are not cyclical. The diagnosis may be unclear from the woman's subjective report, but usually becomes clear when symptom diaries are kept.

Epidemiology

It is difficult to determine the prevalence of premenstrual syndrome in the general population for several reasons: diagnostic criteria have usually been unspecified, enquiries have usually been postal surveys, and the women have been asked to answer retrospective questions. From the literature it seems likely that over 90 per cent of women experience some psychological symptoms premenstrually, but only approximately 10 per cent have symptoms that regularly disrupt their life. Most accounts of premenstrual syndrome include both psychological and physical symptoms. The psychological symptoms include depressed mood, anxiety, irritability, forgetfulness, and loss of libido. Physical symptoms include

Table 15.1 Possible causes of premenstrual syndrome

Physiological
   Disturbance of reproductive hormones (Backstrom and Cartensen 1974; Dalton
      1984)
   Nutritional deficiency: vitamins, minerals, essential fatty acids (Brush 1988)
   Disturbance of endogenous opioids (Reid and Yen 1981)
   Disturbance of the renin angiotensin aldosterone system (Janowski *et al.* 1973)

Psychological
   Variant of affective disorder (Endicott *et al.* 1981)
   Psychological response to the menstrual cue (Osborn and Gath 1990)

Other
   Multifactorial model of premenstrual syndrome (Logue and Moos 1986; Ussher
      1992)

---

bloating, fatigue, tender breasts, appetite change, abdominal pain, and headaches.

The long-term course of premenstrual syndrome is uncertain. It has been suggested that it varies with parity, increasing age, and use of oral contraceptives, but there have been no longitudinal studies.

Aetiology

The main theories are listed in Table 15.1. There have been many suggestions as to the aetiology of premenstrual syndrome. As yet there is no convincing evidence that any of these theories is correct.

Aspects of treatment

There have been many clinical accounts of treatment but few satisfactory controlled trials. It is difficult to interpret the reported findings for two reasons: varying definitions of the syndrome have been used and placebo effects are large.

The placebo effect

It has been found that the placebo response is particularly powerful in double-blind trials of drug treatments for premenstrual syndrome. A 40 per cent response or more can be expected in the first month of treatment. Even higher responses appear to be associated with more invasive treatments, for instance, in a trial of oestrogen implants, there was a 94 per cent placebo response in the first 2 months (Magos *et al.* 1986). This

Table 15.2 Drug treatments for premenstrual syndrome

Hormones	Non-hormonal treatments	Psychotropic drugs
Progesterone	Diuretics	Antidepressants
Progesterone	Mefenamic acid	Lithium
Oestrogen	Pyridoxine	Benzodiazepines
Danazol	Oil of evening primrose	
Bromocryptine		
GnRH agonists		

may explain the diversity of medications that have been reported as effective for premenstrual syndrome. The psychological benefit of participating in a trial (such as being given time, being taken seriously) may be partly responsible for this.

Drug treatments

Few controlled trials have demonstrated drugs to be more effective than placebo. Whilst some women gain significant relief from particular drugs, many try numerous different drugs without benefit. It is important to be aware that many of these treatments, especially hormones, have significant side-effects and some are contraindicated for long-term use. Some of these drugs will now be reviewed under the headings listed in Table 15.2.

Hormones Progesterone, progestogens, and the combined oral contraceptive pill are the most widely used hormones in primary care. Progesterone has been strongly recommended by Dalton (1984), but the evidence is limited to open trials and the theoretical model of progesterone deficiency is unproven (Sampson 1979; Andersch and Hahn 1985; Maddocks *et al.* 1986). Even though controlled trials have found progesterone to be no better than placebo, many women find that progesterone is helpful. Synthetic progestogens are no better than placebo in trials (Dennerstein *et al.* 1986; Sampson *et al.* 1988), but are clinically popular as an alternative to progesterone because they can be taken orally.

For premenstrual syndrome, oestrogen is most commonly used as the combined pill, but satisfactory placebo-controlled trials are lacking and cross-sectional surveys give conflicting results about the influence of the pill on premenstrual syndrome. Various other forms of oestrogen have been evaluated in specialist clinics. Oestrogen implants showed benefit in a trial (Magos *et al.* 1986) but subsequently 10 per cent of the subjects had a hysterectomy. Oestrogen patches, a rapidly reversible form of oestrogen therapy, were found to be superior to placebo in one study (Watson *et al.* 1989).

In specialist practice, use is made of other hormones including danazol, bromocriptine, and gonadotrophin-releasing hormone agonists (GnRH agonists). All these preparations are expensive and carry a high risk of side-effects, hence, they should be used only under close supervision for a few months at a time and should be reserved for women with particularly severe symptoms. GnRH agonists are of general benefit for most symptoms of premenstrual syndrome (Muse 1989), whilst danazol and bromocriptine have most effect on cyclical breast pain.

Non-hormonal treatments   Non-hormonal treatments include diuretics (such as spironolactone) for premenstrual bloating and weight gain (O'Brien *et al.* 1979) and mefenamic acid for pain and fatigue (Mira *et al.* 1986). The dietary supplements pyridoxine and oil of evening primrose are also used. Pyridoxine (Abraham and Hargrove 1980) is widely used, but large doses (>200 mg daily) should be discouraged because of the risk of neuropathy (Schaumburg *et al.* 1983). Oil of evening primrose supplements the fatty acids which are said to be deficient in women with premenstrual syndrome, but trials have not consistently shown benefit for premenstrual syndrome symptoms other than mastalgia (Horrobin 1983).

Psychotropic drugs   Antidepressants are recommended on the assumption that premenstrual syndrome is a form of affective disorder. However, traditional tricyclic antidepressants and monoamine oxidase inhibitors are seldom used for premenstrual syndrome because of the unwanted side-effects. There have been no controlled trials of these drugs for premenstrual syndrome. Recently, however, there has been interest in the use of fluoxetine, a selective serotonin reuptake inhibitor, which specifically increases serotonin levels in the brain. Fluoxetine has relatively few side-effects and appears to produce considerable relief of premenstrual syndrome symptoms compared with placebo (Wood *et al.* 1992; Menkes *et al.* 1992). The trials have been based on small numbers of subjects, but they have led to renewed interest in psychoactive drugs for premenstrual syndrome (see also Chapter 6).

Lithium has been found to be no better than placebo and can have unpleasant side-effects (Steiner *et al.* 1980). Benzodiazepines have been used to reduce anxiety and tension associated with premenstrual syndrome, but are unsuitable because of the risk of dependence (Committee on Safety of Medicines 1988).

Psychological treatments

Psychological factors, such as understanding, education, and support are recognized as important in the treatment of premenstrual syndrome sufferers, but have been little studied (Bancroft and Backstrom 1985). The lack of studies is surprising, because clinical experience suggests that many women would welcome non-drug approaches which allow them to retain more control. Many non-drug treatments have been recommended including psychotherapy, counselling, hypnotherapy, transcendental meditation, and self-help groups. Other treatments have included acupuncture, dietary management, and hypoallergenic environments.

Very few of these approaches have been adequately evaluated. One form of treatment, cognitive therapy, has recently been evaluated in a pilot study in Oxford.

A pilot study of cognitive behaviour therapy for premenstrual syndrome

Aims

The authors have completed a pilot study, in which the main aims were

(i)   to develop a cognitive model for the treatment of premenstrual syndrome;

(ii)   to devise treatment strategies derived from this model;

(iii)   to determine whether such treatment could produce significant improvement in the symptoms of premenstrual syndrome, as compared with no treatment.

A subsidary aim was to characterize the women's psychological and social adjustment.

Cognitive therapy is particularly suitable for premenstrual syndrome both because it is a common-sense approach that is likely to be widely acceptable to women with this condition and because it has been adopted for the management of several forms of functional somatic symptoms. Some preliminary case studies were carried out to establish the feasibility of cognitive therapy for premenstrual syndrome. A cognitive model was then developed for understanding the cognitions and behaviours producing distress amongst women complaining of premenstrual symptoms.

Method

1   A diary measure of premenstrual syndrome was modified from the Moos Menstrual Distress Questionnaire (MMDQ) (Moos 1968a) and validated against the full MMDQ samples of women complaining and those not complaining of premenstrual syndrome. Subjects were drawn from

(i)   obstetrics and gynaecology clinics,

(ii)   a dental surgery list.

2. Treatment techniques were developed in a small series of pilot patients referred for premenstrual syndrome and criteria for inclusion in the main treatment study were validated.

3. In order to establish the main targets for cognitive behavioural intervention, a questionnaire was devised and then validated in premenstrual syndrome sufferers and control subjects. Care was taken to ensure that the beliefs targeted were not confounded by premenstrual syndrome. Analysis of this questionnaire revealed a range of differences in distorted patterns of thinking concerning perfectionism and the importance of being in control emotionally and physically. These findings formed the basis for the subsequent intervention study.

Eighty-four potential subjects were recruited from general practices and gynaecological clinics. Women with overt psychiatric or gynaecological disorder, drug or alcohol abuse, or current use of psychotropic drugs were excluded, but women on current premenstrual syndrome treatments were eligible for the study. The women were required to be regularly menstruating.

Sixty-nine women met the above criteria. These women went on to keep daily symptom diaries for 2 months. On the basis of these diary records, women who had severe cyclical symptoms characteristic of premenstrual syndrome were identified. These women were randomly allocated to one of two groups. One group received individual cognitive therapy immediately (immediate therapy group), whilst the other group (waiting list group) continued keeping diaries for a further two months and then received individual cognitive therapy. Cognitive therapy consisted of 12 sessions over 4 months, each session lasting 1 hour.

Assessments were made before, during, and after treatment. A global rating scale was devised to rate the effects of premenstrual syndrome symptoms in general, as well as in specific areas of life, such as personal relationships, work, and home management. Other measures included standardized ratings of psychiatric morbidity (Beck Depression Inventory, Beck *et al.* 1961; the Present State Examination, Wing *et al.* 1974; Beck Anxiety Inventory, Beck *et al.* 1988), social functioning (SAS-M, Cooper *et al.* 1982), marital functioning (Maudsley Marital Questionnaire, Crowe 1978), life events (Paykel *et al.* 1969), and personality (Eysenck Personality Questionnaire, Eysenck and Eysenck 1975). Details of past history, current complaints and demographic details were recorded in a semi-structured interview carried out by an experienced research interviewer.

The women continued to complete the symptom diary throughout treatment and during the 2-month follow-up. A questionnaire was used to assess changes in attitudes to premenstrual syndrome occurring during therapy.

Results

A diary measure was developed and validated for use in premenstrual syndrome; the results of the validation study were used to develop a prospective diary-based criterion to supplement retrospective self-reported clinical criteria. A measure of distorted thinking was developed and used to investigate premenstrual syndrome; this indicated a characteristic pattern of thinking which was used as the basis for the cognitive therapy used in the outcome study.

Twenty-three women met the inclusion criteria for this study. On random allocation, ten of these women received immediate treatment with cognitive therapy (immediate therapy group), whilst the other 13 women (waiting list group) continued keeping symptom diaries for a further 2 months and then entered treatment. Thus, the waiting list group waited for 4 months before receiving treatment. Analysis of covariance showed that cognitive therapy had significantly beneficial effects compared with waiting (no treatment). Thus, compared with the waiting list group, patients receiving immediate cognitive therapy showed a significant fall in scores for depression, in the global rating of premenstrual syndrome as a problem, and in the level of interference with everyday life. Diary ratings of symptoms showed a similar pattern.

Implications of findings

This preliminary study gave strong evidence that cognitive therapy can be a highly effective treatment for premenstrual syndrome, as compared with no treatment. One of the advantages of cognitive therapy is that it is applied both to the symptoms of premenstrual syndrome and to other factors in the woman's life that may be contributing to those symptoms. The study points to a need for a large-scale controlled clinical trial, which would compare a psychological treatment (such as cognitive therapy) with current methods of treatment, such as prescription of drugs.

Practical guidelines

Guidelines will be reviewed in relation to primary care, specialist gynaecological care, and psychiatric care.

Primary care

Initial assessment   The first step should be to establish whether or not the patient is suffering from premenstrual syndrome as defined by diary ratings of premenstrual symptoms. An attempt should be made to find out why the woman is presenting now. A detailed account should be taken of the patient's premenstrual experiences in the previous 2–3 months and particularly of the most distressing experiences. The doctor should find out the woman's past experience of help seeking, her ideas about the causes of premenstrual syndrome, and her current expectations of treatment.

Unless premenstrual syndrome has been ruled out immediately, the patient should be encouraged to keep a symptom diary. Such a diary can be very valuable because it can aid in diagnosis and can help the woman to work towards a solution of her problems. There are several standard diaries available, which are easy to complete and interpret. It is very important to convince the patient that the diary will be useful and relevant.

Treatment   The patient should be seen again 1 and 2 months after the initial visit. At these visits the diary records should be examined to confirm the diagnosis and also to provide material for discussion. If a woman fails to keep the diary, it can be useful to explore her reasons for doing so. As a result of diary keeping, some women conclude that they do not really have premenstrual problems. For those who do, various approaches to treatment can be used. For example, the diaries can be used to educate the woman about her cycle and the normal range of menstrual experiences. Women can be helped to overcome anxiety and confusion by exploring the normal changes during the month. After the initial diary keeping a management plan should be discussed. Treatment should be kept as simple as possible.

Psychological therapies   Although therapy may be limited by lack of time and specialist expertise, simple procedures can be worthwhile. Examples are counselling, assertiveness training, or anxiety management groups.

Medication   Medication may be appropriate when psychological measures bring no relief or are not acceptable to the patient. Women may request physical treatments in the hope of an easy solution. In general, medication should not be given until diary recordings confirm the diagnosis of premenstrual syndrome. The patient should be advised to take drugs for at least 2 months unless side-effects are troublesome and then to report the results to the doctor.

For general symptoms, pyridoxine and oil of evening primrose are the first choices. These preparations are available without prescription and are safe in normal dose. Many women buy these preparations themselves on the advice of friends. Specific drugs should be considered for specific complaints; for example, mefenamic acid for pain. It may be necessary to prescribe hormones for other gynaecological needs, such as contraception (start with the combined pill) or heavy bleeding (progesterone or progestogens). When premenstrual low mood is the main symptom, especially when there is evidence of current depressive illness or a history of previous depression, an antidepressant such as fluoxetine may be indicated. There is no evidence that other psychoactive drugs are useful for primary premenstrual syndrome.

Self-help groups   Unfortunately most premenstrual syndrome self-help groups are based on the premise that sufferers are ill and need progesterone and should be helped to obtain the latter from sceptical general practitioners. In primary care there is a place for problem-solving premenstrual syndrome groups. Such groups can be run by a practice nurse or health visitor, who encourages the members to discuss fears and misconceptions regarding premenstrual syndrome and also to consider alternative positive and enabling ideas.

Specialist gynaecological care

A few women complaining of premenstrual syndrome require specialist referral. In specialist clinics use may be made of drugs such as oestradiol implants, patches, or gel (with cyclical progestogen), bromocriptine (for mastalgia), danazol, and GnRH agonists.

Specialist psychiatric care

Some women complaining of premenstrual syndrome may benefit from assessment and treatment by a psychiatrist. If psychiatric referral is contemplated it is important to acknowledge and discuss the fears associated with referral. The indications for referral are listed in Table 15.3.

For the psychiatrist, the main task is to ensure that any psychiatric disorder is identified and treated. If psychiatric disorder is treated adequately, the premenstrual symptoms usually subside to a tolerable fluctuation in well-being.

Many psychiatric disorders may present as premenstrual syndrome. They include depressive disorder, anxiety disorder, eating disorders, sleep disorders, alcohol abuse, and personality disorders. Depressive disorder is the most frequent psychiatric disorder associated with premenstrual distress (Gath and Iles 1989).

It is important to be alert to the possibility that premenstrual exacerbation of severe depression may lead to suicide attempts or violence at particular times of the cycle. If premenstrual syndrome appears to be the sole

Table 15.3 Specialist psychiatric clinic

Psychiatric assessment is indicated when
(1) assessment reveals multiple psychological and social stressors;
(2) psychiatric history and the current symptoms resemble those of a previous illness;
(3) psychological problems are dominant (especially suicidal ideas, violent thoughts or actions, or severe anxiety);
(4) premenstrual syndrome may be part of a psychological disorder such as depression;
(5) there is a local psychiatrist or psychologist with a special interest in the treatment of premenstrual syndrome;
(6) there are particular issues associated with premenstrual syndrome requiring expert help, for example previous child sex abuse;
(7) the symptoms are unusual

diagnosis fluoxetine is a suitable drug to use, even if no depression is evident. Drug treatment should be accompanied by psychological measures such as counselling of various kinds.

Conclusion

The essential features of management are careful diary keeping by the patient and assessment by the doctor, together with education, support, and understanding. Any of the available physical treatments may help some women, but it is difficult to predict which patient will respond to each treatment. It is not established that any medication has proven efficacy in controlled trials of women with premenstrual syndrome. The syndrome may be a heterogeneous disorder and any given therapy may be effective for only a proportion of women. Psychological treatments may be beneficial, but they are time-consuming and require commitment from the patient.

The aims of cognitive therapy are to help the woman to change her circumstances and relationships positively and to reduce psychological distress. The pilot study reported in this chapter indicates that cognitive therapy is likely to be an effective and acceptable way of helping women to help themselves.

References

Abraham, G.E. and Hargrove, J.T. (1980). Effects of vitamin B on premenstrual symptomatology in women with premenstrual syndrome: a double blind crossover study. *Infertility*, **3**, 155–65.

American Psychiatric Association (1987). Late luteal phase dysphoric disorder. In *Diagnostic and statistical manual of mental disorders*, (3rd edn). APA, Washington, DC.

Andersch, B. and Hahn, L. (1985). Progesterone treatment of premenstrual tension: a double blind study. *Journal of Psychosomatic Research*, **29**, 489-93.

Backstrom, T. and Cartensen, H. (1974). Estrogen and progesterone in plasma in relation to premenstrual tension. *Journal of Steroid Biochemistry*, **5**, 257-60.

Bancroft, J. and Backstrom, T. (1985). Review: premenstrual syndrome. *Clinical Endocrinology*, **22**, 313-36.

Beck, A.T., Ward, C.H., Mendelson, M., Mock, J., and Erbaugh, J. (1961). An inventory for measuring depression. *Archives of General Psychiatry*, **4**, 561-71.

Beck, A.T., Epstein, N., Brown, G., and Steer, R.A. (1988). An inventory for measuring clinical anxiety: psychometric properties. *Journal of Consulting and Clinical Psychology*, **56**, 893-7.

Brush, M.G. (1988). Vitamins, essential fatty acids and minerals in relation to the aetiology and management of premenstrual syndrome. In *Functional disorders of the menstrual cycle*, (ed, M.G. Brush and E.M. Goudsmit), pp. 69-85. Wiley & Sons, Chichester.

Clare, A.W. (1983). Psychiatric and social aspects of premenstrual complaint. *Psychological Medicine*, **4** (Suppl.), 1-58.

Committee on Safety of Medicines (1988). Benzodiazepine dependence and withdrawal symptoms. *Current Problems*, **21**, 1-2.

Cooper, P., Osborn, M., Gath, D.H., and Feggetter, G. (1982). Evaluation of a modified self-report measure of social adjustment. *British Journal of Psychiatry*, **141**, 68-75.

Crowe, M.S. (1978). Conjoint marital therapy: a controlled outcome study. *Psychological Medicine*, **9**, 623-36.

Dalton, K. (1964). *The premenstrual syndrome*. Charles Thomas, Springfield, IL.

Dalton, K. (1984). *The premenstrual syndrome and progesterone therapy*, (2nd edn). Heinemann Medical Books, London.

Dennerstein, L., Morse, C., Gotts, G., Brown, J., Smith M., Oats, J., and Burrows, G. (1986). Treatment of premenstrual syndrome: a double blind trial of dydrogesterone. *Journal of Affective Disorders*, **11**, 199-205.

Endicott, J., Halbreich, U., Schadt, S., and Nee, J. (1981). Premenstrual changes and affective disorders. *Psychosomatic Medicine*, **43**, 519-29.

Eysenck, H.J. and Eysenck, S.G. (1975). *Manual of the Eysenck personality questionnaire*. Hodder & Stoughton, Sevenoaks, Kent.

Frank, R.T. (1931). The hormonal causes of premenstrual tension. *Archives of Neurological Psychiatry*, **26**, 1053-7.

Gath, D. and Iles, S. (1989). Treating the premenstrual syndrome. *British Medical Journal*, **297**, 237-8.

Horrobin, D.F. (1983). The role of essential fatty acids and prostaglandins in the premenstrual syndrome. *Journal of Reproductive Medicine*, **28**, 465-8.

Janowski, D., Berens, S., Davis, J., and Vanderbilt, U. (1973). Correlations between mood, weight and electrolytes during the menstrual cycle: a renin-aldosterone hypothesis of premenstrual tension. *Psychosomatic Medicine*, **35**, 143-54.

Logue, C.M. and Moos, R.H. (1986). Perimenstrual symptoms – prevalence and risk factors. *Psychosomatic Medicine*, **48**, 388–414.

Maddocks, S., Hahn, P., Moller, F., and Reid, R.L. (1986). A placebo controlled trial of progesterone vaginal suppositories in the treatment of premenstrual syndrome. *American Journal of Obstetrics and Gynaecology*, **3**, 93–9.

Magos, A.L., Brincat, M., and Studd, J.W.W. (1986). Treatment of premenstrual syndrome with subcutaneous oestradiol implants and cyclical norethisterone: placebo controlled study. *British Medical Journal*, **292**, 1629–33.

Menkes, D.B., Taghavi, E., Mason, P.A., Spears, G.F.S., and Howard, R.C. (1992). Fluoxetine treatment of severe premenstrual syndrome. *British Medical Journal*, **305**, 346–7.

Mira, M., McNeil, D., Fraser, I.S., Vizzard, J., and Abrahams, S. (1986). Mefanamic acid in the treatment of premenstrual syndrome. *Obstetrics and Gynaecology*, **68**, 395–8.

Moos, R.H. (1968*a*). The development of a menstrual distress questionnaire. *Psychosomatic Medicine*, **30**, 853–67.

Moos, R.H. (1968*b*). The typology of menstrual cycle symptoms. *American Journal of Obstetrics and Gynaecology*, **103**, 390–402.

Muse, K.N. (1989). Clinical experience with the use of GnRH agonists in the treatment of premenstrual syndrome. *Obstetrics and Gynaecology*, **44**, 317–18.

O'Brien, P.M.S., Craven, D., Selby, C., and Symonds, E.M. (1979). Treatment of premenstrual syndrome by spironolactone. *British Journal of Obstetrics and Gynaecology*, **86**, 142–7.

Osborn, M. and Gath, D. (1990). Psychological and physical determinants of premenstrual symptoms before and after hysterectomy. *Psychological Medicine*, **20**, 565–72.

Paykel, E.S., Myers, J.K., Dienelt, M.N., Klerman, G.L., Lindenthal. J.I., and Pepper. M. (1969). Life events and depression. *Archives of General Psychiatry*, **21**, 753–60.

Reid, R.L. and Yen, S.S.C. (1981). Premenstrual syndrome. *American Journal of Obstetrics and Gynaecology*, **139**, 85–104.

Sampson, G.A. (1979). P.M.S.: a double-blind controlled trial of progesterone and placebo. *British Journal of Psychiatry*, **135**, 209–15.

Sampson, G.A., Heathcote, P., Wordsworth, J., Prescott, P., and Hodgson, A. (1988). Premenstrual syndrome. A double blind cross-over trial of treatment with dydrogesterone and placebo. *British Journal of Psychiatry*, **153**, 232–5.

Schaumburg, H., Kaplan, J., Windebank, A., Vick, N., Rasmus, S., Pleasure, D., and Brown, M.J. (1983). Sensory neuropathy from pyridoxine abuse. *New England Journal of Medicine*, **309**, 445–8.

Slade, P. (1984). Premenstrual emotional changes in normal women: fact or fiction? *Journal of Psychosomatic Research*, **28**, 1–7.

Steiner, M., Haskett, R.F., Osmun, J.N., and Carroll, B.J. (1980). Treatment of premenstrual syndrome with lithium carbonate. *Acta Psychiatrica Scandinavica*, **61**, 96–102.

Ussher, J.M. (1992). Research and theory related to female reproduction: implications for clinical psychology. *British Journal of Clinical Psychology*, **31**, 129–51.

Watson, N.R., Studd, J.W.W., Savvas, M., Garnett, T., and Baber, R.J. (1989). Treatment ot severe premenstrual syndrome with oestrogen patches and cyclical norethisterone. *Lancet*, **2**, 730–2.

Wing, J.K., Cooper., J.E. and Sartorius, N. (1974). *The measurement and classification of psychiatric Symptoms*. Cambridge University Press, London.

Wood, S.H., Mortola, J.F., Chan, Y.F., Moossazadeh, F., and Yen, S.S.C. (1992). Treatment of premenstrual syndrome with fluoxetine: a double blind, placebo controlled, crossover study. *Obstetrics and Gynaecology*, **80**, 339–44.

16 Chronic fatigue, chronic fatigue syndrome, and fibromyalgia

Simon Wessely and Michael Sharpe

In this chapter Drs Sharpe and Wessely discuss the nature of fatigue as a symptom. They then examine the chronic fatigue syndrome emphasizing the arbitrary quality of existing definitions. The aetiology of chronic fatigue syndrome is reviewed and it is concluded that it is a functional syndrome strongly shaped by social and cultural factors. Finally a cognitive behavioural model of the perpetuation of symptoms and disability is described. Practical guidelines for the cognitive behavioural treatment of patients with chronic fatigue syndrome are outlined.

Introduction

Chronic fatigue syndrome exemplifies many of the themes of this book. Fatigue is a common symptom often associated with emotional disorder, distress, and disability. Examination and investigation rarely yields positive findings and the symptoms therefore may be regarded as medically unexplained.

Chronic fatigue has an additional social and political dimension however. One recent journal contribution referred to the 'highly charged, medical, social and political atmosphere' surrounding the subject (Reeves *et al.* 1992) and another the 'proliferation of support groups, and research foundations dominated by patients with the syndrome, and fund raising and lobbying groups' (Charatan 1990). Chronic fatigue syndrome is topical and controversial. 'There is no middle ground when it comes to chronic fatigue' (Lechky 1990). Cheney (1989), a hero of patient organizations, has written that 'we who believe that this is a real disease are almost in a death grip with those forces who would stifle debate, trivialize this problem, and banish patients who suffer from it beyond the edges of traditional medicine' (which means to psychiatry). One medical journalist noted that 'at any dinner party you will find the friend of sufferers, who will either support or hotly dispute this view', usually with 'ferocity' (Collee 1991). Chronic fatigue 'falls into the category of illnesses that cannot be debated dispassionately' (Brodsky 1991). It is this role of personal beliefs interacting with the social and cultural context that gives chronic fatigue syndrome, patients with chronic fatigue, and the doctors who try to help them, special, if unenviable status amongst the functional syndromes.

The problem

What is chronic fatigue?

What exactly is chronic fatigue? Defining chronic is relatively easy — the current consensus is that fatigue can be considered as chronic after 6 months of illness (Holmes *et al.* 1988; Sharpe *et al.* 1991; Schulderberg *et al.* 1992). There is no particular logic for this stipulation, but as it is one of the few non-controversial areas of this subject, we will continue the convention.

What about fatigue? In neurophysiological terms fatigue is the failure to sustain force or power output (Edwards 1981). This is in contrast to weakness, which is the failure to generate force (Edwards 1981). In the field of neuropsychology fatigue can refer to time-related decrements in the ability to perform mental tasks. Fatigue defined in this way can therefore be objectively measured. However, fatigue also refers to a subjective sensation, experienced by the patient, but inaccessible to objective measurement (MacDougall 1899; Muscio 1921) and only appreciable 'second hand' (Berrios 1990). Patients use a variety of terms to describe this elusive but unpleasant feeling: these include the words tiredness, weariness, and exhaustion, as well as fatigue (David *et al.* 1988; Wessely and Powell 1989). To further complicate matters subjective fatigue is unrelated to 'objective' measures of muscle fatigue and endurance (See Wessely and Thomas 1990). Furthermore the experience of fatigue overlaps with other unpleasant sensations such as pain. Thus, although the distinctions between myalgia, fatigue, and weakness are important for doctors, they are often less clear to patients.

Although the problem of definition and measurement may seem academic, this is in fact far from the case. Most patients presenting with chronic fatigue lack any objective abnormality that validates their symptoms, let alone indicates their cause. As other contributors to this volume have noted, the absence of confirmatory evidence of disease commonly poses a problem for the doctor and his or her patient. Those doctors seeking a definitive fatigue test, free from the influence of such ill-defined variables as mood, personality, motivation, cognition, and situation continue to experience frustration. For example, a leading neurobiologist has recently noted the problems in distinguishing post-viral fatigue from affective disorder and concluded that 'one advance that would clarify this issue would be the ability to document weakness in patients objectively' (Kennedy 1991). Not surprisingly this advance remains elusive.

In addition to the absence of laboratory verification many patients with chronic fatigue do not look sick. As with chronic pain (Baszanger 1992), the absence of objective evidence is a fundamental barrier to the normal organization of relationships between sufferer and doctor. One sufferer wrote 'My skin is clear and tanned. I don't have a plaster cast or a broken leg ... people say "you look so well"' (Berrett 1991). Another identified 'looking healthy and strong' as a principal difficulty in dealings with doctors (Finlay 1986).

The size of the problem

Chronic fatigue is a common problem in primary care. Estimates of its prevalence vary (see Lewis and Wessely 1992), but in the UK approximately 10 per cent of general practitice attenders will admit to chronic fatigue (David *et al*. 1990). A Canadian study recently found that 14 per cent of new attenders in general practice complained of fatigue and it was the principal reason for consultation in 7 per cent (Cathebras *et al*. 1992). A variety of conditions can be associated with the complaint, most of them relatively easily diagnosed (for example, anaemia), although for the vast majority of patients physical investigations and examinations are normal (Valdini *et al*. 1989; Lane *et al*. 1990; Gow *et al*. 1991) and a careful psychosocial enquiry more important (Manu *et al*. 1988; Wood *et al*. 1991).

It is a smaller number of patients (perhaps 1 per cent of general practitioner attenders) who suffer from chronic disabling fatigue and no diagnosis other than that of an idiopathic chronic fatigue syndrome who are likely to be referred to hospital (Lewis and Wessely 1992) and it is this group to whom the rest of this chapter is devoted.

What exactly is chronic fatigue syndrome?

Terminology is a minefield. The labels for patients whose symptoms have no adequate medical explanation include historical diagnoses, such as neurasthenia and myalgic encephalomyelitis (ME), diagnoses peculiar to certain medical specialties and influenced by the often arbitrary choice of presenting symptoms, for example fibromyalgia and effort syndrome, and diagnoses that imply particular aetiologies, such as post-viral fatigue syndrome. The nosological status of all these conditions is uncertain (Wessely 1990; Sharpe *et al*. 1991) and we prefer the recently defined broader and aetiological neutral term chronic fatigue syndrome. This was coined by researchers in the USA and Australia (Holmes *et al*. 1988; Lloyd *et al*. 1988). Early attempts to define this syndrome nevertheless proved unsatisfactory and led to substantial revision on both sides of the Atlantic (Sharpe *et al*. 1991; Schulderberg *et al*. 1992). Currently the term chronic fatigue syndrome is used to describe patients who

(1) complain of chronic physical and mental fatigue as well as other symptoms such as muscle pain;

(2)   do not have identifiable organic disease;

(3)   manifest significant disability.

Most of the research cited, as well as our own clinical experience, is based on this broad definition. It is important, however, to be aware that chronic fatigue syndrome is merely an operational definition of a syndrome of uncertain nosological status, which is likely to be aetiologically heterogenous (Sharpe 1992).

Chronic fatigue syndrome and emotional disorder

Like patients with other functional somatic symptoms, patients with severe chronic fatigue suffer considerable psychiatric morbidity. Regrettably each generation of physicians appears to need to discover this afresh and it is even more tragic that this issue continues to fuel the same futile 'organic versus psychological' polemics (Wessely 1991; Shorter 1992). Many studies have confirmed that the majority of those patients seen in specialist centres with a chief complaint of chronic fatigue also fulfil operational criteria for anxiety and depressive disorders (see Abbey and Garfinkel 1990; Kendell 1991; David 1991 for review).

The relationship of emotional disorder to chronic fatigue syndrome is complex (see Abbey and Garfinkel 1990; David 1991; Ray 1991). Emotional disorder may in some cases be a consequence of the illness, but this cannot be the case for many, perhaps the majority of patients, since the prevalence of emotional disorders is greater than that seen in other disabling medical conditions (Wessely and Powell 1989; Katon *et al.* 1991; Wood *et al.* 1991). In other cases the patient may have uncomplicated emotional disorder which has been misdiagnosed as chronic fatigue syndrome. Finally, the possibility that both chronic fatigue syndrome and emotional disorder have a common origin in disturbances of cerebral function has attracted considerable attention (see Wessely 1993).

The physiology and pathology of chronic fatigue

Muscle or brain?   It has always been tempting to speculate that, since fatigue is experienced by many patients as being muscular, it must have a neuromuscular cause. However, the evidence suggests that this is probably not the case. Certainly some ultrastructural abnormalities in muscle have been found, but these are non-specific and unaccompanied by deficits in intermediate metabolism (see Wessely and Thomas 1990). A frequently cited case report in which metabolic abnormalities in muscle metabolism were found using nuclear magnetic spectroscopy (Arnold *et al.* 1984) is exceptional (Wagenmakers *et al.* 1988; Lewis and Haller 1991). Electrophysiological studies are conflicting (Jamal and Miller 1991) and seem unlikely to be of aetiological relevance to the symptom of fatigue (Lloyd *et al*. 1988; Stokes *et al*. 1988). Studies of dynamic muscle function have demonstrated that, apart from evidence of deconditioning, patients with chronic fatigue syndrome have essentially normal muscle strength, endurance and fatiguability (Lloyd *et al*. 1988; Stokes *et al*. 1988; Riley *et al*. 1990; Lloyd *et al*. 1991; Rutherford and White 1991). Lloyd *et al*. (1991) concluded that 'neither poor motivation, nor muscle contractile failure is important in the pathogenesis of fatigue in patients with the chronic fatigue syndrome'.

Patients with chronic fatigue syndrome typically complain of mental as well as physical fatigue. Beard (1880) wrote that 'memory is often temporarily weakened, and consecutive thought and sustained mental activity frequently impossible'. Janet (1919), who singled out psychasthenia from the overburdened concept of neurasthenia, wrote that psychological deficits were the core of the illness. 'Tiredness and a horrible sense of fatigue is caused in psychasthenics by the least physical or psychological effort ... fatigue rapidly affects sensations and perceptions, intellect and movement' (Janet 1919). It seems almost superfluous to note that such symptoms cannot be of neuromuscular origin.

Inactivity; cause or effect? Others have argued that fatigue is not so much the cause of inactivity, but the consequence of it. Riley *et al*. (1990) pointed out that their findings resembled those observed in deconditioned patients (Saltin *et al*. 1968) and Edwards described how such fatigue was explicable in terms of decreased mitochondrial function consequent upon lack of activity (Wagenmakers *et al*. 1988; Edwards *et al*. 1991).

The cellular RNA, cellular protein, and muscle protein synthesis reductions noted in some chronic fatigue syndrome patients (Edwards *et al*. 1991) can be explained by inactivity (Gibson *et al*. 1987). The effects inactivity have been frequently described in the medical literature (Dock 1944; Asher 1947). When considering neurasthenia, Taylor (1907) wrote that 'disuse is as harmful as misuse'. Bed-rest produces muscle wasting, changes in the cardiovascular response to exertion, and consequent intolerance of activity. Other changes include impaired autonomic regulation leading to deficits in postural blood pressure control with dizziness upon standing and also impaired thermoregulation, both of which are common somatic symptoms in chronic fatigue syndrome (see Sharpe and Bass 1992). The degree of inactivity required to produce these changes need not be great: young healthy males lose 20 per cent of muscle strength within 1 week of immobilization (Lamb *et al*. 1965; Muller 1970). Furthermore, inactivity not only increases the sensation of fatigue on exertion but actually reduces the desire to undertake exercise (Zorbas and Matveyev 1986).

Does muscle pain mean muscle disease? One of the consequences of neuromuscular deconditioning is the occurrence of delayed onset post-exertional muscle pain (Klug *et al*. 1989). This results from eccentric contractions, where the muscle lengthens whilst doing work and causes transient local muscle trauma and release of muscle enzymes. This phenomenon is particularly prominent in the untrained person (Editorial 1987). Post-exercise muscle pain, held to be characteristic of chronic fatigue syndrome, should not necessarily therefore be regarded as pathological — it is common to all subjects who engage in activity that requires muscular activity not normally performed in everyday life (Klug *et al*. 1989).

Are patients with chronic fatigue syndrome physically unfit? Almost certainly yes. Studies of subjects with fibromyalgia confirm the clinical impression of deconditioning (Klug *et al*. 1989), as do studies of chronic fatigue syndrome (Riley *et al*. 1990). However, are such changes primary or secondary? The answer is unclear. Similar findings to those in chronic fatigue syndrome can be caused by lack of activity. Certainly chronic fatigue syndrome patients meeting criteria for chronic fatigue syndrome are typically profoundly inactive as a substantial degree of functional impairment is necessary for the diagnosis in all of the current operational criteria. Only one prospective study sheds any light on the matter. In White's (1991) important cohort study of recovery from Epstein–Barr virus, lack of physical fitness in the early weeks after onset of definite Epstein–Barr virus infection was associated with the later development of a fatigue syndrome.

Why then are so many chronically fatigued patients apparently so limited in terms of exercise tolerance? One theory is of a disorder of perception. The study of the perception of effort is a complex endeavour (Mihevic 1981). However, several studies have examined the difference between perceived effort and actual work rate. Investigators from Liverpool measured exercise tolerance and perceived exertion using cycle ergometry (Gibson *et al*. 1993). They found that although the patients with chronic fatigue syndrome reported working at maximum effort, the physiological maximum work rate had not been achieved. Riley *et al*. (1990) also noted that ratings of perceived exertion differed between cases and both normal controls and those with irritable bowel syndrome. Chronic fatigue syndrome patients tended to overrate both their premorbid exercise tolerance arnd their desired exercise tolerance, compared to both normal and irritable bowel syndrome controls. There is thus some evidence suggesting a dissociation between subjective experience of muscle fatigue and physiological fatigue in patients with chronic fatigue syndrome.

Is virus infection the cause of chronic fatigue syndrome?   Clinically many patients with chronic fatigue syndrome report an initial 'viral type' infection — 72 per cent in one recent series (Wessely and Powell 1989) and 91 per cent in another (Petersen *et al*. 1991). This is not a new observation — many Victorian physicians noted that neurasthenia frequently succeeded influenza, typhoid, and other infections (see Wessely 1991). In our own time this observation has been incorporated into the term 'post-viral fatigue syndrome', the currently most popular term for chronically fatigued patients in the UK. However, great caution must be exercised before accepting that infective agents play an important role in the aetiology of chronic fatigue syndromes. The arguments for and against infective aetiologies are described in greater detail elsewhere (Bock and Whelan 1993), but the methodological weaknesses of many studies, the non-specific nature of the association, problems of retrospective bias, absence of links between laboratory and clinical findings, and the lack of congruence between the epidemiology of infections and that of chronic fatigue syndrome, all mean that it is rash to assume that the case for a long lasting post-viral fatigue is proven (Wessely 1992).

What is the prognosis?   The prognosis of chronic fatigue in tertiary care is gloomy. In the Mayo clinic 235 patients with a diagnosis of chronic nervous exhaustion were followed up approximately 6 years later (Macy and Allen 1934). Most remained symptomatic, although precise figures are not given. One hundred and seventy-three cases of neurocirculatory asthenia seen by a single cardiologist were followed up for a mean of 20 years (Wheeler *et al*. 1950). Only 11 per cent asymptomatic, whilst 38 per cent were mildly and 15 per cent severely disabled.

Little has changed. Behan and Behan (1988) wrote that 'most cases do not improve, give up their work and become permanent invalids, incapacitated by excessive fatigue and myalgia'. Hellinger *et al*. (1988) and Gold *et al*. (1990) reported that half the patients referred had significantly improved after 1 year, but half had not and only 6 per cent were symptom free. In a Canadian primary care study over half the patients with fatigue remained so 1 year later (Cathebras *et al*. 1992). Finally, in a systematic follow-up of 144 cases of 'post-viral fatigue' referred to a single infectious disease clinic in Oxford, one of us found that short-term prognosis was poor, although two-thirds had shown some improvement by 4 years (Sharpe *et al*. 1992). However, only 13 per cent considered themselves 'fully recovered', a figure similar to that reported by Wheeler *et al*. (1950) a generation earlier.

Are cognitive factors important in chronic fatigue syndrome?   The majority of patients presenting to a specialist with chronic fatigue believe their illness is due to an external agent, usually an infective one (Matthews *et al.* 1989; Wessely and Powell 1989; Hickie *et al.* 1990). In the UK they may ascribe their illness to putative diseases such as 'ME' and in the USA to chronic fatigue and immune deficiency syndrome (CFIDS). This is the opposite of the situation in primary care (David *et al.* 1990) or in the community (Pawlikowska *et al.* 1994), where most chronically fatigued patients ascribe their condition to psychosocial adversities. There are many possible reasons why patients may adopt this disease attribution. First, many sufferers trace their symptoms to an infective episode. Second, the symptoms of depression and anxiety are similar to those arising after infection (Imboden *et al.* 1959) and both chills and fevers are not uncommon presentations of emotional disorders (Harding *et al.* 1980; Wilson *et al.* 1983). Finally, attribution to a disease for which the person has no responsibility may function to avoid blame for being ill.

The external (non-self) nature of the attribution may have important consequences, irrespective of its accuracy. Some of these are advantageous — 'Symptoms attributed to an external cause are less disabling than symptoms attributed to a personal cause' (Watts 1982). External attribution also protects the patient from the stigma of being labelled psychiatrically ill — 'the victim of a germ infection is therefore blameless' (Helman 1978). Concerning chronic fatigue syndrome specifically 'to attribute the continuing symptoms to persistence of a "physical-disease" is a mechanism that carries the least threat to a person's self-esteem' (Katz and Andiman 1988). 'Patients who suffer from unrelenting fatigue . . . worry that people will think they have a mental problem or a blameworthy characterological weakness of will' (Greenberg 1990). The absence of guilt and the preservation of self-esteem, even in the context of depression, have been noted in patients whose fatigue was attributed to infection (Imboden *et al.* 1959; Powell *et al.* 1990; Webb and Parsons 1991).

There are also disadvantages to such an attribution. It is common knowledge that viruses cannot be treated (Helman 1978) and, thus, this view of aetiology, implicit in the label of 'post-viral fatigue', carries no information about how the sufferer can recover (Wessely *et al.* 1991). Furthermore, attributing chronic fatigue to 'post-viral fatigue', 'ME', and so on, conveys more than a simple statement of aetiology. It also suggests certain beliefs about prognosis and treatment. A few examples from the extensive self-help literature provide a flavour: 'These living viruses are erratic and unpredictable. The prickly-edged ones pierce their way into the body cells. If disturbed by the patient's activity they become as aggressive as a disturbed wasps' nest, and can be felt giving needle-like jabs (or stimulating the nerves to do so) (Dainty 1988). The author, a nurse with chronic fatigue syndrome, continues 'Always remember, until an exciting medical announcement is made, that there is no one drug to cure ME. The only cure is rest and keeping the affected parts of the body rigid so as to improve the body's defences.' Similar sentiments were expressed by another magazine in the following — 'the only hope is that one day some substance will be isolated that has the power to zap the ME virus' and until then 'the most doctors can do is to advise patients to rest, and wait for the ME to go away' (Hodgkinson 1988). All of these opinions may reinforce the despair and helplessness so frequently reported by sufferers. At present the label of chronic fatigue syndrome/ME is frequently associated with a belief that the condition is incurable and that symptoms should be managed by rest. The consequences can be helplessness, increased fatigue, lack of self-confidence, and depression (Powell *et al.* 1990).

Such cognitions must influence not only mood, but also disability. Negative cognitions, such as the beliefs that 'activities that cause an increase in symptoms worsen the disease', 'Activity is impossible in the presence of symptoms', and 'Nothing can be done to hasten recovery except rest' lead to avoidance. Studies of patients with chronic pain suggest that patients who cope with symptoms by avoidance suffer greater disability and more pain than those who cope more actively (Philips 1987). Thus, in both chronic fatigue and chronic pain strategies such as rest, although effective in reducing symptoms in the short-term, are likely to lead to long-term disability.

Both Smith (1989) and Ramsay (1989) use the same words about 'ME' — the disease has 'an alarming tendency to chronicity' (Ramsay 1989; Smith 1989). Sufferers must make 'very significant changes in their life style' (Shepherd 1989). Does this mean that patients are *untreatable* — or do these views themselves influence outcome? Could the perception of 'ME' and related illnesses as incurable become a self-fulfilling prophecy? The factors that may perpetuate illness in patients with chronic fatigue syndrome are listed in Table 16.1.

Table 16.1 Factors which may perpetuate chronic fatigue syndrome

1. Depression and axiety
2. Lack of physical fitness
3. Sleep disturbance
4. Chronic life stresses and difficulties
5. Inaccurate or unhelpful illness beliefs
6. Avoidance of activities

Overview of the evidence concerning treatment

There is now a substantial literature on the treatment of patients with chronic fatigue syndrome. A number of allegedly specific treatments have been proposed to deal with the presumed underlying 'cause' of the abnormal fatiguability. The theory that chronic virus infection was the cause led a trial of the antiviral drug acylovir (Straus *et al.* 1988). Recent formulations of chronic fatigue syndrome involve abnormal immunity and it was inevitable that immunoglobulins would also be tried. Unsurprisingly, the results of these studies have suggested that neither of these agents should be used in the treatment of chronic fatigue syndrome (see Straus 1991; Anon 1991).

Less-specific treatments are at present extremely popular, in particular evening primrose oil and magnesium, both found efficacious in well-publicized, if criticized clinical trials. However, there is no rationale for their use and other studies have been less favourable (McCluskey 1993). The Victorian physician had a vast range of drugs at his disposal, all of which were intended to increase the body's supply of energy. He could also call upon electrical therapy, since, in the age of electricity, the notion that the deficiency of nerve energy could be made up by electrical stimulation was a seductive one (Rabinbach 1990). Most of the substances used now sound absurd to our ears. For example, Althaus (1893), a London neurologist, used a tonic extracted from the brains of young animals to restore brain power. Even in our own time German specialists have used extracts of thymus and spleen as immune stimulants (Hilgers *et al.* 1991), whilst a California physician lists 13 drugs as 'energy improvement treatments' (Goldstein 1990).

The jargon of treatment is an ever-changing parody of contemporary scientific terminology, against a more stable background in which 'The mass media advertising of cures for fatigue over the past century provides a remarkably consistent theme during the midst of social change. Tonics, potions, herbs, vitamins and an incredible array of other substances have been advised as cures for pseudoanergic symptoms' (Karno and Hoffman 1974).

The use of antidepressant drugs

In Chapter 6 Katon outlined the rationale for the use of antidepressant therapy in patients with functional somatic symptoms. The rationale for their use in chronic fatigue is compelling. It is astonishing that at the time of writing there have been two controlled trials of immunoglobulin therapy and none of antidepressant drugs. The evidence supporting the use of antidepressant comes, so far, only from uncontrolled or open studies (Jones and Straus 1987; Lynch *et al.* 1991; Goodnick *et al.* 1992) and a single case study (Gracious and Winser 1991). Current work on possible impairment in serotonergic pathways (Bakheit *et al.* 1992) may suggest the use of serotonin reuptake inhibitors. Two controlled studies of antidepressants have been conducted in patients with the overlapping syndrome of fibromyalgia (Carrette *et al.* 1986; Goldenberg *et al.* 1986) both of which suggested that these drugs have a role in treatment.

Exercise, rest, and chronic fatigue syndrome

For years the mainstay of the non-pharmacological approach to chronic fatigue has been rest. With the description of the first syndrome, neurasthenia, came the rest cure, first described by the charismatic American neurologist, Silas Weir Mitchell. This consisted of enforced confinement to bed, allied with diet, massage, and electrical stimulation. It achieved enormous popularity between 1870 and 1900 (Wessely 1991; Shorter 1992). The rest cure continues to be advocated for chronic fatigue syndrome. An American self-help book contains a chapter entitled 'Rest, rest and more rest' (Feiden 1990), whilst a British equivalent introduces 'aggressive rest therapy' as treatment for ME (Franklin and Sullivan 1989). A popular self-help book tells sufferers that they must only do 'seventy five percent of what you are capable of ... unless you want to plummet down with another relapse soon, you really must follow the rule of doing less than you think you can' (Dawes and Downing 1989).

Although there is no doubting the good faith behind such advice, its long-term wisdom is open to question. Despite innumerable articles advocating rest and stressing the dangers of exercise, there has never been any evidence of neuromuscular damage or deterioration occurring in patients with chronic fatigue syndrome as a result of exercise. On the contrary there is a great deal of evidence documenting the benefits of exercise on both physiological and psychological functioning in patients with a variety of functional somatic symptoms (Dubbert 1992).

Cognitive behaviour therapy and chronic fatigue syndrome

The rationale The model of chronic fatigue syndrome developed in this chapter is different from the simple external agent/disease that directs much of research in this subject. Instead of a disease in which the necessary and sufficient cause is an external agent, usually a virus, we propose a more complex model. The inaccurate and unhelpful beliefs that patients hold lead to unhelpful ways of managing symptoms. Such factors have been claimed as mediators of disability in many illnesses, both physical and psychological (Sensky 1990). Looking specifically at chronic fatigue syndrome, it is plausible that an initial infective trigger or depressive episode may begin a cycle in which the patient's beliefs and fears concerning symptoms and activity fuel avoidant behaviour. A simple version of such a model is illustrated in Fig. 16.1.

The initial symptoms of fatigue and myalgia, which are unpleasant and

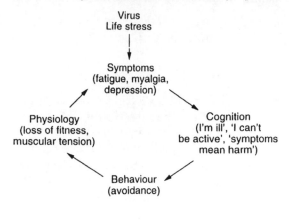

Fig. 16.1 A vicious circle perpetuating chronic fatigue and disability

uncontrollable, together with the attribution of symptoms to a persistent untreatable virus may lead to a state akin to 'learned helplessness' (Powell *et al.* 1990) and, hence, foster disabilit and depression. Avoidance behaviour (which is reinforced by the advice currently offered to patients) sustains symptoms by decreasing activity tolerance and increasing sensitivity to any stimulation. Re-exposure to activity causes more symptoms and more fear. The result is a vicious circle of symptoms, avoidance, fatigue, demoralization, and depression, the clinical picture of chronic fatigue syndrome. A similar role for avoidance in perpetuating symptoms has been implicated for chronic pain (Keefe and Gil 1986; Philips 1987) as well as other symptoms considered in this book.

Such a model implies treatments that differ from those suggested by a simple external agent/disease model. In particular, treatment requires attention to illness beliefs, mood disorder, and behavioural avoidance. According to this view therapeutic success should result from reducing avoidance behaviour, decreasing helplessness, and improving mood. All of these aspects of treatment are already an established part of the management of chronic pain and fibromyalgia. Cognitive behaviour therapy (Chapter 7) potentially provides a means of achieving these aims. A more detailed description of the cognitive behavioural treatment of chronic fatigue syndrome is given elsewhere (Butler *et al.* 1991; Wessely *et al.* 1991; Sharpe 1991; Sharpe 1993; Wessely and Edwards 1993).

Evidence for the efficacy of cognitive behaviour therapy The best evidence for efficacy comes from research into the treatment of patients diagnosed as suffering from fibromyalgia, a condition viewed by many authorities as either synonymous or overlapping with chronic fatigue syndrome. Controlled trials of increased activity in fibromyalgia have shown that exercise retraining leads to reductions in overall symptom scores and pain and also improves sleep (McCain *et al.* 1988; Bennett 1989; Klug *et al.* 1989). In fibromyalgia, unlike chronic fatigue syndrome, there seems to be no dissenting voice from the view that patients should be encouraged to cautiously interrupt the 'cycle of inactivity, fatigue, pain and inactivity' (Bennett 1989; see also Yunus 1988) or that 'the safest and most effective approach seems to be the judicious use of amitriptyline, analgesic agents, an exercise programme, and reassurance that fibromyalgia is not a crippling rheumatic disease or a degenerative neurologic illness' (Dinerman and Steer 1992). Poor compliance with treatment has been noted as a problem, although not perhaps to the same extent as in the treatment of chronic fatigue syndrome. Bell and Bailey (1992) found that nearly half of a sample of patients with fibromyalgia refractory to treatment dropped out of a 12-week ambulatory exercise programme, although the results in those completing the study were encouraging. Most clinicians are now using similar approaches for the management of chronic fatigue syndrome, usually in a pragmatic fashion, rejecting the therapeutic nihilism that has been associated with the diagnosis (Kyle and DeShazo 1992). Others combine a graded exercise programme with psychological counselling (Denman 1990). Few physicians continue to advocate rest as the basis of management.

The authors' own research

The National Hospital study

Butler *et al.* (1991) treated 50 patients seen at the National Hospital for Neurology in London with severe, unexplained fatigue — all of whom fulfilled current criteria for chronic fatigue syndrome and were typical of the severe cases of chronic fatigue syndrome encountered in hospital care. Nearly all thought they had 'ME' and over half were members of a self-help group. The evaluation of treatment was uncontrolled. In addition to chronic behavioural therapy, those fulfilling criteria for major depression were prescribed treatment with dothiepin, a tricyclic antidepressant drug.

The principal obstacle to effective treatment in this trial was refusal. Overall, 18 out of 50 refused the offer of treatment. Treatment refusal was associated with the strength of conviction that the symptoms were due to physical disease and little else. However, of those who accepted, the results were encouraging. Twenty-three (70 per cent) of those starting therapy described themselves as better and the improvements were maintained at 3 months. Using very strict criteria, nine patients could be regarded as symptom free at the end of treatment and a number were able to resume employment after prolonged absence. Treatment response was not influenced by duration of symptoms, but was associated with the strength of attribution of symptoms to an exclusively physical cause. Vereker (1992) reports similar encouraging results and similar obstacles to treatment for children. The long-term outcome is unknown but a 3-year follow-up is now underway. Other investigators have attempted to replicate this result in controlled studies. Hickie and colleagues in Australia recently published a randomized controlled trial of cognitive behavioural therapy in a large sample (Lloyd *et al.* 1993). In the study active treatment was found to be no better than simple clinic attendance and reassurance. However, it would be premature to discount cognitive behavioural therapy as a treatment for chronic fatigue syndrome on the basis of this study because it was given in a brief form and the study confused its evaluation by the concurrent use of immunotherapy.

The Oxford and King's College Hospital studies

We are currently conducting further randomized controlled trials of intensive out-patient cognitive behavioural therapy. In the Oxford trial (Sharpe 1993) consecutive patients who meet criteria for chronic fatigue syndrome are recruited from an infectious disease out-patient clinic. A total of 60 patients have been randomized either to 'treatment as usual' or to cognitive behavioural therapy. Treatment as usual comprises (usually conservative) management by the general practitioner and 'alternative' therapies sought by the patient. The cognitive behavioural therapy consists of 16 1 h sessions of individual cognitive behavioural therapy from a psychiatrist or psychologist given over 4 months. The therapy is based on the cognitive theory of chronic fatigue syndrome as described above and is tailored to the individual. As well as graded increases in activity the therapy addresses the patients' attribution of symptoms to physical disease, negative thinking, and the patient's unrealistic expectations of themselves. Outcome is measured in terms of global ratings, symptom severity, and functional impairment.

Another controlled trial taking place at King's College and Maudsley Hospitals, is comparing a more behaviourally oriented therapy with relaxation therapy. This study is important in controlling for non-specific factors in cognitive behavioural therapy.

Both trials appear to be demonstrating that patients can make considerable gains with psychological treatment aimed at breaking vicious circles of inactivity, dysfunctional cognition, and fatigue, although the superiority of cognitive behavioural therapy to non-specific comparison treatments remains to be proven.

Practical guidelines for the treatment of chronic fatigue syndrome

The doctor–patient relationship

Relationships between doctors and patients have changed considerably in recent years. Shorter (1992) has argued that the rise of media coverage of medicine and the growth of the self-help movement, has led to a decline in medical authority. Certainly patient access to professional information is now greater than ever before. Patient organizations now supply sufferers with digests of professional journals. Such information may have a considerable and often unhelpful influence on patient attributions of illness, which, as described above, can in turn be a major determinant of a patient's willingness to accept psychological treatment. Whatever the reason, a breakdown in the doctor–patient relationship is all too common (David *et al.* 1988).

The doctor who wishes to treat patients with chronic fatigue syndrome must therefore not only be aware of the current research literature, but must also be able to engage patients in a rehabilitative approach. What explanation can be given to the patient — and what can the patient tell their own family and friends? This is an important point, because any improvement that might result from an intervention that is neither virologically or immunologically based may be interpreted by some patients as proof that the problem was 'all in the mind' and be rejected. We emphasize the rehabilitation aspects of treatment and the emphasis on better coping strategies. One possible analogy is 'you have drawn a bad hand at cards, but perhaps you could also play them better'. Another is to compare the treatment of fractures or road traffic accident victims, in which chasing the cause of the accident brings little or no benefit, but sustained attention to rehabilitation is the key to improvement. Whatever strategy is chosen, the principle behind therapy is to return to the patient the responsibility for his or her progress and treatment, without conveying that they were at fault for becoming ill in the first place.

Assessment

The first stage of treatment is a detailed assessment. For the established case assessment should encompass all the dimensions of functional illness (see Chapter 4).

1. A thorough medical examination is required. Most clinicians in this field can now recount 'horror' stories of patients with other, frequently serious, conditions being misdiagnosed as ME. However, the evidence suggests that the combination of physical examination and

basic laboratory tests will detect those needing further investigation (Valdini *et al*. 1989; Lane *et al*. 1990; Ridesdale 1993).

2.   The patient should also be carefully assessed for the presence of emotional disorder. Depression and anxiety are common but may be 'masked'. It is helpful to specifically question the patient about the symptoms of emotional disorder, as well as interviewing an informant.

3.   It is necessary to enquire about the patient's beliefs and fears about their symptoms and how they should be managed. This is best done in a non-judgemental fashion. If the patients interpretations are questioned it must be done with sensitivity. The acceptance of the patient's experience and beliefs as valid is a necessary starting point for a collaborative therapeutic relationship.

4.   An assessment of the patient's functioning and behaviour is essential. It is not unusual to meet subjects who appear relatively free of symptoms, but on enquiry are leading an astonishingly restricted life, often rationalized as 'living within limits'.

5.   The identification of the particular pathophysiological processes underlying the patient's symptoms provides useful information to help the patient to reattribute their symptoms. An enquiry into sleep habits, assessment for hyperventilation, and examination for muscle wasting provide useful clues (Sharpe and Bass 1992).

6.   It is important to interview each patient's partner or spouse for two reasons. First, the beliefs and behaviour of such persons may reinforce any unhelpful illness-related beliefs that the patient holds and, second, it provides a basis for including them in the new approach to the patient's treatment. We therefore involve the patient's partner as often as possible and provide written information for both patient and family.

Aims of treatment

The principal aim of treatment is to reduce functional disability. All treatments have the same intention, but in conventional approaches this is assumed to occur as the inevitable consequence of symptom relief. The approach outlined in this contribution and, indeed, in this book, suggest the alternative approach, that is, increasing activity without waiting for symptoms to diminish. The assumption underlying this approach is that avoidance of activity is a factor perpetuating the symptoms. This is not

Table 16.2 Treatment of chronic fatigue syndrome

Assessment
  Exclude physical disease
  Assess cognitions and behaviours
	Behavioural components
	  Graded increase in activity
	  Relaxation

Engagement in treatment
  Agree formulation of illness
  Agree realistic and valued goals
	Other ingredients
	  Antidepressant medication

Cognitive components
  Education about chronic fatigue syndrome
  Modify attribution for symptoms
  Challenge excessive perfectionism
  Problem solving	

a new idea; a similar approach was first advocated by Waterman (1909), an American neurologist who became disillusioned with the then fashionable 'rest cure'. The stages in treatment are listed in Table 16.2.

The treatment rationale

Before commencing treatment the patient must be persuaded that this approach is at least worth a try. As described elsewhere in this book, the acknowledgement of distress and reality of the patients somatic concerns is fundamental. Patients with chronic fatigue syndrome often come to the consultation with extreme views about the nature of 'physical' and 'mental' illness. Most have already experienced substantial illness delegitimation (Ware 1992), exemplified by being told their symptoms are 'all in the mind' and often recount the experience of meeting doctors who, directly or indirectly, suggested their illnesses were unreal or even malingered. Two possible explanations for the illness are discussed with the patient (see Wessely *et al.* 1991)

1. The conventional view: 'You have a chronic illness in which viral persistence in your muscles is the cause of your symptoms. You must avoid all forms of physical and mental activity in order to prevent further damage. The response to any increase in symptoms must be rest'.

2. The alternative view: 'An acute infection has forced you to become inactive and perhaps also triggered certain biochemical changes in your brain. As a result you experienced intense fatigue, ceased activity, and inevitably become unfit. You now experience symptoms whenever you attempt any activity, but, because of the fear of causing symptoms or a relapse, you never pursue these activities long enough to allow the symptom to subside. These symptoms are real, but do

not reflect continuing infection and with help you can overcome them'.

It is important to point out that the alternative model does not contradict evidence of an organic origin to symptoms — it is based instead on the assumption that the factors that initiate an illness are not necessarily the same as those that perpetuate it. The purpose of treatment is not to replace extreme organic attributions with extreme psychological ones — this would be impractical and also inaccurate (Watts 1982) — but rather to generate a model that encompasses a variety of factors and to demonstrate to the patient that they can influence the course of the illness. The aim is not to find an instant 'cure', but rather to work together on ways of alleviating symptoms. Many patients will have spent a considerable amount of time looking for a specific physical cause for their fatigue in the frustrated hope that this will lead to a solution. The therapist can point this out and suggests that the patient tries the alternative approach of cognitive behavioural therapy for a set period of time (say 3 months). The possible benefits of the 'new' as opposed to the 'old' approach can then be assessed.

The treatment contract

Goals for treatment should be explicitly negotiated and agreed with the patient. Goals should be clearly defined and based on what the patient would realistically like to be able to do in the future. It is important to also explicitly discuss continuing medical investigation and parallel treatments. The continuation of these is likely to be a distraction from the cognitive behavioural therapy.

Treatment issues

Treatment of depression　Depressive disorder merits treatment whether it is considered to be a primary or a secondary problem. Both cognitive behavioural therapy and increasing activity will tend to reduce depression but if it is severe, treatment with antidepressant medication may be considered. The prescription of an antidepressant drug must be accompanied by careful explanation (see Chapter 6).

In-patient versus out-patient　Most patients can be treated as out-patients. However, if the patient is bed-bound, in-patient treatment may be required. There are difficulties in using medical wards for this purpose unless the nurses working on them are trained in behaviour therapy. The principles of treatment are the same as for out-patients but the goals for activity may initially have to be very modest (for example, getting out of bed for meals).

Insurance benefits Problems may also arise if the patient requests a diagnosis the doctor feels is inappropriate or wants certification of permanent invalidity. Whilst many patients are severely disabled, this should not be regarded as a *permanent* state until an adequate trial of treatment has been undertaken. The loss of existing benefits without guarantee of alternative income is a potential obstacle to recovery.

Treatment sessions

Most patients can be treated as out-patients with 1 hour sessions every 1–2 weeks. Typically between five and 20 sessions are required. Each session should begin with setting an agenda. There are usually a number of issues to work on and it is important to cover the essential ones in the time allowed. Once treatment is under way the general approach remains the same. Homework tasks are reviewed and problems discussed. Specific cognitive and behavioural strategies will be focused on during each session and as a general rule it is helpful to stick to one or two problems or items for discussion. New homework tasks are agreed upon, to be carried out before the next session. At the end of each session the patient should be asked to give feedback on their own progress and what they have learned. Behavioural and cognitive interventions are usually employed together, but for clarity they will be described separately.

Behavioural interventions

Behavioural strategies are used to convince the patient that gradual increases in activity can, in fact, be achieved without causing worsening of the illness. The aim is to break the association between symptoms and stopping activity. The emphasis is therefore on practising activities at regular intervals regardless of the occurrence of symptoms. These activities should be consistent with the patient's short-term goals. They may include walking, swimming, domestic tasks, and socializing. Simply prescribing exercise can be counterproductive unless the patient is convinced that such a strategy is at least worth trying.

The activities involved may include virtually no exercise at all — such as getting out of bed for a certain length of time or going to the toilet unaided. It is more important that the initial level of activity is set at a sufficiently low level to be attainable. It may even be necessary to actually restrict activity, since many patients have become caught in a cycle of excessive rest followed by excessive activity on the few 'good days' that result — a 'boom and bust' pattern, also observed in fibromyalgia (Nielson *et al.* 1992).

Tasks are graded in terms of how difficult they are and introduced in stages. During the early stages of treatment the patient may experience an initial increase in symptoms. It is imperative that the therapist predicts this. The symptoms usually decrease in time but may take several days and sometimes weeks. As long as homework is set at a low enough level the patient should be able to tolerate the initial discomfort. Only when symptom reduction and/or increased tolerance to activity has occurred are new targets set.

As important as activity is the planning of rest. Immediate reductions in the amount of rest taken are rarely advised in the early stages. Instead, after a careful functional assessment, usually involving the keeping of a diary, the current pattern of rest is determined. This is averaged over a period of time — a week, for example, and the daily requirement determined. This is then built into the timetable. As with activity, the aim is to rest in a planned and consistent way, rather than it being a response to symptoms. Instead, the goal of the early stages of treatment is to combat the experience of unpredictability of symptoms, so often described by sufferers.

Cognitive interventions

An important cognitive intervention is to provide education about the nature of chronic fatigue syndrome and the cognitive behavioural model. Patients have often read a great deal about the condition, not all of which is either accurate or helpful. The second component is to reduce excessive concern about activity-induced symptoms. Increases in activity are likely to result in a short-term increase in fatigue and other symptoms. The patient may experience thoughts such as 'If I go and do more I'll be unwell for days'. Patients are asked to keep a record of these thoughts and in discussion with the therapist to generate less catastrophic alternatives such as 'I'm bound to feel more fatigued initially as I am not used to exercise, but with practice I will be able to do more'. The evidence for and against this and alternative propositions should be reviewed. If evidence is lacking 'behavioural experiments' can be performed, for example by recording symptoms carefully whilst gradually increasing activity.

Patients may have other non-illness beliefs that can interfere with rehabilitation. These include the tendency to discount any achievement that falls short of their pre-morbid level. These 'all or nothing beliefs' about standards and responsibilities must be questioned if the patient is to be able to pursue consistent and graded increases in activity. Finally, as the patient re-engages with their life it is likely that a number of problems, both old and new, will have to be confronted. Occupational and interpersonal problems may be obstacles to recovery unless successfully managed. Problem-solving techniques (Hawton *et al.* 1989) are useful in this context and consistent with the overall approach of helping the patient to regain control over their own life.

Problems in treatment

Failure to achieve an increase in activity   The most likely reasons for the patient failing to increase their activity level are

(1) too large an increase in activity was planned;

(2) the patient has doubts about the safety or value of the treatment;

(3) there is some other block to increasing activity such as fear of failure.

The problem is best managed by reviewing and revising the targets and eliciting and challenging any inaccurate or exaggerated concerns about the significance of symptoms and implications of failure.

Unwillingness by the patient to accept that psychological factors are relevant to treatment   Patients may express a marked unwillingness to accept any treatment that is perceived to imply that they have psychological problems or psychiatric illness. Clinical experience suggests that the objection to psychological approaches commonly results from a concern that if the illness is labelled as psychological or psychiatric it implies fault. This erroneous belief should be specifically addressed by differentiating between responsibility for becoming ill and responsibility for working toward recovery.

Conclusion

We have argued that chronic fatigue syndromes and fibromyalgia are heterogenous conditions of mixed aetiology strongly associated with and partly explained by emotional disorder, but also with important cognitive, behavioural, pathophysiological, and interpersonal aspects. Chronic fatigue syndrome is currently one of the most topical functional syndromes and the political and social aspects of the illness are particularly salient.

Although a variety of specific agents have been advocated as specific treatments none have been shown to be helpful. A cognitive behavioural approach to rehabilitation is both logical and feasible. The effectiveness of cognitive behavioural therapy compared with other less-specific treatments remains to be demonstrated however.

It is our view that the central issue in the current epidemic of chronic fatigue syndrome is neither viruses nor depression, but views as to what is and what is not a legitimate illness. This same division can be applied to treatment and must be taken into account when 'selling' the approach outlined, which we consider to be the treatment of choice, to the modern consumer of medical care.

References

Abbey, S. and Garfinkel, P. (1990). Chronic fatigue syndrome and the psychiatrist. *Canadian Journal of Psychiatry*, **35**, 625–33.

Althaus, J. (1893). On cerebrine alpha and myelin alpha in the treatment of certain neuroses. *Lancet*, 2 December.

Anon. (1991). Chronic fatigue syndrome — false avenues and dead ends. *Lancet*, **337**, 31–2.

Arnold, D., Bore, P., Radda, G., Styles, P., and Taylor, D. (1984). Excessive intracellular acidosis of skeletal muscle on exercise in a patient with a post-viral exhaustion/fatigue syndrome. *Lancet*, **i**, 1367–9.

Asher, R. (1947). The dangers of going to bed. *British Medical Journal*, **4**, 976–68.

Bakheit, A., Behan, P., Dinan, T., Gray, C., and O'Keane, V. (1992). Possible upregulation of hypothalamic 5-hydroxytryptamine receptors in patients with post-viral fatigue syndrome. *British Medical Journal*, **304**, 1010–12.

Baszanger, I. (1992). Deciphering chronic pain. *Sociology of Health and Illness*, **14**, 181–215.

Beard, G. (1880). *A practical treatise on nervous exhaustion (neurasthenia)*. William Wood, New York.

Behan, P. and Behan, W. (1988). The postviral fatigue syndrome. *CRC Critical Reviews in Neurobiology*, **42**, 157–78.

Bell, M. and Bailey, A. (1992). Refractory fibromyalgia syndrome: efficacy of a comprehensive 12 week ambulatory exercise programme. *Arthritis and Rheumatism*, **35**, R41 (abstract).

Bennett, R. (1989). Physical fitness and muscle metabolism in the fibromyalgia syndrome: an overview. *Journal of Rheumatology*, **16** (Suppl. 19), 28–9.

Berrett, J. (1991). Condemned to live a lonely life. *The Guardian* 6 July.

Berrios, G. (1990). Feelings of fatigue and psychopathology: a conceptual history. *Comprehensive Psychiatry*, **31**, 140–51.

Bock, G. and Whelan, J. (ed) (1993) *Chronic fatigue syndrome*. Wiley, Chichester.

Brodsky, C. (1991). Depression and chronic fatigue in the workplace. *Primary Care*, **18**, 381–96.

Butler, S., Chalder, T., Ron, M., and Wessely, S. (1991). Cognitive behaviour therapy in the chronic fatigue syndrome. *Journal of Neurology, Neurosurgery and Psychiatry*, **54**, 153–8.

Carette, S., McCain, G., Bell, D., and Fam, A. (1986). Evaluation of amitriptyline in primary fibrositis: a double-blind placebo controlled study. *Arthritis and Rheumatism*, **29**, 655–9.

Cathebras, P., Robbins, J., Kirmayer, L., and Hayton, B. (1992). Fatigue in primary care: prevalence, psychiatric comorbidity, illness behaviour and outcome. *Journal of General Internal Medicine*, **7**, 276–86.

Charatan, F. (1990). Chronic fatigue in the US. *British Medical Journal*, **301**, 1236.

Cheney, P. (1989). It's a dirty little war: proponents of a 'psychoneurotic' cause of CIDS try again. *Christopher Street*, **1**, 32–3.

Collee, J. (1991). A doctor writes. *Observer*, 25th August.

Dainty, E. (1988). M.E. and I. *Nursing Standard*, **84**, 49–50.

David, A., Wessely, S., and Pelosi, A. (1988). Post-viral fatigue: time for a new approach. *British Medical Journal*, **296**, 696–9.

David, A., McDonald, E., Mann, A., Pelosi, A., Stephens, D., Ledger, D. and Rathbone, R. (1990). Tired, weak or in need of rest: fatigue among general practice attenders. *British Medical Journal*, **301**, 1199–202.

David, A. (1991). Postviral fatigue syndrome and psychiatry. *British Medical Bulletin*, **47**, 966–88.

Dawes, B. and Downing, D. (1989). *Why M.E.? A guide to combatting post-viral illness*. Grafton, London.

Denman, A.M. (1990). The chronic fatigue syndrome; a return to common sense. *Postgraduate Medical Journal*, **66**, 499–501.

Dinerman, H. and Steere, A. (1992). Lyme disease associated with fibromyalgia. *Annals of Internal Medicine*, **117**, 281–5.

Dock, W. (1944). The evil sequelae of complete bed rest. *Journal of the American Medical Association*, **125**, 1083–5.

Dubbert, P.M. (1992). Exercise in behavioural medicine. *Journal of Consulting and Clinical Psychology*, **60**, 613–18.

Editorial. (1987). Aching muscles after exercise. *Lancet*, **ii**, 1123–5.

Edwards, R.H. (1981). Human muscle function and fatigue. In *Human muscle fatigue: physiological mechanisms*, (ed. R. Porter and J. Whelan), pp. 1–18. Pitman Medical, London.

Edwards, R., Newham, D., and Peters, T. (1991). Muscle biochemistry and pathophysiology in postviral fatigue syndrome. *British Medical Bulletin*, **47**, 826–37.

Feiden, K. (1990). *Hope and help for chronic fatigue syndrome*. Prentice Hall, New York.

Finlay, S. (1986). Don't listen if your GP says it's 'just nerves'. *The Scotsman*, 18 August.

Franklin, M. and Sullivan, J. (1989). *The new mystery fatigue epidemic. M.E. What is it? Have you got it? How to get better*. Century, London.

Gibson, H., Carroll, N., Clague, J., and Edwards, R. (1993). Exercise performance and fatiguability in patients with chronic fatigue syndrome. *Journal of Neurology, Neurosurgery and Psychiatry*, **156**, 993–8.

Gibson, J., Halliday, D., Morrison, W., Stoward, P., Hornsby, G., Watt, P., Murdoch, G., and Rennie, M. (1987). Decrease in human quadriceps muscle protein turnover consequent upon leg immobilisation. *Clinical Science*, **72**, 503–9.

Gold, D., Bowden, R., Sixbey, J., Riggs, R., Katon, W., Ashley, R. *et al.* (1990). Chronic fatigue: a prospective clinical and virologic study. *Journal of the American Medical Association*, **264**, 48–53.

Goldenberg, D.L., Felson, D.T., and Kinerman, H. (1986). A randomized controlled trial of amitriptyline and naproxen in the treatment of patients with primary fibromyalgia. *Arthritis and Rheumatism*, **29**, 131–7.

Goldstein, J. (1990). *Chronic fatigue syndrome: the struggle for health. A diagnostic and treatment guide for patients and their physicians*. Chronic Fatigue Syndrome Institute, Beverly Hills.

Goodnick, P., Sandoval, R., Brickman, A., and Klimas, N. (1992). Bupropion therapy in chronic fatigue syndrome. *Abstracts of the American Psychiatric Association*, Washington, 5 April, pp. 123–4.

Gow, J., Behan, W., Clements, G., Woodall, C., Riding, M., and Behan, P. (1991). Enteroviral RNA sequences detected by polymerase chain reaction in muscle of patients with postviral fatigue syndrome. *British Medical Journal*, **302**, 692–6.

Gracious, B. and Wisner, K. (1991). Nortriptyline in chronic fatigue syndrome: a double blind, placebo-controlled single case study. *Biological Psychiatry*, **30**, 405–8.

Greenberg, D. (1990). Neurasthenia in the 1980s: chronic mononucleosis, chronic fatigue syndrome and anxiety depressive disorders. *Psychosomatics*, **31**, 129–37.

Harding, T., Arango, M., Baltazar, J., Climent, C., Ibrahim, H., Ladrido-Ignacio, L. *et al.* (1980). Mental disorders in primary health care: a study of their frequency and diagnosis in four developing countries. *Psychological Medicine*, **10**, 231–41.

Hawton, K., Salkovskis, P., Kirk, J., and Clark, D. (1989). *Cognitive behaviour therapy for psychiatric problems: a practical guide*. Oxford University Press, Oxford.

Helman, C. (1978). Feed a cold and starve a fever. *Culture, Medicine and Psychiatry*, **7**, 107–37.

Hellinger, W., Smith, T., Van Scoy, R., Spitzer, P., Forgacs, P., and Edson, R. (1988). Chronic fatigue syndrome and the diagnostic utility of Epstein–Barr virus early antigen. *Journal of the American Medical Association*, **260**, 971–3.

Hickie, I., Lloyd, A., Wakefield, D., and Parker, G. (1990). The psychiatric status of patients with chronic fatigue syndrome. *British Journal of Psychiatry*, **156**, 534–40.

Hilgers, A., Krueger, G., Lembke, U., and Ramon, A. (1991). Postinfectious chronic fatigue syndrome; case history of thirty-five patients in Germany. *In Vivo*, **5**, 201–6.

Hodgkinson, L. (1988). M.E. – the mystery disease. *Women's Journal*, November.

Holmes, G.P., Kaplan, J.E., Gantz, N.M., Komaroff, A.L., Schonberger, L.B., Straus, S.E., and *et al.* (1988). Chronic fatigue syndrome: a working case definition. *Annals of Internal Medicine*, **108**, 387–9.

Imboden, J., Canter, A., Cluff, L., and Trever, R.W. (1959). Brucellosis. III. Psychological aspects of delayed convalescence. *Archives of Internal Medicine*, **103**, 406–15.

Jamal, G. and Miller, R. (1991). Neurophysiology of postviral fatigue syndrome. *British Medical Bulletin*, **47**, 815–25.

Janet, P. (1919). *Les Obsessions et la Psychasthenie*, Vol 1. Alcan, Paris.

Jones, J. and Straus, S. (1987). Chronic Epstein–Barr virus infection. *Annual Review of Medicine*, **38**, 195–209.

Karno, M. and Hoffman, R. (1974). The pseudoanergic syndrome. In *Somatic manifestations of depressive disorders*, pp. 55–85. Excerta Medica.

Katon, W., Buchwald, D., Simon, G., Russo, J. and Mease, P. (1991). Psychiatric illness in patients with chronic fatigue and rheumatoid arthritis. *Journal of General Internal Medicine*, **6**, 277–85.

Katz, B. and Andiman, W. (1988). Chronic fatigue syndrome. *Journal of Pediatrics*, **113**, 944–7.

Keefe, F. and Gil, K. (1986). Behavioural concepts in the analysis of chronic pain syndromes. *Journal of Consulting and Clinical Psychology*, **54**, 776–83.

Kendell, R. (1991). Chronic fatigue, viruses, and depression. *Lancet*, **337**, 160–3.

Kennedy, P. (1991). Postviral fatigue syndrome: current neurobiological perspective. *British Medical Bulletin*, **47**, 809–14.

Klug, G., McAuley, E., and Clark, S. (1989). Factors influencing the development and maintenance of aerobic fitness; lessons applicable to the fibrositis syndrome. *Journal of Rheumatology*, **16**, (Suppl. 19) 30–9.

Kyle, D. and DeShazo, R. (1992). Chronic fatigue syndrome: a conundrum, *American Journal of Medical Sciences*, **303**, 28–34.

Lamb, L., Stevens, P., and Johnson, R. (1965). Hypokinesia secondary to chair rest from 4 to 10 days. *Aerospace Medicine*, **36**, 755–63.

Lane, T., Matthews, D., and Manu, P. (1990). The low yield of physical examinations and laboratory investigations of patients with chronic fatigue. *American Journal of Medical Sciences*, **299**, 313–18.

Lechky, O. (1990). Life insurance MDs sceptical when chronic fatigue syndrome diagnosed. *Canadian Medical Association Journal*, **143**, 413–15.

Lewis, G. and Wessely, S. (1992). The epidemiology of fatigue: more questions than answers. *Journal of Epidemiology and Community Health*, **46**, 92–7.

Lewis, S. and Haller, R. (1991). Physiologic measurement of exercise and fatigue with special reference to chronic fatigue syndrome. *Reviews of Infectious Diseases*, **13** (Suppl. 1), 98–108.

Lloyd, A., Hales, J., and Gandevia, S. (1988). Muscle strength, endurance and recovery in the post-infection fatigue syndrome. *Journal of Neurology, Neurosurgery and Psychiatry*, **51**, 1316–22.

Lloyd, A., Gandevia, S., and Hales, J. (1991). Muscle performance, voluntary activation, properties and perceived effort in normal subjects and patients with the chronic syndrome. *Brain*, **114**, 85–98.

Lloyd, A., Hickie, I., Brockman, A., Hickie, C., Wilson, A., Dwyer, J., and Wakefield, D. (1993). Immunologic and psychologic therapy for patients with chronic fatigue syndrome: a double-blind, placebo-controlled trial. *American Journal of Medicine*, **94**, 197–203.

Lynch, S., Seth, R., and Montgomery, S. (1991). Antidepressant therapy in the chronic fatigue syndrome. *British Journal of General Practice*, **41**, 339–42.

McCain, G., Bell, D., Mai, F., and Holliday, P. (1988). A controlled study of the effects of a supervised cardiovascular fitnes training program on the manifestations of primary fibromyalgia. *Arthritis and Rheumatism*, **31**, 1135–41.

McCluskey, D. (1993). Pharmacological treatments to the theory of chronic fatigue syndrome. In *Chronic fatigue syndrome*, (ed. G. Bock and J. Whelan) pp. 280–87. John Wiley, Chichester.

MacDougall, R. (1899). Fatigue. *Psychological Review*, **6**, 203–8.

Macy, J. and Allen, E. (1934). Justification of the diagnosis of chronic nervous exhaustion. *Annals of Internal Medicine*, **7**, 861–7.

Manu, P., Matthews, D., and Lane, T. (1988). The mental health of patients with a chief complaint of chronic fatigue: a prospective evaluation and follow-up. *Archives of Internal Medicine*, **148**, 2213–17.

Matthews, D., Manu, P., and Lane, T. (1989). Diagnostic beliefs among patients with chronic fatigue. *Clinical Research*, **37**, 820A.

Mihevic, P. (1981). Sensory cues for perceived exertion: a review. *Medicine Science Sports Exercise*, **13**, 150–63.

Muller, E. (1970). Influence of training and of inactivity on muscle strength. *Archives of Physical Medicine and Rehabilitation*, **51**, 449–52.

Muscio, B. (1921). Is a fatigue test possible? *British Journal of Psychology*, **12**, 31–46.

Nielson, W., Walker, C., and McCain, G. (1992). Cognitive behavioral treatment of fibromyalgia syndrome: preliminary findings. *Journal of Rheumatology*, **19**, 98–103.

Pawlikowska, T., Chalder, T., Hirsch, S.R., Wallace, P., Wright, D.J.M., and Wessely, S. (1994). Population based study of fatigue and psychological distress. *British Medical Journal*, **308**, 763–77.

Petersen, P., Schenck, C., and Sherman, R. (1991). Chronic fatigue syndrome in Minnesota. *Minnesota Medicine*, **74**, 21–6.

Philips, H. (1987). Avoidance behaviour and its role in sustaining chronic pain. *Behaviour Research and Therapy*, **25**, 273–9.

Powell, R., Dolan, R., and Wessely, S. (1990). Attributions and self esteem in depression and the chronic fatigue syndrome. *Journal of Psychosomatic Research*, **34**, 665–73.

Rabinbach, A. (1990). *The human motor: energy, fatigue and the origins of modernity*. Basic Books, New York.

Ramsay, M. (1989). Introduction. In *Living with ME; a self-help guide*, (ed. C. Shepherd), pages xiii–iv. Heinemann, London.

Ray, C. (1991). Chronic fatigue syndrome and depression: conceptual and methodological ambiguities. *Psychological Medicine*, **21**, 1–9.

Reeves, W., Pellett, P., and Gary, H. (1992). The chronic fatigue syndrome controversy. *Annals of Internal Medicine*, **117**, 343.

Ridsdale, L. (1993). Tired all the time. *British Medical Journal*, **303**, 1490–91.

Riley, M., O'Brien, C., McCluskey, D., Bell, N., and Nicholls, D. (1990). Aerobic work capacity in patients with chronic fatigue syndrome. *British Medical Journal*, **301**, 953–6.

Rutherford, O. and White, P. (1991). Human quadriceps strength and fatigability in patients with post-viral-fatigue. *Journal of Neurology, Neurosurgery and Psychiatry*, **54**, 961–4.

Saltin, B., Blomqvist, G., Mitchell, J., Johnson, R.L., Wildenthal, K. and Chapman, C.B. (1968). Response to exercise after bed rest and after training. *Circulation*, **38** (Suppl. 7), 1–78.

Schluederberg, A., Straus, S., Peterson, P., Blumenthal, S., Komaroff, A., Spring, S. *et al.* (1992). Chronic fatigue syndrome research: definition and medical outcome assessment. *Annals of Internal Medicine*, **117**, 325–31.

Sensky, T. (1990). Patients' reactions to illness. *British Medical Journal*, **300**, 622–3.

Sharpe, M. (1991). Psychiatric management of PVFS. *British Medical Bulletin*, **47**, 989–1005.

Sharpe, M. (1992). Fatigue and chronic fatigue syndrome. *Current Opinion in Psychiatry*, **5**, 207–12.

Sharpe, M. (1993). Non-pharmacological approaches to treatment. *Chronic fatigue syndrome*, pp. 298–317. Chichester.

Sharpe, M. and Bass, C. (1992). Pathophysiological mechanisms in somatization. *International Review of Psychiatry*, **4**, 81–97.

Sharpe, M.C., Archard, L.C., Banatvala, J.E., Borysiewicz, L.K., Clare, A.W., David, A.S., and *et al.* (1991). A report – chronic fatigue syndrome: guidelines for research. *Journal of the Royal Society of Medicine*, **84**, 118–21.

Sharpe, M., Hawton, K., Seagroatt, V., and Pasvol, G. (1992). Follow up of patients with fatigue presenting to an infectious diseases clinic. *British Medical Journal*, **305**, 347–52.

Shepherd, C. (1989). *Living with ME: a self-help guide*. Heinemann, London.

Shorter, E. (1992). *From paralysis to fatigue: a history of psychosomatic illness in the modern era*. Macmillan, New York.

Smith, D. (1989). Myalgic encephalomyelitis. In 1989 *members reference book*, (ed. Royal College of General Practitioners), pp. 247–50. Sabre Crown Publishing, London.

Stokes, M., Cooper, R., and Edwards, R. (1988). Normal strength and fatigability in patients with effort syndrome. *British Medical Journal*, **297**, 1014–18.

Straus, S. (1991). Intravenous immunoglobulin treatment for the chronic fatigue syndrome. *American Journal of Medicine*, **89**, 551–3.

Taylor, J. (1907). Management of exhaustion states in men. *International Clinics*, **17**, 36–50.

Valdini, A., Steinhardt, S., and Feldman, E. (1989). Usefulness of a standard battery of laboratory tests in investigating chronic fatigue in adults. *Family Practice*, **6**, 286–91.

Vereker, M. (1992). Chronic fatigue syndrome: a joint paediatric–psychiatric approach. *Archives of Disease in Childhood*, **67**, 550–5.

Wagenmakers, A., Coakley, J., and Edwards, R.H.T. (1988). The metabolic consequences of reduced habitual activities in patients with muscle pain and disease. *Ergonomics*, **31**, 1519–27.

Ware, N. (1992). Suffering and the social construction of illness: the delegitimation of illness experience in chronic fatigue syndrome. *Medical Anthropology Quarterly*, **6**, 347–61.

Waterman, G. (1909). The treatment of fatigue states. *Journal of Abnormal Psychology*, **4**, 128–39.

Watts, F. (1982). Attributional aspects of medicine. In *Attributions and psychological change*, (ed. C. Antaki and C. Brewin), pp. 135-55. Academic Press, London.

Webb, H. and Parsons, L. (1991). Chronic PVFS in the neurology clinic. In *Post-viral fatigue syndrome*, (ed. R. Jenkins and J. Mowbray), pp. 233-9. John Wiley, Chichester.

Wessely, S. (1990). The natural history of chronic fatigue and myalgia syndromes. In *Psychological disorders in general medical settings*, (ed. N. Sartorius, D. Goldberg G. de Girolamo, J.A. Costa e Silva, Y. Lecrubier, and H. Wittchen), pp. 82-97. Hans Huber, Bern.

Wessely, S. (1991). The history of the postviral fatigue syndrome. *British Medical Bulletin*, **47**, 919-41.

Wessely, S. (1992). Chronic fatigue syndrome: current issues. *Reviews in Medical Microbiology*, **3**, 211-6.

Wessely, S. (1993). The neuropsychiatry of chronic fatigue syndrome. In *Chronic fatigue syndrome*, (ed. G. Bock and J. Whelan), pp. 212-37. John Wiley, Chichester.

Wessely, S. and Edwards, R.H.T. (1993). Fatigue. In *Neurological rehabilitation*, (ed. R. Greenwood, M. Barnes, T. McMillan, and C. Ward), pp. 311-25. Churchill Livingstone, Edinburgh.

Wessely, S. and Powell, R. (1989). Fatigue syndromes: a comparison of chronic 'postviral' fatigue with neuromuscular and affective disorders. *Journal of Neurology, Neurosurgery and Psychiatry*, **42**, 940-8.

Wessely, S. and Thomas, P.K. (1990). The chronic fatigue syndrome ('myalgic encephalomyclitis' or 'postviral fatigue'). In *Recent advances in neurology*, Vol. 6, (ed. C. Kennard), pp. 85-132. Churchill Livingstone, Edinburgh.

Wessely, S., Butler, S., Chalder, T., and David, A. (1991). The cognitive behavioral management of the postviral fatigue syndrome. In *Postviral fatigue syndrome*, (ed. R. Jenkins and J. Mowbray), pp. 305-34. John Wiley, Chichester.

Wheeler, E., White, P., Reed, E., and Cohen, M. (1950). Neurocirculatory asthenia (anxiety neurosis, effort syndrome, neurasthenia). *Journal of the American Medical Association*, **142**, 878-89.

White, P. (1991). The post-infectious fatigue syndrome. *Abstracts of the Annual Meeting of the Royal College of Psychiatrists*, Brighton, 5 April, p. 79.

Wilson, D., Widmer, R., Cadoret, R., and Judiesch, K. (1983). Somatic symptoms: a major feature of depression in a family practice. *Journal of Affective Disorders*, **5**, 199-207.

Wood, G., Bentall, R., Gopfert, M., and Edwards, R. (1991). A comparative psychiatric assessment of patients with chronic fatigue syndrome and muscle disease. *Psychological Medicine*, **21**, 619-28.

Yunus, M. (1988). Diagnosis, etiology and management of fibromyalgia syndrome. an update. *Comprehensive Therapy*, **14**, 8-20.

Zorbas, Y.G. and Matveyev, I.O. (1986). Man's desirability in performing physical exercises under hypokinesia. *International Journal of Rehabilitation Research*, **9**, 170-4.

17 Chronic pelvic pain

Lesley Glover and Shirley Pearce

In this chapter Drs Glover and Pearce begin by describing the prevalence of pelvic pain and the associated cost to health services. An aetiological model of pelvic pain is outlined in which pathophysiological processes in the pelvis (which include abnormal venous congestion) interact with psychological factors to produce the sensation of pelvic pain. A preoccupation with disease explanations for the pain, increased attention to the somatic sensations, and the acquisition of 'pain behaviours', may all then act to perpetuate a syndrome of chronic pelvic pain.

The authors argue that the assessment and management of patients with chronic pelvic pain presents particular problems and requires special skills. A therapeutic approach using cognitive behavioural techniques is outlined. Finally, the advantages and pitfalls of a group intervention for this problem are described.

Introduction

Pelvic pain is one of the most common symptoms reported by women attending gynaecology clinics (Beard and Pearce 1989) and has been estimated to cost the NHS £163 million per year (0.6 per cent of total expenditure) (Beard and Pearce 1992). Any effective psychological treatment is likely therefore to have the potential to lead to cost savings, as well as to reductions in the patients' pain and disability.

Pelvic pain and pelvic pathology

Gillibrand (1981) found that of 331 women presenting with pelvic pain only 37 per cent had any identifiable pathology. Even when pelvic abnormalities are detected, it is not always possible to demonstrate a causal association between these and the pain complaints. Many cases of chronic pelvic pain may therefore be regarded as functional.

Pelvic pain and psychological factors

A number of studies have attempted to identify the psychological factors associated with unexplained or functional pelvic pain. One approach has been to compare patients with unexplained chronic pelvic pain with patients without pain, using psychometric tests or psychiatric interviews. However, the results of this approach have been discrepant. Gidro-Frank *et al.* (1960) and Benson *et al.* (1959) reported a higher incidence of psychiatric problems in women with unexplained pelvic pain, whereas others (for example, Castelnuovo-Tedesco and Krout 1970) did not.

Because it has been recognized that the long-term experience of pain may have psychological consequences, whatever the underlying organic pathology, more recent studies have compared patients with functional pelvic pain to patients with chronic pain of an equivalent duration that is clearly attributable to organic disease. Such a study was carried out by Pearce (1989) who found no difference on measures of mood and personality between women with and without organic disease.

Some differences did emerge however on other psychological measures. For example, women experiencing pain in the absence of identified disease were found to have higher disease conviction scores on the modified Illness Behaviour Scale (Pilowsky and Spence 1975). There was also a trend for those without organic disease to have higher hypochondriasis scores, suggesting that these women may be more concerned about their physical state and, hence, monitor bodily sensations more closely than those with disease. Significantly, women without disease reported higher rates of serious illness and death in family members. Although such exposure is not sufficient to cause unexplained pelvic pain, (since many of the illnesses and deaths had occurred several years before the onset of the pain), it does suggest that exposure to serious illness may influence attitudes, causing closer monitoring of one's own bodily sensations and well-being. Given certain other conditions, such as a tendency to venous congestion, this may lead to the reporting of symptoms.

Other studies have suggested that certain sexual experiences and attitudes may influence the likelihood of a presentation with pelvic pain. Gross *et al.* (1980) identified early traumatic sexual experiences (incest) in nine out of 25 patients with chronic pelvic pain. However, Petrucco and Harris (1982) found that 72 per cent of women with undiagnosed chronic pain were orgasmic and reported no sexual problems. More systematic investigation is required before concluding that sexual behaviour and experience play an etiological role.

Pathophysiology — the role of pelvic venous congestion

Beard *et al.* (1989) have suggested that the endocrine control of ovarian function may be disturbed by stress. This view is based on the observation that 54 per cent of women with pelvic pain due to congestion were found to have polycystic ovaries (Adams *et al.* 1990). It was backed up by the observation that suppression of ovarian function by medroxyprogesterone acetate significantly improved pelvic blood flow (Reginald *et al.* 1989) and that oophorectomy resulted in relief from pelvic pain in women with demonstrable congestion (Beard and Reginald 1990).

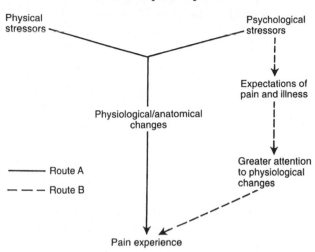

Fig. 17.1 A model for pelvic pain in which the pain experience may be due to physiological changes (Route A) or changes in pain perception and behaviour (Route B)

A model of chronic pelvic pain

The model presented in Fig. 17.1 proposes that there are a group of women who develop pain associated with pelvic congestion. It is suggested that these women have a biological predisposition to develop changes in pelvic blood flow with the experience of stress and that these changes are either greater in magnitude or take longer to return to baseline levels than those in normal women. Exposure to psychological stressors will therefore produce changes in the pelvic vasculature which lead, over time, to the development of chronically dilated pelvic veins. In these patients psychological factors play a direct causal role (Route A in Fig. 17.1).

Although current evidence supports the existence of a venous abnormality in some women with otherwise unexplained pelvic pain, there are women who report pain in the absence of any such observable underlying physiological changes. In such cases psychological factors may play an indirect role in the development of pain by altering the perception of physiological changes so that they are perceived as pain (Route B in Fig. 17.1). Hence, it is proposed that the abnormal sensory afferent activity from the pelvis is more likely to be reported as painful by women who are closely monitoring their physiological state, possibly because they are concerned about illness in general or pelvic dysfunction in particular. The experience of pain then leads to 'pain behaviour' which may be reinforced and maintained by social factors (Fordyce 1982). Feedback loops may also arise at several of these levels of pain experience, for example being in pain is likely to direct further attention to the pelvis and lead to increased preoccupation with and expectation of pain.

Psychological interventions in women with pelvic pain

Specific gender issues in pelvic pain

While a number of issues discussed here are relevant to the treatment of patients with all types of chronic pain, there are some that are specific to women with pelvic pain. Pelvic pain is located in the reproductive organs and is therefore linked with beliefs relating to femininity and sexuality, as well as with attitudes to women's bodies. Attributions about pelvic pain may differ from those about pains in other sites: women learn from an early age to expect certain aspects of gynaecological functioning to be painful. These attributions and expectations are likely to influence their responses to the pain (for a full discussion of gender issues in gynaecological pain see Erskine and Pearce (1991)).

The experience of previous medical treatment may also be of special relevance in pelvic pain. A woman with pelvic pain may have undergone repeated vaginal examination or even pelvic surgery. As a consequence she may feel that this intimate part of her body has become public and that decisions about it have been removed from her control.

The assessment interview

The first assessment interview with a woman presenting with gynaecological pain can be difficult both for the psychologist and for the patient. Many women will have been through a succession of lengthy investigations and failed treatments before being told that no further medical treatment can be attempted. The referral to the psychologist may have been made with minimal explanation. As a result, the woman is likely to feel ambivalent about the appointment. Her first words and gestures may reveal puzzlement, apprehension, hopelessness, irritation, or even hostility. It is also possible that negative or mixed feelings may be hidden under outward politeness or compliance and it is important that this is dealt with early in the interview. Here, the values and communication skills of the therapist play a crucial role. The process of counselling women in pain rests on the same foundations of respect, genuineness, and empathy which underlie any effective form of helping (Rogers 1961). These values need to be translated into the kind of sensitive and accurate listening skills which facilitate the expression of doubts, as well as hopes about the likely benefits of counselling (Egan 1986).

Patients are often ambivalent about psychological interventions. The traditional view of pain as either 'real' and 'in the body' or 'unreal' and

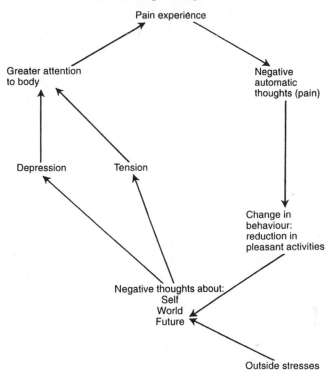

Fig. 17.2 A model of the role of psychological factors for use in treatment

'in the mind' may lead some patients to see the offer of psychological treatment as implying an accusation of malingering or madness. The fear of being labelled in this way needs to be acknowledged and discussed (see Chapter 5.

Once the process of engagement has been achieved, an outline of the model of pain shown in Fig. 17.2 can be very useful, especially if the woman's own experience of pain is used to provide examples. The aim is to move the woman on from her view of pain as a unitary, physiological process which is outside her control, towards a multidimensional model which can accommodate a psychological interaction. This allows hopelessness about cure to begin to give way to a new hope of rehabilitation. Failure to initiate this all-important process of 'reappraisal' can often render subsequent efforts at management fruitless.

Developing the interview

Once a shared model of pain is at least tentatively agreed, it is easier to take a case history. This should include attention to past episodes of pain as well as to the psychosexual history. In some patients it may be possible to begin a functional analysis of the pain in the first session. This includes an assessment of any precipitating factors or aggravating factors, the temporal and situational determinants of pain episodes, and an exploration of the attributions and reactions of both the patient and significant others to these episodes. Indeed, all those components of pain described by Karoly (1985) should he investigated.

The response of a partner or significant other may be one of the factors maintaining the pain and interviewing the partner or significant other can be important. We also often ask the woman to keep a pain diary (for example, Erskine and Williams 1989) before the next session; this can pave the way for more detailed discussions of fluctuations of pain in relation to psychosocial changes and also provides a useful baseline to explore the impact of any future intervention. Karoly (1985) gives a full and critical account of multilevel assessment.

It is important to explore the woman's own goals for treatment and it is not uncommon for these to change over the course of the assessment. For example, if the pain and pain management emerge as the main focus, a cognitive behavioural approach is likely to be the treatment of choice (see below). However, the presenting pain problem may become less salient as other problem areas such as depression, marital conflict, eating disorder, or a history of sexual abuse are revealed. In such cases nondirective counselling, cognitive therapy, marital therapy, or psychodynamic counselling may become appropriate, either as an alternative or as an adjunct to pain management.

In the following sections we will review the existing literature concerning specific psychological approaches for the management of pelvic pain, both on an individual and group basis. We will also present an outline of some of the practical issues we consider important with this client group.

Review of specific psychological interventions

Cognitive behavioural treatment

A prerequisite for any intervention is a credible model. We have found the model of pelvic pain presented in Fig. 17.2 to be more persuasive and relevant to chronic pelvic pain patients than the Gate Control Theory of pain (Melzack and Wall 1965), which is often used in general pain treatment programmes.

Beard *et al.* (1977) were among the first to describe psychological approaches to chronic pelvic pain. They presented anecdotal evidence that some women responded well to relaxation training. Unfortunately this was not a controlled study so the specific benefits of relaxation training could not be assessed. Most subsequent studies also had methodological shortcomings (Pearce *et al.* 1982; Petrucco and Harris 1982).

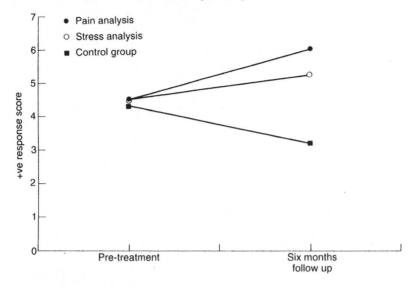

Fig. 17.3 Gynaecologists' ratings of pain in a controlled trial of two psychological interventions

The most recent controlled studies have used cognitive behavioural therapy. These interventions, some of which are described below, are structured, time limited, and include the planning of behavioural tasks. The results of two recent controlled trials of cognitive behavioural therapy provide firmer evidence that psychological interventions can be effective in the management of chronic pelvic pain, particularly in the long-term. In the first study Pearce (1986) compared stress analysis and pain analysis with a minimal intervention control group. Women allocated to the 'stress analysis' group received cognitive behavioural stress management as well as relaxation training; discussion of the pain was discouraged and the focus of counselling was directed towards current concerns other than the pain. By contrast, the 'pain analysis' group were asked to closely monitor their pain and any associated antecedent and consequent events. This therapy aimed to identify patterns associated with pain episodes and to teach alternative strategies for avoiding or reducing pain. In addition, graded exercise programmes were instituted and spouses were encouraged to become involved in these. A range of measures was used to assess outcome: these included ratings of mood, pain intensity, and behavioural disruption, as well as 'blind' ratings by the gynaecologist of the extent to which the patient was affected by her pain. At 6 months follow-up, both treatment groups were significantly better than controls on all measures of outcome (see Fig. 17.3 and 17.4).

The second study (Farquar *et al.* 1990) examined the possibility of

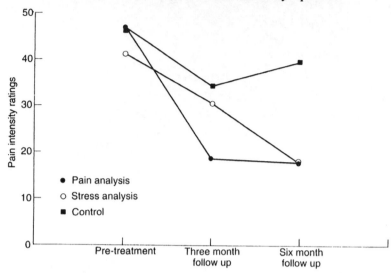

Fig. 17.4 Ratings of pain intensity in a controlled trial of two psychological interventions

integrating psychological treatment with pharmacological control of vascular congestion. This study was a randomized controlled investigation of psychological intervention and provera (medroxyprogesterone), a drug which suppresses ovarian activity, both alone and in combination. Four treatment groups were compared: provera alone, provera plus psychotherapy, placebo alone, and placebo plus psychotherapy. A number of outcome measures were recorded: pre-treatment, post-treatment, and at 3, 6, and 9 months' follow-up. In the short-term clear benefits of provera, given either alone or combined with psychotherapy, emerged. There was a tendency immediately post-treatment for women in the provera and psychotherapy group to do less well than those receiving provera alone. This result may suggest that the demands of psychological treatment (during which the stress management and pain coping strategies are being learnt), detract from the short-term benefits of provera. This trend is reversed at long-term follow-up: at 9 months although all groups had improved the provera plus psychotherapy group experienced significantly more 'pain-free days' than the other treatment groups (see Fig. 17.5).

These findings suggest an important interaction between psychological and pharmacological treatments. In particular, patients who reported reductions in pain effected by provera early in treatment were better able to learn the cognitive pain management strategies which formed part of the psychological treatment. This observation provides further support for the view that pain should be assessed and treated at both psychological and physical levels.

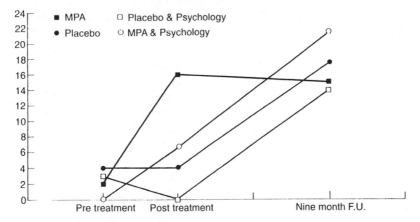

Fig. 17.5 Number of pain-free days in a controlled trial of psychological and medroxy progesterone treatment

Cognitive behavioural treatment: practical guidelines

On the basis of both clinical experience and on an examination of the literature concerning the treatment of chronic pain in general, we suggest that a cognitive behavioural intervention for chronic pelvic pain should include the following components.

1. The identification of goals. These should be agreed through discussion and be as specific as possible. These goals are likely to include an increase in the patient's activities, including hitherto avoided activity. They will also include the development of coping strategies to deal with identified current stressors. Stressors may derive from relationships, from the home or working environment, or from intra-psychic processes. Intrapsychic processes that cause difficulties to the woman include negative expectations and attributions about reproductive functioning, poor body image, and poor self-esteem.

2. Making a treatment contract (usually verbal) which includes the number of expected sessions, session duration, and treatment methods. Relief of pain intensity should be avoided as a goal or endpoint. However, the distress caused by pain can be minimized and patients should expect to feel in greater control of their pain by the end of therapy.

3. Relaxation training through progressive muscular relaxation or self-hypnosis is an important technique for reducing the effects of stress. We use tapes to enhance home practice. After a few weeks of daily

practice the relaxation can be applied to daily life and especially to pain episodes.

4. A graded, individual exercise programme. In a hospital setting it is sometimes possible to liaise with a physiotherapist. Failing this, a simple walking or swimming programme can be safely introduced, if need be in consultation with the medical referrer or general practitioner. The principle of pacing *all* activity needs to be emphasized (see also Chapter 16). Some patients need gentle restraint from excessive effort, while others may need encouragement to exercise. Bed-rest should be discouraged as a coping measure, while other forms of rest can be used as a time-limited reward for previous activity.

5. The identification and discussion of new strategies to cope with current stressors. Assertiveness training and anxiety management may both help the women avoid stressors or reduce their impact.

6. The teaching of cognitive pain coping strategies. This involves:

   (i) the identification of negative or 'automatic' thoughts used in anticipation of or during a pain episode and the substitution of more adaptive self-statements (for example, Beck *et al.* 1979);

   (ii) the practice of additional strategies such as focusing on an engrossing pleasant image or distracting mental activity (for example, making lists or mental arithmetic).

   Pearce and Erskine (1989) give a fuller account of these techniques. To be successful, these strategies need to be carefully devised and planned with the patient and, above all, practised.

7. Setting weekly 'homework' tasks which enable the woman to progress towards her goals and generalize achievements made during sessions.

8. Inviting the spouse or significant other to become a source of support for the patient in implementing the components above. This usually means educating the partner or friend about the programme and tactfully alerting him or her to their potential to be either a powerful reinforcer of pain behaviour or a facilitator of new and more adaptive behaviours.

The relevance of each of these different components will obviously vary between patients. It is important therefore to tailor the programme to the individual woman's needs.

Specific problems in the treatment of pelvic pain

The following topics may have to be addressed in the treatment of this group of patients

1. Women with chronic pelvic pain often, though not always, experience pain on intercourse. As a consequence anxiety about intercourse may occur and it may be avoided. The patient's partner may also become afraid of harming his spouse and marital difficulties may ensue. It is important therefore to address sexual topics and to attempt to find acceptable compromises for both partners. Interviewing the couple together may be helpful to encourage them to discuss possible solutions.

2. Some women with chronic pelvic pain will have a history of sexual abuse which may not be revealed until treatment is underway. If abuse is disclosed a decision must be made as to how to manage the disclosure. Within the framework of a pain management programme there is not time to address these issues adequately. If a good therapeutic relationship has been established however, it is desirable to address this topic within that relationship; if possible extra sessions should be arranged to do this. If the patient is in group treatment then one of the group facilitators should provide individual support to a patient who has disclosed abuse. Continuity of care is recommended, but this may be difficult to provide if resources are limited. If a long-term intervention addressing abuse is indicated then the patient should be referred for appropriate treatment.

Despite evidence that the psychological approaches outlined here can be an effective means of managing pain (see Chapter 7) (Germaine and Freedman 1985; Pearce 1986), there are still too few pain clinics or departments of gynaecology in the UK which employ or liaise with a psychologist. We would like to see a time when psychologists are an accepted part of a multidisciplinary gynaecological team. Ideally the psychologist would see all patients immediately after their initial meeting with the gynaecologist to assess the impact of the pain on the woman's life. This interview would take approximately 30 min and would improve the quality of the assessment. The presence of a psychologist at this stage would also facilitate psychological intervention in the longer term. While the joint approach may not be practical in all clinical settings, investing time in psychological assessment in the early stages of clinic attendance may prove economical in the longer term. It will also help to overcome the current dichotomy between medical and psychological approaches to the treatment of pelvic pain.

Group intervention for women with chronic pelvic pain

The efficacy of group intervention has been demonstrated in patients with mixed chronic pain syndromes (Pearce and Erskine 1989; Turner and Jensen 1993). For patients suffering from pelvic pain, trials of treatment have concentrated on the application of individual therapy. However the efficacy of a group intervention for pelvic pain has been examined in a recent pilot project (J. Petrak, L. Glover, T. Sichel, and B. Hedge, submitted)

The treatment group met fortnightly for six sessions of 1.5 h each. The women's needs were assessed using questionnaires and the following topics were identified for inclusion in the treatment:

(1)   medical information;

(2)   coping with pain;

(3)   stress management;

(4)   counselling.

The group was supervised by two psychologists. Each group session dealt with a specific topic which was presented in the opening 30 min. of the session by a pre-arranged speaker. In the first session the model discussed earlier (see Fig. 17.2) was introduced and at subsequent meetings information was presented and discussed in the context of that model. Meetings were structured, with approximately half the time assigned to the speaker and half to discussion. The initial membership was six, but two patients left during the course of the group. Standardized measures of mood and pain as well as specific questions relating to use of pain coping strategies were recorded before and after the study. Questions about the group were included in the 'post-intervention' questionnaire.

At the time of the post-group evaluation, group members had increased both the number and frequency of pain coping strategies and increased their belief in the efficacy of these strategies. They had greater confidence in their ability to control and to cope with the pain, despite exhibiting no significant reductions in depression, anxiety, or general pain measures. The group members response to the post-group questionnaire indicated two main themes.

1.   The women's desire to meet other women in a similar position and their relief at having done so.

2.   The women's request for more information from the clinic about treatment trials and treatment options.

We consider that a number of other important issues were raised by this pilot study which have not been adequately addressed in the general pain literature. These include the following.

1. Selection of patients. Of the two women who left during the course of the group, one was waiting for her first appointment at the clinic and the other for a hysterectomy. Thorough assessment of group members is necessary to ensure that not only are they open to the idea of psychological strategies for coping with their pain, but also that they are all at a similar stage of treatment.

2. Content of the educational component. While it is important to provide information to help women understand the nature of their condition and its treatment, it is important not to foster unrealistic expectations. A balance must be achieved between psychological and medical information. This would enable women to develop coping skills and strategies, while also providing reassurance about the causes and possible consequences of their pain.

3. Role of support versus skills acquisition. A group such as the one described above provides a combination of support and skills training. While the women found that sharing experiences was very valuable, it is not clear whether simply sharing experiences in the setting of a pain treatment group is therapeutic or whether it can reinforce negative pain-related cognitions and behaviour.

4. Individual versus group intervention. As yet no studies have compared these two types of intervention.

Only limited conclusions can be drawn from this uncontrolled pilot study. However, it is likely that group-based interventions could be a cost-effective way of making limited psychological resources available to these patients and we hope that future process and outcome research on treatments for chronic pelvic pain devotes more attention to this approach (see also Chapter 10 for a discussion of group treatments).

Conclusions

A model of chronic pelvic pain is described which involves a putative pathophysiological mechanism (pelvic venous congestion). This contributory factor may interact with psychological and other factors to lead to the experience of pelvic pain. Cognitive behavioural techniques have been shown to be effective in the management of this disorder, both individually and as an adjunct to pharmacological treatment. Group psychological treatment offers promise to patients with this chronic, distressing, and costly disorder.

References

Adams, J., Reginald, P.W., Franks, S., Wadsworth, J., and Beard, R.W. (1990). Uterine size and endometrial thickness and the significance of cystic ovaries in women with pelvic pain due to congestion. *British Journal of Obstetrics and Gynaecology*, **97**, 583-7.

Beard, R.W. and Pearce, S. (1989). Gynaecological pain. In *The textbook of pain*, (2nd edn), (ed. P.D. Wall and R. Melzack), pp. 466-82. Churchill Livingstone, London.

Beard, R.W. and Pearce, S.A. (1992). Cost of pelvic pain. Letter to *The Times*.

Beard, R.W. and Reginald, P.W. (1990). Chronic pelvic pain. In *Gynaecology*, (ed. R. Shaw). Churchill Livingstone, London.

Beard, R.W., Belsey, E.N., and Liberman, J. (1977). Pelvic pain in women. *American Journal of Obstetrics and Gynaecology*, **128**, 566-70.

Beard, R.W., Reginald, P.W., and Pearce, S. (1989). Psychology and somatic factors in women with pain due to pelvic congestion. In *Mechanisms of physical and emotional stress*, (ed. G.P. Chrousos, D.L. Loriaux, and P.W. Gold), pp. 413-21. Plenum Press, New York.

Beck, A.T., Rush, A.J., Shaw, B.F., and Emery, G. (1979). *Cognitive therapy of depression*. Guilford Press, New York.

Benson, R., Hanson, K., and Matarazzo, J. (1959). Atypical pelvic pain in women: gynaecologic and psychiatric considerations. *American Journal of Obstetrics and Gynaecology*, **77**, 806-23.

Castelnuovo-Tedesco, P. and Krout, B.M. (1970). Psychosomatic aspects of chronic pelvic pain. *International Journal of Psychiatric Medicine*, **1**, 109-26.

Egan, G. (1986). *The skilled. helper*. Brooks/Cole Publishing Co, California.

Erskine, A. and Pearce, S. (1991). Pain in gynaecology. *Counselling and communication in health care*, pp. 177-91 (ed. H. Davis and L. Fallowfield). John Wiley & Sons Chichester.

Erskine, A. and Williams, A.C. de C. (1989). Chronic pain. In *Health psychology*, pp. 427-42 (ed. A.K. Broome). Chapman and Hall, London and New York.

Farquar, C M., Rogers, V., Franks, S., Pearce, S., Wadsworth, J., and Beard, R.W. (1990). A randomised controlled trial of medroxyprogesterone acetate and psychotherapy for the treatment of pelvic congestion. *British Journal of Obstetrics and Gynaecology*, **6**, 1152-62.

Fordyce, W.E. (1982). A behavioural perspective on chronic pain. *British Journal of Clinical Psychology*, **21**, 1-12.

Germaine, L.M. and Freedman, R.R. (1985). Behavioural treatment of menopausal hot flushes. Evaluation by objective methods. *Journal of Consulting and Clinical Psychology*, **52(b)**, 1072-9.

Gidro-Frank, L., Gordon, T., and Taylor, H.C. (1960). Pelvic pain and female identity. *American Journal of Obstetrics and Gynaecology*, **79**, 1184-202.

Gillebrand, P.N. (1981). *The investigation of pelvic pain*. Communication at the

Scientific Meeting on 'Chronic pelvic pain — a gynaecological headache'. Royal College of Obstetrics and Gynaecologists, London.

Gross, R.J., Doer, H., Caldirola, P., Guzinski, G., and Ripley, H.S. (1980). Borderline syndrome and incest in chronic pain patients. *International Journal of Psychiatry in Medicine*, **10**, 79–86.

Karoly, P. (1985). The assessment of pain: concepts and procedures. In Karoly, P. (ed.) *Measurement strategies in health psychology*, pp. 461–515. Wiley, New York.

Melzack, R. and Wall, P.D. (1965). Pain mechanisms: a new theory. *Science*, **150**, 971–9.

Pearce, S. (1986). *Chronic pelvic pain: a psychological investigation*. Unpublished PdD thesis, University of London.

Pearce, S. (1989). The concept of psychogenic pain. An investigation of psychological factors in chronic pelvic pain. *Current Psychological Research and Reviews*, **6**, 16–21.

Pearce, S. and Erskine, A. (1989). Chronic pain. In *The practice of behavioural medicine*, (ed. S. Pearce and J. Wardle J.), pp. 83–111. The British Psychological Society and Oxford University Press, Oxford.

Pearce, S., Knight, C.K., and Beard, R.W. (1982). Pelvic pain — a common gynaecological problem. *Journal of Psychosomatic Obstetrics and Gynaecology*, **1**, 12.

Petrucco, O.M. and Harris, R.D. (1982). A psychological and venographic study of women presenting with non-organic pelvic pain. Paper presented Eighth New Zealand Congress, Auckland, New Zealand.

Pilowsky, I. and Spence, N.D. (1975). Patterns of illness behaviour in patients with intractable pain. *Journal of Psychosomatic Research*, **19**, 279–87.

Reginald, P.W., Adams, J., Franks, S., Wadsworth, J., and Beard, R.W. (1989). Medroxyprogesterone acetate in the treatment of pelvic pain due to venous congestion. *British Journal of Obstetrics and Gynaecology*, **96**, 1148–52.

Rogers, C. (1961). *On becoming a person*. Constable, London.

Turner, J.A. and Jensen, M.P. (1993). Efficacy of cognitive therapy for chronic low back pain. *Pain*, **52**, 169–77.

18 Chest pain and palpitations

Christopher Bass and Richard Mayou

In this chapter Drs Bass and Mayou draw attention to the high prevalence of complaints of non-cardiac chest pain and benign palpitations in different medical settings. They also point out the important covariation between these symptoms and other functional complaints and describe the poor outcome in terms of continued symptoms and disability. The contribution of pathological, physiological, and psychological factors to aetiology is reviewed. Emotional disorders (especially symptoms of anxiety and panic) occur in a proportion of patients but many have no conspicuous psychiatric morbidity.

The importance of *early* intervention following medical assessment and reassurance is emphasized in order to prevent the development of secondary handicap. Early intervention is particularly important in patients with chest pain and normal coronary arteries, as this subgroup has been shown to have high rates of psychiatric morbidity and functional disability.

Both pharmacological and psychological treatments are described and the essential components of cognitive behavioural treatment, which has been shown to be effective in controlled studies, are outlined. This treatment has potential in both individual and group settings and the authors describe a brief self-help intervention administered by trained cardiac nurses which sets an important precedent in the management of patients with functional somatic symptoms.

Introduction

This chapter describes the clinical characteristics of patients with functional chest pain and palpitations, proposes a multifactorial interactive aetiological model, and suggests practical approaches to treatment.

The problem

Chest pain

Community-based studies (Hannay 1978; Von Korff *et al.* 1988; Murabito *et al.* 1990) have consistently found that chest pain is common in the general population and that the prevalence of chronic symptoms is also surprisingly high. For example, in a questionnaire study of adult enrollees of a large health maintenance organization, in which respondents were asked to report only pain problems that had lasted a whole day or had occurred several times in a year, the prevalence of chest pain in the previous 6 month period was 12 per cent (Von Korff *et al.* 1988). A higher proportion of chest pain patients had sought treatment in the previous 6 months (35 per cent) than had patients with pain in other areas, for example headache, abdominal pain, facial pain.

Chest pain and palpitations are commonly reported in all surveys of patients in *primary care* (for example, Shepherd *et al.* 1966; Kroenke and Mangelsdorff 1989), but only a minority are ever given a specific organic diagnosis. Moreover, the distinction between angina and non-cardiac chest pain is often difficult to make in primary care and it is probable that angina is often erroneously overdiagnosed on the basis of the history and non-invasive investigations. However, it is uncommon for the diagnosis of angina to be missed (Cannon *et al.* 1988).

There is now considerable evidence concerning non-cardiac chest pain in hospital settings. Chest pain is a very frequent cause of attendance at *emergency departments* and high proportions of patients are reassured that investigations are normal and discharged (Wulsin and Yingling 1991; Karlson *et al.* (1994)). The long-term outcome for such attenders in terms of cardiac disease is excellent, but there is evidence that many continue to experience symptoms and to suffer disability (Roll *et al.* 1992).

Unexplained chest pain is also common in *cardiac clinics*. For example, in a study of 94 consecutive referrals to a cardiac clinic for chest pain or palpitations, just over half the patients were diagnosed as not having ischaemic heart disease or any other significant physical disorder (Mayou *et al.* 1994). The characteristics of these patients with 'non-cardiac' symptoms are shown in Table 18.1. Psychiatric disorder was more common than in the general population and one-third were rated as suffering from psychiatric disorder, either anxiety or depression. A number of patients had been taking cardiac drugs before referral, some had been told that they had heart disease and a number had previously attended emergency departments and out-patient clinics for chest pain. There have also been many reports of *in-patients* with chest pain and normal coronary arteries (Beitman *et al.* 1989; Chambers and Bass 1990).

Outcome of non-cardiac chest pain

In the general population most chest pain is transient. However, in the Framingham study 32 per cent of subjects with 'non-anginal chest discomfort' still reported symptoms 2 years later, but the risk of ischaemic heart disease was not increased. Studies of patients referred to cardiologists for non-cardiac chest pain have revealed that many continue to report symptoms and disability despite medical reassurance (Channer *et al.* 1987). For example, in the Oxford study (Mayou *et al.* 1994) only a minority of these patients said that they were fit and without symptoms 6 months later. The

Table 18.1 Characteristics of new patients (see Mayou *et al.* 1994) referred to a cardiac clinic with presenting symptoms of chest pain or palpitations and assessed as 'non-cardiac'. Figures are percentages.

Cardiologists' assessment	Chest pain	Palpitations
Physical factors		
Chest wall	33	–
Oesophagus	10	–
Other	15	–
Not known	42	–
Awareness of tachycardia	–	33
Awareness of ectopics	–	67
Hyperventilation	21	33
Psychiatric consultation	30	39
History		
Previous consultation for 'nerves'	15	56
Model for heart disease (in relatives or others)	26	11
Cardiac drugs	41	33
Cardiac diagnosis	18	–
Research ratings		
Psychiatric disorder	38	50

majority still had symptoms, did not feel reassured, and described effects on everyday life (Table 18.2). Many were dissatisfied with medical care, especially that received in general practice and much less satisfied than other patients who were diagnosed as having heart *disease*. This poor outcome changed little during the following 2.5 years. At the final 3 year review 70 per cent reported that they had suffered symptoms in the last 3 months, symptoms which were frequently described as both severe and moderately or very distressing. There was no overall improvement in mood and 65 per cent had attended their general practitioners in the previous 3 months, although none were currently attending out-patients. Patients with chest pain but a negative exercise test also have a poor outcome: two-thirds continue to report pain 1 month after the test (Channer *et al.* 1987).

Patients who have had negative coronary angiography have an especially poor outcome. Follow-up studies of patients with chest pain and normal coronary arteries have consistently found that despite a good physical outcome approximately three-quarters (range 64–100 per cent) report persistent pain, half regard their lives as significantly disabled, and others report emotional distress and continue to use cardiac and other medical resources. In a recent long-term follow-up study Potts and Bass (1993) found that much of the physical symptoms and psychological distress detectable 1 year after angiography (Bass *et al.* 1983) persisted for as long as 11 years in spite of further medical attention. Of the 40 patients

Table 18.2 Consecutive referrals to a cardiac clinic: outcome of 'non-cardiac' group (62 per cent) at 6 months

Outcome	Per cent
Improved (self-report)	59
Symptoms in last month	76
Limitation of activity	20
Effect on work	26
Effect on walking	24
Reassured	
No	39
Partially	46

with normal or near-normal coronary arteries interviewed atter 11 years, 22 (55 per cent) had at least one current psychiatric diagnosis (Potts and Bass 1994).

Prevalence of palpitations

Patients with medically benign palpitations have attracted much less attention. In the Oxford follow-up study the general picture for the smaller number of patients who presented with palpitations was similar to those with non-cardiac chest pain (Mayou *et al.* 1994). The cardiologists thought that all patients were 'excessively aware' of their cardiac rhythm, either tachycardia or associated ventricular ectopics. As with the patients with chest pain, panic attacks were commonly diagnosed at psychiatric assessment. These findings are in accordance with studies by Barsky (1992, 1994) of patients attending for 24 h EEG recording. He was able to demonstrate excessive awareness of cardiac rhythm as compared with control subjects.

Overlap with other functional syndromes

Although this chapter is primarily concerned with the two commonly overlapping complaints of chest pain and palpitations, it is important to be aware that functional syndromes are extremely heterogeneous. That is to say, patients with chest pain and palpitations are particularly likely to report symptoms of breathlessness and fatigue. Indeed, for many years patients with atypical non-cardiac chest pain were given the designation 'effort syndrome', because their bodily complaints were aggravated by exercise. In addition symptoms such as fatigue, abdominal pain, or nausea may also be reported.

Many patients satisfying diagnostic criteria for effort syndrome between

Table 18.3 Prevalence of panic disorder in different settings

Setting	Prevalence (%)
General population[a]	1–3
Primary care[a]	6–10
Psychiatric out-patients[b]	8–12
Cardiac out-patients[c]	10–15
Treadmill exercise clinic[d]	20–30
Normal coronary angiograms[e]	30–45

[a]Katon (1989, p. 17). [d]Bass *et al.* (1988).
[b]Wing and Pryce (1976). [e]Bass and Wade (1984), Katon *et al.* (1988).
[c]White (1934).

World Wars I and II now satisfy current diagnostic criteria for chronic fatigue syndrome (Sharpe *et al.* 1991). Similarly, some patients with atypical non-cardiac chest pain satisfy diagnostic criteria for primary fibromyalgia (Pellegrino 1990). This co-relation between various functional somatic complaints has been demonstrated in primary care by Kirmayer and Robbins (1991).

Relationship to emotional disorders

It is common for aetiology to be multicausal with an interaction between physical, psychological, and social factors. However, an emphasis on the psychological and social contributions to aetiology is not to claim that psychiatric disorder can always be diagnosed. Only a minority of patients who present to family doctors with atypical chest pain are suffering from anxiety or depressive disorders, although rates are higher among those referred for specialist assessment in cardiac clinics, especially those who have normal coronary angiograms (Table 18.3). In the Oxford follow-up study, patients with benign palpitations were more likely than those with chest pain to be diagnosed as suffering from panic disorder (Mayou *et al.* 1994).

Ford (1987) reviewed the association between chest pain and psychiatric illness in the Epidemiological Catchment Area (ECA) study and found that 2.5 per cent of patients complained of medically unexplained chest pain. Patients with chest pain were four times as likely to have panic disorder, three times as likely to have phobic disorder, and twice as likely to have major depression as controls without chest pain.

It is often difficult to apply criteria for somatoform disorders. Chest pain and palpitations can occur as part of somatization disorder, and in a study of 41 patients satisfying research criteria for somatization disorder Smith *et al.* (1986) found that cardiovascular symptoms (chest pain, breathlessness, and palpitations) were among the most frequently reported.

Previous episodes of panic and phobic avoidance can also often be elicited in patients diagnosed as having this chronic, polysymptomatic disorder. Patients with hypochondriasis may also report atypical, non-cardiac chest pain, when the complaint may be accompanied by the belief that the heart is in some way irreparably damaged. Hypochondriacal complaints, especially exaggerated fears about heart disease, are not uncommon in patients with both panic disorder and somatization disorder.

Implications from epidemiology

It is apparent that very large numbers of people suffer from chest pain and palpitations. Although many patients have an excellent outcome following medical assessment and reassurance, a minority do less well and describe continuing symptoms, disability, and worry about heart disease and they make considerable demands on health services.

These findings suggest that there is a need to:

1. Improve routine care by more detailed explanation of non-cardiac causes and giving patients greater opportunity to express their fears.

2. Provide extra help for a minority of patients. Intervention should occur *early* in the course of the disorder, before secondary handicaps have had time to develop. For example, routine review 4–6 weeks after either a negative exercise test or angiogram would enable those with persistent symptoms to be identified at a relatively early stage and offered appropriate help. There is evidence that treatment of these patients can be beneficial and this will be described later in the section on management.

Aetiology

Although this chapter is primarily concerned with treatment, it is important to have a grasp of the multitude of possible aetiological factors that can contribute to non-cardiac chest pain. This calls for an adequate knowledge of gastroenterology, rheumatology, and the pathophysiology of anxiety, if the results of complex investigations and the meaning or relevance of any physical signs are to be understood.

Specific causes

Of the many non-cardiac causes of chest pain the most important are oesophageal spasm and dysmotility (Richter *et al.* 1987), musculoskeletal chest wall pain (Wise *et al*. 1992), referred pain from the thoracic spine (Epstein *et al*. 1979), hyperventilation, and psychiatric disorder.

Although a strong case has been made for the importance of *oesophageal reflux and spasm* or 'nutcracker' oesophagus in non-cardiac chest pain (especially those with chest pain and normal coronary arteries; see Ward *et al*. 1987) the link between this organic abnormality and chest pain is not always robust. For example, Peters *et al*. (1988) showed only 36 per cent of 92 episodes of pain occurred at the same time as the oesophageal abnormality) and the vasodilator nifedipine was no more effective than placebo in improving pain in patients with nutcracker oesophagus (Richter *et al*. 1987).

Musculoskeletal abnormalities are often unsuspected causes of chest pain. Their exact prevalence is unknown, but they have been noted in up to 10 per cent of patients presenting with chest pain (Wolf and Stern 1976). There is an important association between these disorders (often referred to as costochondral syndrome or costosternal syndrome) and emotional disorders: Benson and Zavala (1954) reported that two-thirds of such patients were convinced that they had serious heart disease. More recently Wise *et al*. (1992) studied 100 patients with chest pain referred for assessment by a rheumatologist. All had undergone coronary angiography, which revealed no greater than 25 per cent narrowing of coronary diameter. Sixty-nine patients had chest wall tenderness, but typical chest pain was evoked by palpation in only 16. Tender areas were not found in a control group of 25 patients with arthritis but no symptoms of chest pain. A diagnosis of primary fibromyalgia was made in only five of the 100 patients, including two of the 16 in whom chest palpation reproduced pain. This suggests only a small degree of overlap between patients with non-cardiac chest pain and fibromyalgia. Possible causes of chest pain in these patients include repeated trauma from coughing, respiratory disease, or sudden movements, which produce small tears in the sternocostal ligaments. Careful physical examination of the chest wall for evidence of localized or diffuse chest wall tenderness should therefore be an important part of the assessment of these patients.

Although *hyperventilation* has been commonly reported in patients with non-cardiac chest pain (Evans and Lum 1977; Channer *et al*. 1985), doubt has been expressed about its importance as an aetiological factor. It does, however, provide a plausible link between anxiety and chest pain, as well as to other physical symptoms. This anxiety can lead to over-breathing (Magarian 1982) and, thence, to alkalosis, which may in turn cause coronary artery spasm (Rasmussen *et al*. 1986) or perhaps increased microvascular tone.

Exercise-induced hyperventilation is known to be more common in patients with chest pain and normal coronary arteries than in those with coronary artery disease (Chambers *et al*. 1988) and may be responsible for some of the observed association between chest pain and exercise in these patients. Furthermore, hyperventilation can cause ECG changes resembling ischaemia (Lary and Goldschlager 1974), so exercise-induced hyperventilation could be responsible for some of the positive exercise ECGs encountered in patients with normal coronary arteries.

Hyperventilation may also exert effects by other mechanisms which do not involve the heart. For example, it is known to be capable of inducing oesophageal spasm (Rasmussen *et al.* 1986), and it may bring about chest pain via fatigue or cramp in overworked intercostal muscles (Chambers and Bass 1990) or by aggravating pre-existing chest wall disorders such as fibrositis (Wise *et al.* 1992; see below). The precipitation of chest pain by breath holding or breathing with a deliberately overinflated chest supports such a possibility (Bass 1990).

Despite the possible linking mechanisms, hyperventilation is unlikely to be a complete explanation; hyperventilation provocation tests reproduce pain in fewer than half the cases (Evans and Lum, 1977; Bass *et al.* 1991) and the test–retest reliability is low (Lindsay *et al.* 1991). Furthermore, there are other ways in which psychiatric morbidity could be causally linked to chest pain. Anxiety may increase skeletal muscle tone, for example and lead to spasm or fatigue in the musculature of the thorax. It is also known to cause oesophageal dysmotility in healthy normals (Young *et al.* 1987) and may therefore cause or aggravate dysmotility-induced chest pain in patients with non-cardiac chest pain. It is reasonable to conclude that hyperventilation is an epiphenomenon in the aetiology of chest pain, that is, it is secondary to anxiety. Indeed, non-cardiac chest pain is unlikely to have a single causal explanation (see below).

A multicausal interactive model of non-cardiac chest pain and palpitations

The results of the studies described above suggest that several possible causes co-occur. This was recently demonstrated by Cooke *et al.* (1991), who performed oesophageal monitoring and PH monitoring, exercise tests with end-tidal pCO_2 measurement, and ratings of psychiatric morbidity in patients with chest pain and normal coronary arteries. Fifty-eight per cent had two or more abnormalities and oesophageal abnormalities co-existed with hypocapnia in one-third and with psychiatric morbidity in one-quarter. Abnormal physiological and psychiatric findings were not associated with descriptions of pain as 'typical' or 'atypical'.

Although this interesting study was carried out on a group of patients who had undergone invasive investigations, the results confirm both the heterogeneity and overlap. Indeed, they suggest that any attempt to link psychiatric abnormalities and presenting physical symptoms of chest pain using unitary causal explanations is fruitless.

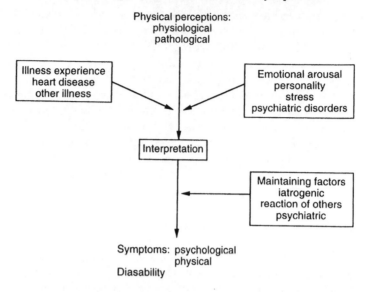

Fig. 18.1   An aetiological model for non-cardiac chest pain and palpitations

The central feature of the model in Fig. 18.1 is the concept that subjective symptoms, physical and psychological, are the result of patients' interpretation (or misattribution) of somatic perceptions (Chambers and Bass 1990; Mayou 1984). These underlying perceptions may be due to minor physical pathology, excessive awareness of normal physical and bodily processes such as palpitations or to hyperventilation. They may also be due to the somatic consequences of anxiety or other primary psychiatric disorder. The cardiologist Wood (1941) recognized this 50 years ago and emphasized the importance of chest wall pain, hyperventilation, oesophageal sensations, and other physical causes and the way that these interacted with psychological factors.

We have already emphasized the importance of psychosocial variables in making it more likely that individuals will misinterpret bodily sensations as more threatening than is, in fact, the case. These include the following:

1. Illness knowledge and experience, that is, knowledge of heart disease and other illnesses, family history of heart disease, models of heart disease in friends and neighbours, general experience of doctors, and satisfaction with medical care.

2. Concern, worry and autonomic arousal, all of which are more common than diagnosable psychiatric disorders. Once the symptoms are established, they may be maintained or reinforced by the patient's persistent awareness of the minor physical perceptions or by other

factors, such as secondary anxiety and panic, the reaction of friends and relatives, and the reaction and actions of doctors. Each of these factors may lead a patient who has suffered temporary chest discomfort to experience prolonged overconcern.

3. Patients recovering from myocardial infarction or cardiac surgery also frequently worry about medically insignificant aches and pains and atypical non-cardiac chest pain, palpitations, and breathlessness are all very common in this group of patients.

Management

Chest pain is frequently transient and medical assessment and straightforward reassurance are often effective. Patients with more persistent complaints require further treatment. This may involve further general discussion or occasionally specific treatment of one of the medical causes described in the previous section. A variety of specific treatments have been suggested for patients with persistent complaints and disability but who do not have any specific treatable physical problem. We review these in the following section and thereafter describe the Oxford research which has concentrated on the development and application of cognitive behavioural treatments.

Drug treatments

The choice of drug treatment depends on the underlying psychiatric disturbance. Medication may be used either in conjunction with other psychological treatment methods or as the sole form of treatment. The most important drugs are tricyclic antidepressants, monoamine oxidase inhibitors (MAOIs), beta blockers, and benzodiazepines.

Tricyclic antidepressants These drugs are indicated for those patients in whom chest pain and palpitations are accompanied by either depressed mood or panic attacks. There is evidence from a recent multinational study that imipramine is of benefit in patients with panic episodes that are accompanied by predominantly cardiorespiratory symptoms (Briggs *et al*. 1993). Cannon *et al*. (1994) recently demonstrated that imipramine reduced the frequency of chest pain in patients with normal coronary arteries by 50 per cent, and that this improvement occurred independently of the drug's effect on psychiatric morbidity. The authors suggested that imipramine may have a visceral analgesic effect.

Because these patients may be especially sensitive to the side-effects of these drugs it is usually advisable to start with a small dose, for example dothiepin 25 mg at night, gradually increasing to 50 mg daily by the end of the first week. Thereafter, the dose should be increased by 25 mg increments every 3 days up to 150–200 mg per day. It is important to tell the patient not to expect any marked change in mood for at least 2 or 3 weeks. Panics should also be blocked at this dosage, but if the patient continues to panic then the dose should be increased to 250 mg or even 300 mg per day if necessary (see Chapter 6).

Monoamine oxidase inhibitors (MAOIs)   Because chest pain and palpitations are very common in patients with panic episodes, drugs which block panics have enormous potential in the treatment of these disorders. Although there have been no controlled trials of MAOIs in patients with functional cardiovascular complaints, these drugs, particularly phenelzine, are particularly useful when the symptoms of panic, avoidance, anergia, irritability, and mild depression accompany the cardiovascular complaints (Bass and Kerwin 1989).

There is considerable evidence to suggest that patients with anxiety (with or without panic) and somatic symptoms (the most common of which are cardiorespiratory) show good therapeutic response to phenelzine compared with placebo (Liebowitz *et al.* 1988).

Benzodiazepines   The risks of dependence and withdrawal symptoms limit the use of these drugs in the treatment of patients with functional chest pain and palpitations. In spite of this, Beitman *et al.* (1988) have recently shown in an open trial of alprazolam that seven out of eight chest pain patients without ischaemic heart disease and with panic disorder experienced a 50 per cent or greater reduction in panic frequency as well as decreases in anxiety and depression. Clearly, further controlled trials need to be carried out before claims are made about the efficacy of this drug, which, like the older benzodiazepines, carries the risk of dependence and withdrawal symptoms (Tyrer 1989).

Beta blockers   Sympathetically mediated symptoms such as chest pain, palpitations, trembling, and sweating respond to beta blockers (Tyrer 1976). Although the drugs only act peripherally on specific symptoms, they may reduce subjective anxiety indirectly because of the interaction between the physiological and cognitive components of anxiety. Patients with tachycardia in excess of 90 per minnute may also benefit from beta blockade, the dose of which should he titrated against the pulse rate, for example metoprolol 50–100 mg/day.

Breathing retraining

We have already pointed out that hyperventilation is a particularly power-ful mechanism for the production of sensations that are subsequently misinterpreted. Although the contribution of breathing retraining as a therapeutic procedure in patients with panic attacks has probably been overstated, there is evidence that this treatment can play an important part in the management of some patients with non-cardiac chest pain, regardless of whether this is accompanied by symptoms of panic (Bass 1994). One study that demonstrated the efficacy of breathing retraining in patients with functional cardiac symptoms was recently carried out by DeGuire *et al.* (1992). These authors used three methods of breathing retraining, at differing levels of complexity:

(1) guided breathing retraining;

(2) guided breathing retraining with physiological monitoring of thoracic and abdominal movement plus peripheral temperature;

(3) guided breathing retraining with physiological monitoring of thoracic abdominal movement, peripheral temperature, and end-tidal CO_2.

These were compared with a no treatment control group to determine the effectiveness of breathing retraining on modifying respiratory physiology and reducing functional cardiac symptoms in subjects with signs associated with the hyperventilation syndrome. Of 41 subjects studied, 16 were diagnosed as having mitral valve prolapse.

The results demonstrated that all three methods of breathing retraining were equally effective in modifying respiratory physiology and reducing the frequency of functional cardiac symptoms. The two factors that were thought to contribute to treatment success were:

(1) reduction in respiratory rate;

(2) the subject's perception that treatment had generalized and that paced diaphragmatic breathing was being maintained.

That is to say, the patient's perception of being able to maintain paced diaphragmatic breathing was a strong predictor of treatment success. It is also worth noting that the authors found that subjects with mitral valve prolapse responded as well to treatment as did those without.

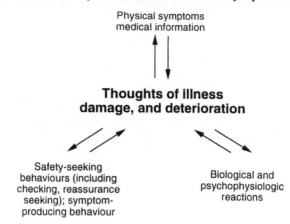

Fig. 18.2　The interaction between thoughts of danger, attention, behaviour, and physiologic responses in the maintenance of cardiac concern. (Reproduced with permission from Salkovskis 1992.)

Cognitive behavioural treatment

According to cognitive theory, events do not give rise to anxiety; anxiety is caused by the person's interpretation of these events as threatening. In other words, people become anxious when they believe that danger is imminent or when they consciously perceive a threat. Someone suddenly noticing palpitations without an obvious cause would *only* become anxious if these were interpreted as a sign of a heart condition. The degree of anxiety relates to how strongly the beliefs of danger are held, how serious the danger is believed to be, and how much it is believed that one could cope with or escape from the perceived danger.

　　The cognitive theory of chest pain associated with anxiety is based on the observation that these patients have an enduring tendency to misinterpret sensations in the chest region as a sign of serious illness. Once this key misinterpretation occurs, thoughts of threat and danger interact with other responses, as illustrated in Fig. 18.2 (Salkovskis 1992) and Chapter 7.

The Oxford studies – cognitive behavioural therapy

Referrals from general practice

This first study (Klimes *et al.* 1990) showed that psychological treatment using cognitive behavioural techniques was effective in the treatment of non-cardiac chest pain. Thirty-one patients with persistent non-cardiac pain were entered into a controlled trial of cognitive behavioural therapy. The mean duration of pain was 4.7 years. Patients were randomized to

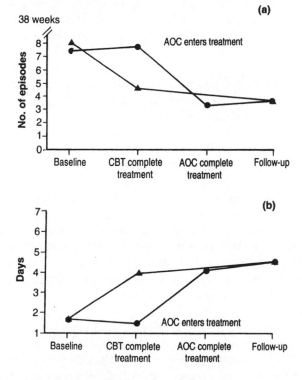

Fig. 18.3 The pattern of changes in measures of (a) episodes of chest pain per week and (b) numbers of days per week without pain. (CBT = cognitive behavioural treatment; AOC = assessment-only controls). (Reprinted with permission from Klimes *et al.*, 1990).

either immediate treatment or to a control group which involved assessment only. Treatment involved teaching patients how to anticipate and manage symptoms and the modification of inappropriate health beliefs. The mean number of sessions was 7.2. There were significant reductions in chest pain, limitations and disruption of daily life, autonomic symptoms, distress, and psychological morbidity in the treated group as compared with the control group who were unchanged. The assessment-only control group were treated subsequently and showed comparable changes. Improvements were fully maintained by both treated groups at 4–6 months follow-up (Fig. 18.3).

The stages of treatment were as follows (initiated in chronological order over the course of four to eleven sessions).

1. Functional analysis of complaints, an explanation of why psychological treatment was being offered, and an introduction to progressive muscular relaxation.

2. The main focus was on the role of breathing; forced over-breathing was used to demonstrate how easily 'real' unpleasant sensations can be induced. Learning of slow-paced breathing and control was introduced.

3. An introduction to distraction (focusing attention away from symptoms and associated worrying) and to monitoring the relationship of chest pain to mood and activity.

4. Beginning to apply skills (relaxation, slow-paced breathing, and distraction) and to monitor effects on pain.

5. Review and management of any maintaining factors, for example morbid health beliefs. Use of exposure to counteract avoidance of exertion, response prevention methods to counter checking (for example, repeated pulse-taking) and other reassurance-seeking behaviours, pacing activities to control unrealistic demands, cognitive challenge of residual beliefs about organic illness, and problem-solving for social problems.

The treatment was acceptable to all patients, even those who were sceptical about the significance of psychological factors in the aetiology of their complaints. The patients were assured that their physical state could, if necessary, be reassessed at the completion of treatment. Two patients referred with diagnoses of non-cardiac chest pain were diagnosed as suffering from ischaemic heart disease during the follow-up stage of the study. One man was reassessed by the cardiac clinic and the diagnosis changed to angina; the other suffered a myocardial infarct during follow-up, having reported improvement during treatment. Both reported that they had found treatment helpful and it is evident that psychological treatment of anxiety and atypical symptoms can be acceptable to those in whom there is diagnostic uncertainty.

Psychological treatment in the cardiac clinic

A recent study has evaluated cognitive behavioural methods in successive patients reassured by cardiologists in the cardiac clinic, or following negative coronary and geography. Table 18.4 shows the follow-up of 150 consecutive patients at 6 weeks. Approximately 40 per cent were assessed and thought to be suitable for treatment, but 14 refused, either because they or their family did not think that behavioural treatment would be useful or because they felt that they could now manage to make changes themselves without further help. More than one-quarter of subjects either turned down the offer of assessment or made an appointment and did not

Table 18.4 Assessment of 137 consecutive patients with non-cardiac chest pain and recruitment for a controlled trial of a cognitive behavioural treatment

Refused 6-week assessment	22
Did not attend 6-week assessment	17
Assessed not suitable:	
Major depression	1
No chest pain in last month	22
Chest pain less than 1 per week	17
Assessed:	
Refused study	14
Pilot	7
Treatment trial	37
Total	137

attend. A number of these patients said that they no longer had chest pain or any disability, but several had significant problems but did not see attendance as being worthwhile or convenient. Outcome for those in the treatment group was excellent and significantly better than the controls. This replication of the previous findings in a clinic sample is encouraging.

A major conclusion from the study was that many patients felt dissatisfied and uncertain with didactic medical reassurance and wanted more opportunity for discussion, an explanation of their symptoms, and advice on how to cope with returning to full activities and with any further symptoms. We believe that these patients benefited from our assessment and that they would have been particularly responsive to similar help at an earlier stage. Only a minority of patients are likely to require specialist extra treatment.

These patients can also be treated in group settings. In a recent study of patients with chest pain and normal coronary arteries S. Potts (personal communication) found significant reductions in both the severity and frequency of chest pain episodes, as well as reductions in the use of nitrates, ratings of anxiety, and disability.

Self-help following coronary angiography

We have recently begun a controlled trial of self-help intervention for patients with chest pain who have had negative coronary angiograms. The intervention consists of explanation, handout and cassette, and telephone follow-up, administered by a cardiac nurse immediately following the results of the angiogram and before discharge from hospital. This procedure is popular with many patients because it answers their questions and needs and because it is provided by a ward cardiac nurse who works closely with the cardiologist.

Guidelines

The multicausal interactive model actually helps us to understand aetiology by stressing minor physical problems and also individual beliefs, personality, and circumstances. It also points to ways in which medical intervention could reduce distress and disability by modifying the patient's interpretations of his/her symptoms.

Initial assessment and care

On first presentation it is necessary to consider the specific causes of chest pain and also to elicit the patient's attitudes and beliefs. If angina or other specific physical causes can be excluded, it is appropriate to reassure the patient. Such reassurance will include an explanation of aetiology which emphasizes the role of minor physical and psychological factors. It is also essential that the patient has an opportunity to ask questions and raise particular anxieties. The patient should be asked to return to the clinic if there are continuing symptoms.

Review of persistent symptoms

If symptoms continue more detailed assessment is necessary. This will include reviewing the possibility of a physical cause and the role of psychological factors. The assessment may lead to more detailed advice about anxiety management. For example, monitoring of daily symptoms may reveal avoidance of certain activities that may require the introduction of a graded activity programme.

At this stage it is helpful to consider the specific treatments discussed in the previous sections. Difficulties frequently arise because of an uncertainty about the diagnosis and the remaining possibility of heart disease. Specialist cardiological referral may well be necessary to clarify the diagnosis. The patient should be aware that heart disease is being considered but that this is only one of several possible diagnoses.

Preparing the patient for psychological referral

Before specialist psychological treatment can begin it is important to 'prepare' the patient and explain the reasons for referral. General practitioners and members of the cardiology staff may need to be informed of the most appropriate ways of preparing a patient for referral for psychological treatment. This may be explained as follows: 'I think it is possible that emotional factors or stress may be aggravating or contributing to your chest pain/palpitations, etc. I have a colleague who has a lot of experience in helping patients with this kind of problem. Would you like to arrange for him/her to make you an appointment?'

Two other factors need to be addressed before psychological treatment can begin. These are

(1) providing a plausible alternative explanation for the pain;

(2) withdrawing cardiac medication.

The first is necessary because the patient will want to know the rationale for psychiatric referral. The explanation should be congruent with the patient's socio-cultural background and should provide new information, not merely an explanation that 'investigations were normal so there is nothing to worry about'. It might be appropriate, for example, to explain to the patient that the pain is aggravated by 'stretching or tensing of the chest wall muscles'. The patient is more likely to accept this explanation if palpation of the chest wall reveals an area of tenderness and if this tender area becomes more painful after a number of simple manoeuvres; for example, breath-holding, walking up a flight of stairs. Psychological treatment can only proceed after these stages have been negotiated. The treatment can be supervised by a psychiatrist or psychologist, but the best solution might be direct access to help from a specialized nurse or counsellor based within the cardiac clinic (Mayou 1993).

Withdrawing cardiac medication

If the patient with non-cardiac chest pain has been taking anti-anginal medication before referral the psychiatrist or psychologist, then this medication should be gradually withdrawn. This phase of management requires skilful handling, because in effect the therapist is inviting the patient to negotiate the transition from a 'sick' to a 'healthy' mode of living. This may be difficult in a patient who has already adjusted to the life of an invalid. Attempting to 'undiagnose' angina is beset with problems (Dart *et al.* 1983): prolonged unemployment and receipt of welfare payments increase the chance of the patient remaining in the sick role.

Management of patients with more chronic symptoms

In patients with more chronic and enduring symptoms of non-cardiac chest pain and/or palpitations who have developed secondary handicaps, the most important (and difficult) part of treatment is engagement (see

Chapter 5). This requires clinical skills and a supportive, non-adversarial style of interviewing.

The content of treatment depends on the maintaining factors. For example, patients with chronic chest pain and/or palpitations with stable premorbid personalities and adjustment require different management from those in whom the somatic complaints are part of a chronic, polysymptomatic disorder, for example somatization disorder. In the latter 'damage limitation' is a more realistic therapeutic goal and the management should be coordinated with the patient's general practitioner (see Chapter 21).

References

Barsky, A.J. (1992). Palpitations, cardiac awareness, and panic disorder. *American Journal of Medicine*, **92**(1A), 31–4.

Barsky, A.J., Cleary, P.D., Sarnie, M.K., and Ruskin, J.N. (1994). Panic disorder, palpitations and the awareness of cardiac activity. *Journal of Nervous and Mental Disease*, **182**, 63–71.

Bass, C. (1990). Functional cardiorespiratory syndromes. In *Somatization: physical symptoms and psychological illness*, (ed. C. Bass), p. 171. Blackwell Scientific Publications, Oxford. pp. 171–206.

Bass, C. (1994). Management of patients with hyperventilation-related disorders. In *Behavioural and psychological approaches to breathing disorders*, (ed. R. Ley and B. Timmons), pp. 149–55. Plenum, New York.

Bass, C. and Kerwin, R. (1989). Rediscovering monoamine oxidase inhibitors. *British Medical Journal*, **298**, 345–6.

Bass, C., Wade, C., Hand, D., and Jackson, G. (1983). Patients with angina with normal and near normal coronary arteries: clinical and psychosocial state 12 months after angiography. *British Medical Journal*, **287**, 1505–08.

Bass, C., Chambers, J.B., Kiff, P., Cooper, D., and Gardner, W.N. (1988). Panic anxiety and hyperventilation in patients with chest pain: a controlled study. *Quarterly Journal of Medicine*, **69**, 949–59.

Bass, C., Chambers, J.B., and Gardner, W.N. (1991). Hyperventilation provocation in patients with chest pain and a negative treadmill exercise test. *Journal of Psychosomatic Research*, **35**, 83–7.

Beitman, B.D., Basha, I.M., Trombka, L.H., Jayaratna, M.A., Russell, B.D., and Tarr, S.K. (1988). Alprazolam in the treatment of cardiology patients with atypical chest pain and panic disorder. *Journal of Clinical Psychopharmacology*, **8**, 127–9.

Beitman, B.D., Mukerji, V., Lamberti, J.M., Schmid, L., DeRosear, I., Kushner, M. *et al.* (1989). Panic disorder in patients with chest pain and angiographically normal coronary arteries. *American Journal of Medicine*, **63**, 1399–403.

Benson, E.H. and Zavala, D.C. (1954). Importance of the costochondral syndrome in evaluation of chest pain. *Journal of the American Medical Association*, **156**, 1244–6.

Briggs, A.C., Stretch, D.D. and Brandon, S. (1993). Subtyping of panic disorder by symptom profile. *British Journal of Psychiatry*, **163**, 201–9.

Cannon, P.J., Connell, P.A., Stockley, I.H., Garner, S.T. and Hampton, J.R. (1988). Prevalence of angina assessed by a survey of prescription for nitrates. *Lancet*, **1**, 979–81.

Cannon, R.O., Quyyumi, A.A., Mincemoyer, R., Stine, A.M., Gracely, R.H., Smith, W.B. *et al.* (1994). Imipramine in patients with chest pain despite normal coronary angiograms. *New England Journal of Medicine*, **330**, 1411–7.

Chambers, J.B., Bass C. (1990). Chest pain and normal coronary anatomy: review of natural history and possible aetiologic factors. *Progress in Cardiovascular Diseases*, **33**, 161–84.

Chambers, J.B., Kiff, P.J., Gardner, W.N., Jackson, G., and Bass, C. (1988). Value of measuring end-tidal partial pressure of carbon dioxide as an adjunct to treadmill exercise testing. *British Medical Journal*, **296**, 1281–84.

Channer, K.S., Papouchado, M., James, M., and Rees, J.R. (1985). Anxiety and depression in patients with chest pain referred for exercise testing. *Lancet*, **ii**, 820–3.

Channer, K.S., James, M.A., Papouchado, M., and Russell Rees. J. (1987). Failure of a negative exercise test to reassure patients with chest pain. *Quarterly Journal of Medicine*, **63**, 315–21.

Cooke, R.A., Chambers, J.B., Anggiansah, A., Henderson, R.A., Sowton, E., and Owen, W. (1991). Chest pain and normal coronary arteries: a clinical evaluation with oesophageal function tests, exercise ECG, end-tidal CO_2 measurement and psychiatric scores. *European Heart Journal*, **12** (Suppl.), p. 103.

Dart, A.M., Alban Davies, H., Griffith, T., and Henderson, A.H. (1983). Does it help to undiagnose angina? *European Heart Journal*, **4**, 461–3.

DeGuire, S., Gevirtz, R., Kawahara, Y., and Maguire, W. (1992). Hyperventilation syndrome and the assessment of treatment for functional cardiac symptoms. *American Journal of Cardiology*, **70**, 673–7.

Epstein, S.E., Gerber, L.H., and Borer, J.S. (1979). Chest wall syndrome: a common cause of unexplained cardiac pain. *Journal of the American Medical Association*, **241**, 2793–8.

Evans, D.W. and Lum, L.C. (1977). Hyperventilation: an important cause of pseudoanigina. *Lancet*, **1**, 155–7.

Hannay, D.R. (1978). Symptom prevalence in the community. *Journal of the Royal College of General Practitioners*, **28**, 492–9.

Karlson, B.W., Wiklund, I., Bengtson, A., and Herlitz, J. (1994). Progress and symptoms one year after discharge from the emergency department in patients with acute chest pain. *Chest*, **105**, 1442–7.

Katon, W., Hall, M.L., Russo, J., Cormier, L., Hollifield, M., Vitaliano, P.P., and Beitman, B.D. (1988). Chest pain: relationship of psychiatric illness to coronary angiographic results. *American Journal of Medicine*, **84**, 1–9.

Kirmayer, L.J. and Robbins, J.M. (1991). Functional somatic symptoms. In *Current concepts of somatization: research and clinical perspectives.* (ed. L. Kirmayer and J. Robbins), pp. 79–106. American Psychiatric Press, Washington.

Klimes, I., Mayou, R.A., Pearce, M.J., Coles, L., and Fagg, J.R. (1990). Psychological treatment for atypical chest pain: a controlled evaluation. *Psychological Medicine*, **20**, 605–11.

Kroenke, K. and Mangelsdorff, D. (1989). Common symptoms in ambulatory care: incidence, evaluation, therapy and outcome. *American Journal of Medicine*, **86**, 262-8.

Lary, D., Goldschiager, N. (1974). Electrocardiographic changes during hyperventilation resembling myocardial ischaemia in patients with normal coronary arteries. *American Heart Journal*, **87**, 383-90.

Liebowitz, M.R., Quitkin, F.M., Stewart, J.W. *et al*. (1988). Antidepressant specificity in atypical depression. *Archives of General Psychiatry*, **45**, 129-36.

Lindsay, S., Saqi, S., and Bass, C. (1991). The test retest reliability of the hyperventilation provocation test. *Journal of Psychosomatic Research*, **35**, 155-61.

Magarian, G.J. (1982). Hyperventilation syndromes: infrequently recognised common expressions of anxiety and stress. *Medicine*, **61**, 219-43.

Mayou, R. (1989). Atypical chest pain. *Journal of Psychosomatic Research*, **33**, 393-404.

Mayou, R. (1992). Patients' fears of illness: chest pain and palpitations. In *Medical symptoms not explained by organic disease*, (ed. F. Creed, R. Mayou, and A. Hopkins). pp. 25-33. Royal College of Psychiatrists and Royal College of Physicians, London.

Mayou, R. (1993). Management of atypical non-cardiac chest pain. In *Psychological treatment in disease and illness*, (ed. M. Hodes and S. Moorey), pp. 101-13. Gaskell and The Society for Psychosomatic Research, London.

Mayou, R.A., Bryant, B., Clark, D., and Forfar, C. (1994). Referrals to a cardiac clinic for chest pain or palpitations. *British Heart Journal*, **72**, 548-53.

Murabito, J.M., Anderson, K.M., Kannel, W.B., Evans, J.C., and Levy, D. (1990). Risk of coronary heart disease in subjects with chest discomfort. The Framingham Study. *American Journal of Medicine*, **89**, 297-302.

Pellegrino, M.J. (1990). Atypical chest pain as an initial presentation of primary fibromyalgia. *Archives of Physical Medicine and Rehabilitation*, **71**, 526-8.

Peters, L., Maas, L., Petty, D., Dalton, C., Penner, D., Wu, W. *et al*. (1988). Spontaneous non-cardiac chest pain: evaluation by 24-hour ambulatory oesophageal motility and Ph monitoring. *Gastroenterology*, **94**, 878-86.

Potts, S. and Bass, C. (1993a). Psychosocial outcome and use of medical resources in patients with chest pain and normal or near-normal coronary arteries: a long term follow up study. *Quarterly Journal of Medicine*, **86**, 583-93.

Potts, S. and Bass, C. (1994). Chest pain with normal coronary arteries: psychological aspects. In *Angina pectoris with normal coronary arteries (syndrome X)*, (ed. J.C. Kaski). pp. 65-88. Kluwer, Norwell, MA.

Rasmussen, K., Ravnbaek, J., Funch-Jensen, P., and Gagger, J.P. (1986). Oesophageal spasm in patients with coronary artery spasm. *Lancet*, **1**, 174-6.

Richter, J.E., Dalton, C.B., Bradley, L.A., and Castell, D.O. (1987). Oral nifedipine in the treatment of non-cardiac chest pain in patients with the nutcracker oesophagus. *Gastroenterology*, **93**, 21-8.

Roll, M., Kollind, M., and Theorell, T. (1992). Five year follow up of young adults visiting an emergency unit because of atypical chest pain. *Journal of Internal Medicine*, **231**, 59-65.

Salkovskis, P. (1992). Psychological treatment of non-cardiac chest pain: the cognitive approach. *American Journal of Medicine*, **92** (Suppl. 5A), 114-21.

Savage, D.D., Devereux, R.B., Garrison, R.J., Castelli, W.P., Anderson, S.J., Levy, D. *et al.* (1983). Mitral valve prolapse in the general population. 2. Clinical features: the Framingham study. *American Heart Journal*, **106**, 577–81.

Sharpe, M., Archard, L., Banatvala, J., Borysiewicz, L.K., Clare, A.W., David, A., *et al.* (1991). Guidelines for research in chronic fatigue syndromes. *Journal of the Royal Society of Medicine*, **84**, 118–21.

Shepherd, M., Cooper, B., Brown, A.C., and Kalton, G. (ed.) (1966). *Psychiatric illness in general practice*. Oxford University Press, Oxford.

Smith, G.R., Monson, R.A., and Ray, D.C. (1986). Patients with multiple unexplained symptoms. *Archives of Internal Medicine*, **146**, 69–72.

Tyrer, P. (1976). *The role of bodily feelings in anxiety*. Oxford University Press, London.

Tyrer, P. (1989). Treating panic. *British Medical Journal*, **298**, 201.

Von Korff, M., Dworkin, S.F., Le Rosche, L., and Kruger, A. (1988). An epidemiologic comparison of chest pain complaints. *Pain*, **32**, 173–83.

Ward, B., Wu, W.C., Richter, J.C. *et al.* (1987). Long term follow up of patients with non-cardiac chest pain: is diagnosis of esophageal etiology helpful? *American Journal of Gastroenterology*, **82**, 215–18.

Wise, C.M., Semble, E.L., and Daiton, C.B. (1992). Musculoskeletal chest wall syndromes in patients with non-cardiac chest pain: a study of 100 patients. *Archives of Physical Medicine Rehabilitation*, **73**, 147–9.

Wolf, E. and Stern, S. (1976). Costosternal syndrome. *Archives of Internal Medicine*, **136**, 189–91.

Wood, P. (1941). Da Costa's syndrome (or effort syndrome). *British Medical Journal*, **i**, 767–72, 805–11, 845–51.

Wulsin, L.R. and Yingling, K. (1991). Psychiatric aspects of chest pain in the emergency department. In *Unexplained chest pain*, (ed. J. Richter, B. Beitman, and R. Cannon), pp. 1175–88. W.B. Saunders, Philadelphia.

Young, L.D., Richter, J.E., Anderson, K.O. *et al.* (1987). The effects of psychological and environmental stressors on peristaltic oesophageal contractions in healthy volunteers *Psychophysiology*, **24**, 132.

PART 5 SPECIAL POPULATIONS

19 The management of functional somatic symptoms in children

M. Elena Garralda

Professor Garralda points out that children whose powers of expression are more limited than those of adults, are likely to express distress as in the form of somatic symptoms. She cites evidence of the frequency of such problems both in the general population and in primary care, as well as in specialist paediatric and child psychiatry clinics. Whilst functional somatic symptoms in children generally have a good prognosis, they may be persistent and often cause distress to both the children and their families. In many aspects the aetiology and management of functional somatic symptoms in children differs little from that in adults but in children the family is of particular importance.

It is noted that many children can be managed satisfactorily in primary and paediatric care by means of explanation and reassurance, although a proportion require more intensive help. The regrettable lack of good research evidence about the effectiveness of specific treatment methods means that these have to be chosen on clinical experience alone. Practical guidelines for treating children and their families are outlined.

Introduction

The most common functional somatic symptoms in children are aches and pains. Other fairly common symptoms include tiredness, dizziness or blackout, and loss of limb function. As the communication of distress is regarded as a fundamental aetiological factor in functional somatic symptoms (Lloyd 1986) it is not surprising that such symptoms are particularly common in childhood, since children have immature cognitive and verbal skills and a limited vocabulary for emotional expression. A special feature of functional somatic symptoms in childhood is the importance of family attitudes, which may influence the emphasis placed on physical symptoms by the child, determine whether medical help is sought, and influence cooperation with subsequent treatment.

One important category of functional symptoms that will not be discussed in this chapter is *factitious illness*. In childhood this term refers to cases in which a parent's actions (for example, poisoning and suffocation) result in physical symptoms in the child, who is then taken to health care professionals for investigation and treatment. These problems are rare but increasingly recognized. A case has been made for understanding factitious illness as an exaggerated need on the part of the parents to consult doctors and is related to disturbed parenting (Eminson and Postlethwaite 1992).

The problem

Before considering the treatment of functional somatic symptoms in children their occurence and aetiology will be briefly reviewed.

Epidemiology

Recent epidemiological studies of children and adolescents have found that the parents of 11 per cent of girls and 4 per cent of boys aged 12–16 years either report recurrent distressing somatic symptoms in their child or perceive them children as sickly (Offord *et al.* 1987). Enquiry of adolescents reveals that ten per cent of adolescents describe frequent or persistent symptoms. These are more common in girls and headaches and poor sleep are the most frequent problems (Aro *et al.* 1987).

Most epidemiological research has focused on specific symptoms, particularly abdominal pain and headache (Goodman and McGrath 1991). These studies have found that over 10 per cent of children in the general population report recurrent abdominal pains severe enough to affect their daily activities (Apley and Naish 1958; Faull and Nicol 1986; Golding and Butler 1986; Zuckerman *et al.* 1987). Occasional headaches occur in as many as 50 per cent of schoolchildren (Hockaday 1982) and migraine in some 4–5 per cent of 12 year olds (Bille 1962; Oster 1972; Zuckerman *et al.* 1987).

It is also common for children to report more than one functional symptom at a time. In a recent study of schoolchildren and adolescents 50 per cent reported at least one somatic symptom, 15 per cent four or more symptoms, and 1 per cent more than 12 (Garber *et al.* 1991). There is considerable variation in the degree of distress and disability associated with functional somatic symptoms, but in only a minority of cases are they associated with either substantial impairment of function or prolonged absence from school (Collin *et al.* 1985). The epidemiology of somatization in children and adolescents has been reviewed by Campo and Fritsch (1994).

Primary care and paediatric clinics   Children with functional somatic symptoms represent a considerable proportion (some 8–10 per cent) of attenders in primary care (Starfield *et al.* 1980). A presentation with functional symptoms is particularly common at stressful periods, such as early primary school years and early adolescence (Schor 1986). More persistent symptoms, most commonly stomach pains and headaches do occur however and these children tend also to be frequent users of school and other medical facilities (Christensen and Mortensen 1975; Lewis *et al.* 1977; Lewis and Lewis 1989). The symptom of chronic fatigue in particular is believed to be common, especially in adolescence, but as yet there have been no satisfactory epidemiological studies (see Chapter 16).

When clinicians are asked to identify children in whom the presentation of a somatic problem is strongly influenced by psychological factors, the rate obtained is one in five of children attending in primary care and nearly one in two of children attending general paediatric clinics (Bailey *et al.* 1978; Garralda and Bailey 1987, 1990). The psychological factors involve stress related to school adjustment in the child (that is, children not performing up to expectations) and a family style of focus on physical symptoms and frequent surgery attendance (Garralda and Bailey 1987).

Psychiatric clinics The majority of children presenting with functional symptoms are seen in primary care or in secondary paediatric care and few are referred to child psychiatry. Apley (1975) considered that only approximately in one in ten children seen in his hospital paediatric clinic required referral to child psychiatry, mainly because of excessive anxiety and depression in the *parents*. In a report of children with problems severe enough to require child psychiatric in-patient treatment, Livingston *et al.* (1988) found that 8 per cent had functional somatic symptoms, but in every case these problems were accompanied by other psychiatric disorders.

Association with psychiatric disorder

The majority of children with functional symptoms do *not* have associated psychiatric disorders. However, psychiatric disorder, most commonly depression, is commonly found in association with functional somatic symptoms, particularly in cases severe enough to lead to be referred for paediatric or psychiatric consultation (Garralda and Bailey 1990; Garralda 1992*a*). Children who present to paediatricians with functional somatic symptoms tend to be described as having particular characteristics; these include temperamental rigidity, sensitivity, and families characterized by illness, maternal mental distress, and a particularly close mother–child relationship.

Epidemiological surveys have consistently found a link between recurrent abdominal pains and behavioural problems, the nature of which varies according to the age of the child. In younger children stomach aches are linked to dependency and fearfulness (Zuckerman *et al.* 1987). In schoolchildren with problems severe enough to require paediatric admission, a third have been considered to have a psychological disorder (Crossley 1982), typically manifest as inhibition, fearfulness, and over-controlled

behaviour. In adolescents there may also be special links between functional somatic symptoms and depression (Wasserman *et al.* 1988). The
association with psychological dysfunction is probably less significant for
headaches than for abdominal pains and the majority of children with
headaches do not have behavioural problems.

Not surprisingly, children who require assessment and treatment by
child psychiatrists, usually for conversion syndromes, have higher rates of
associated psychiatric disorders. But even in these cases psychiatric disturbance is only found in approximately half (Leslie 1988).

Aetiology

Why do children develop functional somatic symptoms? Their aetiology
is not well understood but a number of factors in both child and family
are considered to be relevent. It is not clear, however, whether these factors are primary or merely secondary to the functional symptoms
themselves. Nor is it clear which factors or combinations of factors are
essential for functional symptoms to occur.

The factors that perpetuate the symptoms once they have developed are
of particular importance when planning therapeutic interventions. These
appear to be similar in all samples studied, whether minor problems in the
general population or severe disorders seen in child psychiatric clinics.
These are listed in Table 19.1 and have recently been reviewed by the
author (Garralda 1992*a*).

The lack of a medical explanation does of course not necessarily mean
that symptoms are an expression of psychiatric dysfunction. It is entirely
possible that future research will discover underlying physiological anoma-
lies. There is, for example, suggestive evidence that inflammatory bowel
changes and abnormalities of gastric electrical rhythm may be present in
some children with unexplained abdominal pains (van der Meer *et al.* 1990;
Cucchiara *et al.* 1992). A psychological contribution should only be identified therefore when there is positive evidence. Examples are when there
is a close time relationship between a likely stresser and the somatic symptoms or when the severity of the physical handicap is out of proportion
to the established pathophysiology and there is also associated psychiatric
disorder.

Review of the evidence

It must be recognized that most episodes of functional somatic symptoms
do not come to medical attention and are effectively dealt with by the
parents. It is clear from general population surveys that parents of young
children with abdominal pains — and the same is likely to apply to other

Table 19.1 Contributory factors

---

1. Physical conditions, for example an accident causing limb injury, a gastrointestinal upset, or a viral infection tend to feature as precipitating factors
2. Associated psychiatric disorder, especially emotional disorder
3. Concern over academic performance, in some cases with covert school refusal
4. Characteristic child personality features, for example conscientiousness and obsessionality, enhanced sensitivity, insecurity, and anxiety
5. A history of severe family health problems sometimes involving considerable handicap and symptomatology similar to that in the child
6. Concurrent gross family psychopathology in a minority, especially:
    (i) high academic and behavioural expectations from the children;
    (ii) emotional closeness and decreased emotional expressiveness in family interactions;
    (iii) marked concern over parenting
7. In severe cases:
    (i) hostility to psychological explanations and lack of trust in medical interventions;
    (ii) sexual abuse

---

functional symptoms — are well aware that the pain may be related to 'nerves' or worries about school and that the child may be using the pain to avoid something he or she finds difficult (Faull and Nicol 1986). Most parents report that their child tends to be reluctant to go to school when having a 'tummy ache'. The common parental reactions are either to play the symptom down so that the child learns to cope and forget about it or to comfort and reassure the child and to try to find out the cause. Analgesic medication is often given and it is common for parents or young children to provide some sort of psychological relief, such as a 'magic rub'.

There has been very little research into the treatment of functional symptoms in childhood and the following sections are therefore based to a great extent on descriptive clinical accounts. The few attempts at systematic evaluation of interventions have usually been based on small numbers of children and have involved a combination of several treatment components so that it is difficult to tease out the essential therapeutic elements. The following sections outline work done at various levels of care (namely primary care, paediatric out-patients, and psychiatric out- and in-patients care) and highlight what may he regarded as good clinical practice.

Treatment in primary care

We know little of what general practitioners do for children presenting at their surgeries with functional symptom but there are indications that these children are given more follow-up appointments than other attenders and that they are more often referred to secondary services (Garralda and Bailey 1987). A survey of General Practitioners in London found that children and adolescents presenting with combined physical and psycho-social problems were commonly prescribed medication (this occurred in half the cases). In approximately 20 per cent of children or adolescents reassurance, an opportunity to ventilate the problem, and/or advice to the mother were provided (Bailey *et al.* 1978).

Although the exact nature of these supportive interventions by doctors in primary care is uncertain, it seems likely that the *style* of intervention affects parental satisfaction. Work with young mothers in health clinics has documented the superiority of statements reflecting empathy and encouragement, over the simple expression of support (Wasserman *et al.* 1984). Mothers value such assurance highly and they feel that they learn from advice provided during consultations (Cunningham-Burley and Irvine 1987).

There is evidence indicating that parental child-rearing attitudes can be modified by advice and training provided in child health supervision sessions (Cullen, 1976; Gutelius *et al.* 1977) and that this has beneficial effects on the child's behaviour. It may also be helpful for functional symptoms. Furnell and Dutton (1986) described a primary care intervention for children with toddlers' diarrhoea and associated behavioural difficulties, which included counselling for parental anxiety about environmental stress, together with training in consistent and effective management of childhood behaviour using operant conditioning principles. The intervention was generally effective with the diarrhoea stopping in two-thirds of the children after a mean of 2 months treatment. The mothers' ratings of the children's behaviour also improved significantly. Improvement was maintained at 6 months follow-up. This uncontrolled study is interesting in illustrating a parallel reduction in somatic and behavioural symptoms.

A different approach to increasing confidence in parenting was taken by Benson and Turk (1988) who offered group therapy to mothers who frequently presented both themselves and their children to primary care services. Although only based on a group of ten mothers, this study found a reduction in consultation rates and suggested that the mothers were able to learn better coping strategies.

Treatment in paediatric services

Clinicians have outlined helpful approaches for use in the hospital paediatric clinic (Apley 1975; Valman 1982; Lask and Fosson 1989). The main components are summarized in Table 19.2. Joint paediatric and psychiatric management can be helpful, as, for example, in the management of chronic fatigue (Vereker 1992).

Table 19.2 Clinical management in paediatric clinics

1. Show interest in the child's entire background from the first consultation
2. Investigate and exclude organic disease confidently early on
3. Convince parents that organic disease has been ruled out
4. Encourage parents to release the emotional tension by sympathetic discussion of topics about which they feel strongly
5. Friendly and tactful guidance to help modify harmful aspects of the child's environment (for example, excessive emotional or academic demands on the child)
6. Avoid questioning the child's truthfulness about the symptom
7. If there is a school attendance problem
    (i) firm support to help the child return to school;
    (ii) discuss and alleviate school problem
8. Attention to any associated emotional disorders
9. Psychiatric referral when appropriate.

Specific treatments for abdominal pains and headaches

Treatments for specific problems such as abdominal pains and headaches have been devised for use in the community, school, primary care, and out-patient paediatric settings. Whereas non-specific advice by primary care doctors is not seen as helpful by mothers of children with recurrent abdominal pains (Faull and Nicol 1986), helping parents to understand the links between psychological and physical pain is (Wasserman *et al.* 1988). Apley (1975) noted improvements in the majority of children with recurrent abdominal pains treated in his paediatric out-patient clinic by psycho-therapeutically informed interventions aimed at identifying specific anxieties in both parents and children and at pointing out the associations between pain and stress. He also reported earlier resolution of symptoms and fewer recurrences in treated than in non-treated cases.

Comparable results have been reported in small studies using cognitive behavioural techniques. Finney *et al.* (1989) treated children with recurrent abdominal pains referred to primary care-based paediatric psychology services by a combined therapy of self-monitoring of pain, limiting the attention given to the symptom, use of relaxation and dietary fibre supplementation, and encouraging the child to participate in routine activities. The results indicated improvements in pain symptoms and reduced school absences. Sanders *et al.* (1989) used a comparable treatment in children with recurrent abdominal pains referred by paediatrician, family physicians, or self-referrals and found that the treatment group tended to improve more quickly than a non-treatment group. In a further study, (Sanders *et al.* 1994) a cognitive behavioural family intervention was found to be superior to standard paediatric care.

Studies in both schools and in paediatric out-patient clinics have shown that tension headaches can be substantially improved by relaxation training (Larsson 1992). In several studies of adolescents this approach was superior to an attention only control and effective whether administered at the clinic or as a home-based self-administered treatment (Larsson and Mellin 1988). However, McGrath *et al.* (1988) failed to report a superiority of relaxation over 'placebo' discussions in young adolescents with headaches severe enough to lead to referral to paediatric neurology clinic. Attending a clinic and receiving brief reassurance was often sufficient to bring relief.

Further research is therefore required to examine the relative advantages and disadvantages of the different approaches and to define the essential therapeutic ingredients.

Practical guidelines

Assessment

Factors which raise the suspicion that psychological factors are playing a part in clinical somatic presentations are not dissimilar to those alerting adult clinicians and include the following.

1. A time relationship between a likely stress and physical symptoms. Examples include stomach aches which occur selectively before the child is due to start for school in the morning or asthma precipitated by parental arguments. Detailed enquiry is required about what makes the symptoms better or worse and questions concerning worries and stresses at school or at home should be included. It is important to establish whether school attendance is being affected by the symptom.

2. Severity of handicap out of keeping with the established patho-physiology. This can be a fine clinical judgement to make and for more severe cases depends on good and ongoing paediatric–psychiatric liaison.

3. The presence of concurrent psychiatric disorder. This can also affect compliance with medical treatments and have an adverse effect on the medical symptoms.

4. The characteristic child, family, and illness factors described above (Table 19.1). These should be considered carefully as they contribute to the diagnosis of a functional component to the physical symptoms and to definition of target areas for treatment.

5. The degree and nature of the parental concern about the child's symp-

toms. It is well established that parents often attend surgeries with their children for reasons that are not initially apparent and which require gentle exploration during the consultation (Bass and Cohen 1982).

The paediatric clinic

The majority of children with functional symptoms who are seen by paediatricians do not require referral to psychiatric clinics. This means general practitioners and paediatricians need to develop skills in the recognition and management of the associated psychological aspects. Graham and Jenkin (1985) have helpfully summarized these as follows.

1. An awareness of the relevant psychosocial factors, including ascertainment of who is chiefly concerned about the child's symptoms, as well as skills in interviewing children with and without their parents.

2. Advice on simple behavioural techniques for minor behavioural problems, for example tantrums, oppositional symptoms, and separation anxiety.

3. Counselling skills to help families deal with stresses, for example maternal depression, loss of confidence in the ability to parent, and over-concerns over school and development.

4. A knowledge of family dynamics and an ability to recognize problems such as those involved in marital breakdown, over-concern, and over-protection of the child.

5. Skills to determine when referral for a psychiatric opinion is called for.

Out-patient psychiatric treatment

Referral to child psychiatry is indicated when:

(1) there is diagnostic uncertainty about the relevance of psychological factor;

(2) there is associated psychiatric disturbance;

(3) there are major family problems affecting resolution of the symptoms;

(4) when the child fails to respond to paediatric treatment.

The following general principles have been found to be helpful.

1. Close and parallel attention to physical and psychiatric symptoms, including good paediatric–psychiatric liaison.

2. Intervention with the family to help them to change their focus from physical to psychological issues, at a pace the family can cope with.

3. Emphasis on school attendance and, if required, school return at a carefully judged point in treatment.

4. Facilitating emotional expression and the development of techniques to deal with anxiety and psychological distress in the child can be helpful adjuvant techniques.

5. Specific techniques such as relaxation can be useful for specific symptoms, such as headaches and generally for stress management.

6. Family involvement is of particular relevance. Functional symptoms in children are often associated with particularly close family relationship and with intense involvement by the parents in the child's condition. Developing an alliance and a common purpose with parents is often a major aspect of treatment.

7. The majority of children can be effectively treated as out-patients either at the paediatric clinic or at the psychiatric clinic, but the length of treatment may vary from a single out-patient session to long-term therapy. Occasionally in-patient treatment is required, often in paediatric wards under conjoint paediatric–psychiatric supervision. When the psychiatric aspects are most prominent then admission to a psychiatric in-patient unit is advised.

In-patient psychiatric treatment

Psychiatric in-patient treatment is indicated when the severity of the problem is such that it causes major physical, emotional, or social handicap, for example in children who are unable to leave home or bed because of the severity of the pains, tiredness, or loss of limb function. It can also be helpful when parent–child separation is required in order to break a dysfunctional pattern of over-close relationships which impedes the child's attempts to develop sufficient confidence to cope with anxiety and with functional symptoms. It may also be indicated when the child has a profound depressive or anxiety state.

Many of the therapeutic principles outlined above also apply to the in-patient treatment of severe cases. Descriptive studies indicate that such treatment can result in substantial improvements for a considerable number of cases. A special characteristic is the use of the admission itself as a curative agent. It is important not to take a punitive approach towards the child, nor to enter into a contest of wills (Grattan-Smith *et al.* 1988), but to use the child's wish for discharge from hospital to motivate him or her to want to get better. Leslie (1988) has argued from her work with children exhibiting conversion hysteria that although the child is reluctant to stop being ill, he or she may be even more reluctant to remain in hospital indefinitely. For some severely incapacitated cases treated in paediatric wards, discussion of the possibility of transfer to a psychiatric unit at a well-chosen point in treatment can lead to remarkable improvements (Garralda 1992*b*). In Leslie's sample of children with conversion syndromes, the use of combined paediatric–psychiatric or purely psychiatric in-patient admission resulted in symptom resolution within 3 months of starting treatment in 85 per cent of the sample. More modest but still encouraging results are reported by other groups (Grattan-Smith *et al.* 1988).

The treatment of severely incapacitated cases can be challenging to both paediatric and child psychiatric services. Dubowitz and Hersov (1976) suggested that the three essentials of management in these cases are to limit further investigations to the essential minimum, to institute quickly a programme of graded physical rehabilitation if motor dysfunction is involved, and to treat the underlying psychological problems. Some of the clinical strategies used in addressing specific aetiological factors are described in more detail below.

Management strategies

Associated physical problems The degree to which families will accept the contribution of psychological factors varies considerably. As with adult patients, it can be helpful to draw a distinction between physical factors that precipitated the illness and the possible role of psychological factors in perpetuating it (Butler *et al.* 1991). When changing the emphasis from the physical to the psychological, the aims are to win the confidence of the child and family and to persuade nursing, medical staff, and parents that making the child feel that others believe they are 'putting it on' is unhelpful, and will increase resistance to treatment. It is more helpful to explain to the child that 'worries and muddles play tricks with the body and produce physical symptoms' (Leslie 1988).

A sense of hope is conveyed by explaining that the contributory psychological factors are both identifiable and treatable and the approach suggested offers the best chance of recovery. It is often helpful to combine psychological with physical treatments as part of a gradual process of changing the emphasis; for example, physiotherapy can be employed for disorders of motor function.

It is important to be aware that when the tendency to provide somatic explanations for symptoms of emotional distress is a strong family characteristic, periods of increased stress may result in renewed functional symptomatology. Psychological treatment may therefore precipitate worsening of symptoms if it is proceeding at a pace which is too swift for the child and family.

Symptoms of depression and anxiety Mood changes of depression and anxiety are common and on occasions flatness of affect and withdrawal are prominent. It can be difficult to ascertain whether the depressive symptoms preceded or followed the onset of somatic symptoms. Although this issue may be important in determining parental perceptions of the relationship between physical and psychological symptoms, it is not an essential consideration in the treatment of the depression. Although the available evidence has failed to show beneficial effects for antidepressants in childhood and adolescent depression (Gadow 1992), clinical practice suggests that these drugs may be helpful in children with severe withdrawal and depression and lead to improvements in mood and eating habits, which in turn help the child develop a more positive attitude towards symptoms and treatment (Garralda 1992b). Relaxation exercises or the prescription of a tranquillizer (for example, thioridazine in small doses for short periods) can sometimes be helpful in treating associated anxiety.

Personality Children with somatization tend to be described as temperamentally fussy, keen on certain routines, and rigid. In addition, they are commonly seen as not communicating their feelings and distress easily to others and, thus, less able to use this means of gaining relief from the usual life stresses.

In treatment it is helpful to discuss the child's personality with the family and explore ways in which it may have caused difficulties in coping with stress and illness. For the child this can be an unwelcome discussion, because it exposes a weakness which he or she may regard as shameful and unacceptable. Parents may share these feelings. Consequently it is important that the therapist creates a non-critical atmosphere in which these issues can be constructively addressed.

Academic expectations A further characteristic commonly displayed by children with somatization is the presence of parental high expectations. Some of these children are in fact high achievers (Lask 1986). In this context the additional stress of a viral illness or of a mild injury has a dual effect. On the one hand, it leads to missing school and the consequent need to work to catch up to the previous high level of academic achievement, on the other, it curtails activity, relieves pressure, and gives comfort without the need to discuss the stresses. The child is put in a situation where nothing less than a high level of functioning is acceptable, yet it is not within reach any more. Giving in to illness may provide a way out of this dilemma and bring welcome comfort from others.

Reluctance to attend school, overt or covert, is often found in the previous histories of children with functional symptoms. Assessment of school attendance and of any possible school stresses, whether related to academic expectations or to social adjustment and peer relationships, should therefore be a part of the assessment procedure. Some children fervently deny school stress at early stages in treatment but may become more open when they develop trust for the therapist. Plans need to be made for decreasing such stresses and for a gradual return to school after recovery.

Family health problems and preoccupation with illness Families of children with functional symptoms may have had experience of chronic illness in other family members who have exhibited symptoms similar to those of the affected child. Families may also report examples where medical interventions have been unhelpful or misguided and where they feel that important conditions have not been identified. They have consequently developed a mistrust of medical intervention. In these cases it seems that the family may have become over-sensitized to somatic concerns, although they may not themselves accept this. In treatment it is often quite difficult to draw helpful parallels between these preoccupations and the child's somalization. The positive family history is useful for the clinician at the diagnostic stage but, in the author's experience, it is seldom a helpful topic for therapeutic exploration.

Family emotional closeness and decreased emotional expressiveness Emotional closeness between family members and a tendency not to communicate freely on emotional issues can be quite striking in many families. Minuchin *et al.* (1975) have used terms such as enmeshment, overprotectiveness, and lack of conflict resolution to describe these family characteristics and have ascribed a prominent role to them in the aetiology of functional somatic symptoms. It is important that parents do not perceive discussion of their family as critical or incriminating, as this may lead to a defensive reaction and hostility to therapy.

It is more useful to recognize and respect, rather than to challenge, the close nature of family relationships and to acknowledge that this closeness can slow and limit the process of establishing a therapeutic alliance with an outsider to the family unit, such as the therapist. A helpful strategy for addressing family communication on emotional issues is to discuss with the family how they detect or recognize cues indicating distress in other family members and how they provide mutual comfort. Parents may be given direct advice to use terms and explanations involving emotions in order to help the child feel that it is acceptable and desirable to use an emotional vocabulary and to communicate distress. Establishing a therapeutic alliance with parents is crucial in helping children shift his/her attitudes concerning somatic symptoms and the expression of distress. The process is slow because children are often in a state of heightened anxiety at the start of treatment. The knowledge that treatment aims to reduce the prominence of the physical symptoms may be only partially appealing and may also fill them with apprehension and anxiety. Support, encouragement, and firmness from parents in the face of considerable distress in the child are all required to resolve the initial difficult phase, before the underlying limitations in emotional expression can be usefully addressed.

Sexual abuse   Sexual abuse is a contributory factor in some children with somatization. It may be more frequent than has been recognized in the past in severe withdrawal states (Lask *et al.* 1991) and perhaps also in children with less severe problems. When sexual abuse is established as a stressor, procedures need to be set into motion to ensure the child's protection. In some instances this may mean care away from the family.

Family or individual treatments   Conjoint family assessment and treatments are almost always required as part of treatment. Systematic evaluation of the effects of a family approach to functional symptoms is lacking, but family therapy techniques have been found to be helpful in the treatment of other psychologically influenced somatic problems such as asthma (Lask and Matthe 1979; Gustafsson *et al.* 1986).

Individual work with the child also has a place in treatment. Adolescents may benefit from sharing underlying anxieties independently from their parents in individual therapy sessions aimed at helping them understand the psychological processes involved. They may also be assisted to develop helpful cognitive and relaxation strategies to deal with their anxieties.

Conclusion

The management of functional somatic symptoms in children is still largely based on clinical insights rather than systematic research. There is, however, considerable evidence concerning the frequency, nature, and associations of these problems that leads to basic principles of intervention. The way is open for systematic research into the treatment of what are common and potentially handicapping symptoms in children. This is an area in which increasing psychiatric involvement should result in considerably improved treatment outcomes.

References

Apley, J. (1975). *The child with abdominal pains*, (2nd edn). Blackwell Scientific, Oxford.

Apley, J. and Naish, N. (1958). Recurrent abdominal pains: a field survey of 11,000 school children. *Archives of Disease in Childhood*, **33**, 1656-70.

Aro, H., Paronen, O., and Aro, S. (1987). Psychosomatic symptoms among 14 to 16 year old Finnish adolescents. *Social Psychiatry*, **22**, 171-6.

Bailey, V., Graham, P. and Boniface, D. (1978). How much child psychiatry does a general practitioner do? *Journal of the Royal College of General Practitioners*, **28**, 621-6.

Bass, L.W. and Cohen, R.L,. (1982). Ostensible versus actual reasons for seeking pediatric attention: another look at the parental ticket of admission. *Pediatrics*, **70**, 870-4.

Benson, P. and Turk, T. (1988). Group therapy in a general practice setting for frequent attenders: a controlled study of mothers with pre-school children. *Journal of the Royal College of General Practitioners*, **38**, 539-41.

Bille, B. (1962). Migraine in children. *Acta Paediatrica*, **51** (Suppl. 136), pp. 1-51.

Butler, S., Charder, T., Ron, M., and Wessely, S. (1991). Cognitive behavioural therapy in the chronic fatigue syndrome. *Journal of Neurology, Neurosurgery and Psychiatry*, **54**, 153-8.

Campo, J.U. and Fritsch, S.L. (1994). Somatization in children and adolescents. *Journal of American Academy of Child and Adolescent Psychiatry*, **33**, 1223-33.

Christensen, M.F. and Mortensen, O. (1975). Long-term prognosis in children with recurrent abdominal pain. *Archives of Disease in Childhood*, **50**, 110-14.

Collin, C., Hockaday, J.M., and Waters, W.E. (1985). Headache and school absence. *Archives of Disease in Childhood*, **60**, 245-7.

Crossley, R.B. (1982). Hospital admissions for abdominal pain in childhood. *Journal of Royal Society of Medicine*, **75**, 772-6.

Cucchiara, S., Riezzo, G., Minella, R., Pezzolla, F., Giorgio, I., and Auricchio, S. (1992). Electrogastrography in non-ulcer dyspepsia. *Archives of Disease in Childhood*, **67**, 613-17.

Cullen, K.J. (1976). A six-year controlled trial of prevention of children's behaviour disorders. *Journal of Pediatrics*, **88**, 662-6.

Cunningham-Burley, S. and Irvine, S. (1987). Practice research. 'And have you done anything so far?' An examination of lay treatment of children's symptoms. *British Medical Journal*, **295**, 700-2.

Davison, I.S., Fault, C., and Nicol, A.R. (1986). Research note: Temperament and behaviour in six-year-olds with recurrent abdominal pain: a follow-up. *Journal of Child Psychology and Psychiatry*, **27**, 539-44.

Dubowitz, V. and Hersov, L. (1976). Management of children with non-organic (hysterical) disorders of motor function. *Developmental Medicine and Child Neurology*, **18**, 358-68.

Eminson, D.M. and Postlethwaite, R.J. (1992). Factitious illness: recognition and management. *Archives of Disease in Childhood*, **67**, 1510-16.

Faull, C. and Nicol, A.R. (1986). Abdominal pain in six-year-olds: an epidemiological study in a new town. *Journal of Child Psychology and Psychiatry*, **27**, 251-60.

Finney, J.W., Lemanek, K.L., Cataldo, M.F., Katz, H.P., and Fuqua, R.W. (1989). Pediatric psychology in primary health care: brief targeted therapy for recurrent abdominal pain. *Behaviour Therapy*, **20**, 283-91.

Furnell, J.R.G. and Dutton, P.V. (1986). Alleviation of toddler's diarrhoea by environmental management. *Journal of Psychosomatic Research*, **30**, 283-8.

Gadow, K.D. (1992). Pediatric psychopharmacotherapy: a review of recent research. *Journal of Child Psychology and Psychiatry*, **33**, 153-95.

Garber, J., Walker, L.S., and Zeman, J. (1991). Somatization symptoms in a community sample of children and adolescents: further validation of the Children's Somatization Inventory. *Psychological Assessment: A Journal of Consulting and Clinical Psychology*, **3**, 588-95.

Garralda, M.E. (1992*a*). A selective review of child psychiatric syndromes with somatic presentation. *British Journal of Psychiatry*, **161**, 759-73.

Garralda, M.E. (1992*b*). Chronic fatigue syndrome in childhood. A discussion of psychopathological mechanisms. *European Child and Adolescent Psychiatry*, **1**, 111-18.

Garralda, M.E. and Bailey, D. (1987). Psychosomatic aspects of children's consultations in primary care. *European Archives of Psychiatry and Neurological Sciences*, **236**, 319-22.

Garralda, M.E. and Bailey, D. (1990). Paediatric identification of psychological factors associated with general paediatric consultations. *Journal of Psychosomatic Research*, **34**, 303-12.

Golding, J. and Butler, N.R. (1986). Headaches and stomach aches. In *From birth to five,* **9**, 130-40 (ed. N.R. Butler and J. Golding). Pergamon Press. Oxford.

Goodman, J.E. and McGrath, P.J. (1991). The epidemiology of pain in children and adolescents: a review. *Pain*, **46**, 247-64.

Graham, P. and Jenkins, S. (1985). Training of paediatrician for psychosocial aspects of their work. *Archives of Disease in Childhood*, **60**, 777-80.

Grattan-Smith, P., Fairley, M., and Procopis, P. (1988). Clinical features of conversion disorder. *Archives of Discase in Childhood*, **63**, 408-14.

Gutelitts, M.F., Kirsch, A.D., MacDonald, S., Brooks, M.R., and McErlean, T. (1977). Controlled study of child health supervision: behavioral results. *Pediatrics*, **60**, 294-304.

Gustafsson, P.A., Kjellman, N.I.M., and Cederblad, M. (1986). Family therapy in the treatment of severe childhood asthma. *Journal of Psychosomatic Research*, **30**, 369-74.

Hockaday, J.M. (1982). Headache in children. *British Journal of Hospital Medicine*, **27**, 383-91.

Larsson, B. (1992). Behavioural Treatment of somatic disorders in children and adolescents. *European Child and Adolescent Psychiatry*, **1**, 68-81.

Larsson, B. and Mellin, L. (1988). The psychological treatment of recurrent headache in adolescents — short-term outcome and its prediction. *Headache*, **28**, 187-95.

Lask, B. (1986). The high-achieving child. *Postgraduate Medical Journal*, **62**, 143-5.

Lask, B. and Fosson, A. (1981). *Childhood illness: the psychosomatic approach.* John Wiley, Chichester.

Lask, B. and Matthew, D. (1979). Childhood asthma. A controlled trial of family psychotherapy. *Archives of Disease in Childhood*, **55**, 116-19.

Lask, B., Britten, C., Kroll, L., Magagna, J., and Tranter, M. (1991). Children with pervasive refusal. *Archives of Disease in Childhood*, **66**, 866-9.

Leslie, S.A. (1988). Diagnosis and treatment of hysterical conversion reactions. *Archives of Disease in Childhood*, **63**, 506-11.

Lewis, C.E. and Lewis, M.A. (1989). Educational outcomes and illness behaviours in participants in a child-initiated care system: a 12-year follow-up study. *Pediatrics*, **84**, 845-50.

Lewis, C.E., Lewis, M.A., Lorimer, A., and Palmer, B.B. (1977). Child-initiated care: the use of school nursing services by children in an 'adult-free' system. *Pediatrics*, **60**, 499-507.

Livingston, R., Taylor, J.L., and Crawford, S.L. (1988). A study of somatic complaints and psychiatric diagnoses in children. *Journal of the American Academy of Child and Adolescent Psychiatry*, **27**, 185-7.

Lloyd, G.G. (1986). Psychiatric syndromes with a somatic presentation. *Journal of Psychosomatic Research*, **30**, 113-20.

McGrath, P.J., Humphreys, P., Goodman, J.T., Keene, D., Firestone, P., Jacob, P., and Cunningham, S.J. (1988). Relaxation prophylaxis for childhood migraine: a randomized placebo-controlled trial. *Developmental Medicine and Child Neurology*, **30**, 626-31.

Minuchin, S., Baker, L.M., Rosman, B.L., Liebman, R., Milman, L., and Todd, T.C. (1975). A conceptual model of psychosomatic illness in children. *Archives of General Psychiatry*, **32**, 1031-8.

Offord, D.R., Boyle, M.H., Szatmari, P., Rae-Grant, W.I., Links, P.S., Cadman, D.T., *et al.* (1987). Ontario child health study. II. Six-month prevalence of disorder and rates of service utilization. *Archives of General Psychiatry*, **44**, 833-6.

Oster, J. (1972). Recurrent abdominal pain, headache and limb pains in children and adolescents. *Pediatrics*, **50**, 429-36.

Sanders, M.R., Rebgetz, M., Morrison, M., Bor, W., Gordon, A., and Dadds, M. (1989). Cognitive-behavioral treatment of recurrent nonspecific abdominal pain: an analysis of generalization, maintenance, and side effects. *Journal of Consulting and Clinical Psychology*, **57**, 294-300.

Sanders, M.R., Shepherd, R.W., Cleghorn, G., and Woolford, H. (1994). Treatment of recurrent abdominal pain in children: a controlled comparison of cognitive behavioural family intervention and standard paediatric care. *Journal of Consulting and Clinical Psychology*, **62**, 306-14.

Schor, E.L. (1986). Use of health care services by children and diagnoses received during presumably stressful life transitions. *Pediatrics*, **77**, 834-41.

Starwell, B., Gross, E., Woodl, M., Pantwell, R., Allen, C., Gordon, B. *et al.* (1980). Psychosocial and psychosomatic diagnoses in primary care of children. *Pediatrics*, **66**, 159-67.

Valman, B. (1982). *The ABC of 1 to 7*. British Medical Association, London.

van der Meer, S.B., Forget, P.P., and Arends, J.W. (1990). Abnormal small bowel permeability and duodenitis in recurrent abdominal pain. *Archives of Disease in Childhood*, **65**, 1311-14.

Vereker, M. (1992). Chronic fatigue syndrome: a joint paediatric–psychiatric approach. *Archives of Diseases of Childhood*, **67**, 550-5.

Wasserman, R.C., Barriatua, R.D., Carter, W.B., and Lippincott, B.A. (1984). Pediatric clinician's support for parents makes a difference: an outcome based on analysis of clinician patent interaction. *Pediatrics*, **74**, 1047-63.

Wasserman, A.L., Whitington, P.F., and Rivara, F. (1988). Psychogenic basis for abdominal pain in children and Adolescents. *Journal of American Academy of Child and Adolescent Psychiatry*, **27**, 179-84.

Zuckerman, B., Stevenson, J., and Bailey, V. (1987). Stomach aches and headaches in a community sample of preschool children. *Pediatrics*, **79**, 677-82.

20 The treatment of somatic symptoms in the elderly

Jane Pearce and Charles Morris

The diagnosis and management of somatic symptoms in the elderly has attracted little attention. However, Drs Pearce and Morris show that there is considerable evidence that such symptoms are at least as common as in younger people and are often associated with considerable disability and use of medical resources.

The high prevalence of physical disease in the elderly makes assessment difficult and means that an interaction of behavioural, physical and psychological factors is extremely common. Presentation and course are also substantially affected by social circumstances and by the reaction of families, friends, and other carers. Adequate assessment and treatment depend upon the giving of full weight both to physical and psychological factors as well as to social influences.

There is little evidence concerning the effectiveness of specific treatment of functional somatic symptoms in the elderly, but it appears that methods that are effective in younger people are equally helpful in the elderly. The authors emphasize that most problems can be managed in primary care with relatively simple techniques and that it is especially important to pay attention to physical, psychological, and social factors from the outset.

Introduction

This chapter is concerned with the management of older people with functional somatic symptoms (that is, people in their seventh decade of life and above). Although the elderly suffer the same psychological disorders as younger people, there are additional factors operating in later life which influence both the nature of the symptoms and their presentation. They include the development of physical disease with its consequent disability and handicaps, changes in social situation and family relationships, and the inevitable approach of death. Because of these factors the treatment techniques discussed in other chapters may require modifications if they are to be used successfully in the treatment of older people.

The medical problems in the elderly, whether physical or psychological, are often (if not always) multifactorial in aetiology. Appreciation of this fact is essential in planning management. Thus, somatic symptoms may be explained entirely by organic disease, partially by disease, and partially by functional disorder or they may be entirely functional in origin. All three categories are common but it is the middle group who are likely to present the most difficult management problems and it is on this problem that we shall concentrate.

The degree to which any non-life-threatening disease 'should' limit activity is by no means easy to determine. To quote Murphy (1982), 'With lesser degrees of illness, it is not always possible to make an objective judgement about severity since time spent at home recuperating in the sick role varies so much according to the mood, habits, expectations and personality'. The degree of handicap is determined by many factors outside the individual's control, such as medical attitudes to old people, the expectations of the person's family, and the organization of the 'caring services'.

Gurland (1976) has described many of the difficulties in age-related research and emphasized the difficulties involved in assessing physical symptoms in an older population, particularly when large scale surveys are carried out by relatively inexperienced interviewers. The diagnosis of physical disease is complicated and potentially inaccurate in the elderly (see below; Fairweather and Campbell 1991) and the same applies to psychiatric illness, for example it has been suggested that the symptom pattern of depression differs between those aged below 65 and the more aged elderly (Fogel and Fretwell 1985; Newmann *et al.* 1991). Studies of physical symptoms in the elderly therefore require stringent and skilful assessments, and their conclusions need particularly careful analysis.

Epidemiology

What somatic symptoms occur in an elderly population? Self-perception of being in 'good health' declines with age, although there is disagreement about the extent of this decline. Victor (1991) found that 46 per cent of 64–69-year-olds and only 27 per cent of over 85 years reported their health as good, but Copeland *et al.* (1986) reported that 86 per cent over 65 years rated their health as excellent or good (excluding those with mental illness). Such statements by older people as 'At my age I should be looked after' and 'I'm too old to change' should not be regarded as normal, as most older people are remarkably resilient in the face of increasing disabilities (Little 1992).

However, community surveys do reveal a high prevalence of symptomatic complaints in older age groups (Bergmann 1992). In one such study, 28 per cent of males and 43 per cent of females aged 65–74 years reported experiencing painful joints in the month prior to questioning (Cox *et al.* 1987) and the General Household Survey found that 57 per cent of over 75 years reported a long-standing illness which limited their activities. Furthermore, when 'disability' (as opposed to 'illness') is examined, those over 60 years constitute 75 per cent of the most severely disabled and 14 per cent of men over 75 years old are housebound by disability (Martin *et al.* 1988). The same survey found that 14 per cent of males and 20 per cent of females aged 65–74 years described an episode of acute physical illness in the 14 days prior to interview and these proportions increased to 18 and 23 per cent respectively in those over 75 years (OPCS 1988). Earlier studies reported an increased prevalence of ill-health in the elderly with days of restricted activity per year, long-standing physical illness, mean number of chronic conditions per person, and functional restriction all increasing with age (OPCS 1982).

It is difficult to determine to what extent the non-specific symptoms described in epidemiological surveys are 'functional', but it is reasonable to conclude the parallel increases with age. There is also some evidence that somatic complaints differ in *type* between age groups. For example, von Korff *et al.* (1988) found that survey respondents over 65 years of age suffered more back pain (males only) but less headache, facial pain, and abdominal pain than younger respondents. Conversely, the experience of back pain in women and of chest pain in both sexes were no different in the two age groups. In a similar survey of randomly selected households, Crook *et al.* (1984) found persistent pain complaints to be more common in the older age groups with 80-year-olds having four times the rate of 30-year-olds and one and a half times that of 60-year-olds. Both these studies reported more pain complaints in the retired, separated, and widowed. There is no systematic information about the prevalence of functional complaints in elderly primary care attenders. It appears that general practitioners manage most patients with unexplained somatic symptoms probably without recourse to specialist services. They refer a minority to specialists, the choice of which depends on the severity and probable cause of the symptoms. The path of referral may also be influenced by the nature of associated complaints, the attitudes of the general practitioner, and the ease of access to the different medical specialties. A given patient may, in different places, be referred to geriatricians, psychiatrists, or other specialized physicians. For example, in an area with no specific geriatric medical provision more patients with unexplained physical symptoms are likely to be referred to the psychogeriatrician, even though this deprives the patient of a specialist physical assessment.

Neither are there adequate studies indicating the prevalence rates of functional somatic symptoms in elderly patients attending hospital clinics, although elderly patients have been noted in cardiac clinics (Beitman *et al.* 1990) and among internal medicine referrals (Barsky *et al.* 1991).

Age-related aetiological factors

The most difficult patients to understand and manage are those in whom multiple factors contribute to the clinical presentation, each of which may partially explain the symptoms. The main problem in assessing the elderly therefore is in deciding on the balance of aetiological factors, in particular the extent to which physical disease explains the complaints and disability. We will use the term 'age-related aetiological factors' to refer to those factors which are of particular significance in later life. These factors will sometimes interact with attributes present throughout life, such as personality and childhood experience. We shall not attempt to discuss these lifelong factors.

Physical disease   The special characteristics of physical disease when it occurs in the older person include multiple pathology, non-specific or insidious presentation, rapid deterioration if untreated, and a high incidence of secondary complications (Evans 1992). In addition, similar clinical presentations may have quite different causes. For example, a patient with pneumonia may not present with pleuritic chest pain, cough, and pyrexia but with 'confusion' or 'gone off her legs'. Fairweather and Campbell (1991) elegantly discuss the difficulties in diagnosis in old age and attribute this to the effects of both multiple aetiology and the 'degradation of clinical information'. Multiple aetiology (as distinct from multiple pathology) makes diagnosis more complex as several, possibly minor, aetiological processes can interact to produce an apparently single disorder and presentation. Thus, many common clinical problems, such as falls or urinary incontinence, usually have a multiple causation (Lipsitz *et al.* 1986; Campbell *et al.* 1985, 1989).

'Degradation of clinical information' refers to the imprecise nature of clinical information derived, for example, from the physical examination and investigation, of older patients. Interpretation of findings is made even more difficult by the usual practice of defining 'normal ranges' for investigations with regard to younger age groups, since what is considered 'mildly abnormal' in a younger adult may not be abnormal in an older person. The clinical errors of either failing to make a diagnosis when a disease is present or making a diagnosis when a disease is not present occur twice as often in the elderly as in younger patients (Fairweather and Campbell 1991).

Combined physical and psychiatric illness   Depressive and anxiety symptoms are strongly related to physical health. Vetter *et al.* (1986) found that of those aged over 70 years with no physical disability, 3 per cent had depressive symptoms and 7 per cent anxiety symptoms, whilst the proportions in those with severe disability rose to 20 and 40 per cent respectively. Depressive illness in the elderly is associated with chronic poor health (Murphy 1982; Dover and McWilliam 1992) and increased mortality, even after physical illness is controlled for (Murphy *et al.* 1988). In those with both mental and physical disorders, depression (and not physical illness) may be the strongest predictor of somatic discomfort (Rozzini *et al.* 1988) and of disability (Wells *et al.* 1989).

Psychiatric disorder is more frequent in physically ill elderly people than in the general population, be they chronic geriatric in-patients (Sadavoy *et al.* 1990; Shah *et al.* 1992), day hospital attenders (Turrina 1992), or acutely ill in-patients (Bergmann and Eastham 1974; Schukit *et al.* 1975; O'Riordan *et al.* 1989; Ramsay *et al.* 1991).

Somatic symptoms and psychiatric illness

Depressive disorder It has been suggested that older patients with depressive illness exhibit more somatic symptoms than the younger depressed patient and that hypochondriacal symptoms may precede and dominate the apparent mood change (Lewis 1934; Alarcon 1964). Alarcon (1964) maintained that the majority of those with depression and prominent physical symptoms had not suffered lifelong health concern but developed their symptoms as a result of depressive illness, whilst the minority with long-standing somatic symptoms reported a change in intensity or in the nature of the symptoms with the onset of depression. McDonald (1973) agreed that 'increasing age produces a somatisation of neurotic presentation'. However, other more recent authors have found no difference in symptom profiles between younger and older patients with major or minor depression (Blazer *et al.* 1987; Copeland *et al.* 1987; Downes *et al.* 1988; Kramer-Ginsberg *et al.* 1989; Oxman 1990). A cross-cultural comparision found no differences between Liverpool and Zaragoza, Spain (Dewey *et al.* 1993).

The authors believe that most depressed elderly patients present in very similar ways to younger patients, although a few older people may be reluctant to acknowledge low mood and may present with more florid nihilistic ideas concerning bodily functions.

Emotional disorders It is widely believed that hypochondriacal symptoms are a prominent feature of neurotic disorder. Bergmann (1971) found that over 30 per cent of elderly 'neurotics' identified in a community survey exhibited hypochondriasis and that the proportion was the same in both chronic and late-onset groups. There were equal numbers of men and women among subjects identified as neurotic and physically ill, in contrast to a preponderance of women amongst the physically well, suggesting that these may form two different aetiological groups. Lindesay (1991*a,b*) reported an association between hypochondriasis and phobic disorder, suggesting that 12 per cent of elderly people with phobic disorder have unexplained physical symptoms (that is, symptoms not accounted for by anxiety or known physical disease). In addition, he found that the commonest precipitant for late-onset agoraphobia was physical illness, particularly cardiac or respiratory disorders. Again this demonstrates a close interplay between psychiatric and physical disorder in the elderly.

Beitman *et al.* (1990) studied cardiology patients with chest pain but no evidence of coronary artery disease. They found that one-third of their sample of 27 patients over 65 years old satisfied diagnostic criteria for panic disorder and that the age of onset ranged from 62 to 83 years. All were widowed compared with only 40 per cent of those without panic disorder. The phenomenology of the disorder in those over 65 years was no different from that seen in a younger sample.

Somatoform disorders　　The applications of the subcategories of somatoform disorder have proved problematic in the elderly and have received little attention. In particular, clinicians have been reluctant to diagnose conversion disorder because of the high risk of occult physical disease.

In the Epidemiological Catchment Area project, Swartz *et al.* (1989) estimated somatization disorder (full and abbreviated criteria) to be actually less prevalent in the over 65 years age group than in 45–64 year olds.

We see three major disadvantages of definitions of hypochondriasis as defined in DSM-IV. First, it requires 'preoccupation with the fear of having, or the belief that one has, a serious disease' but in many elderly patients with unexplained physical symptoms such preoccupation is a less important feature (and may even be absent) than disability or handicap. For example, the patient who presents with reluctance to get out of bed rather than concern over symptoms (see below). Hence, a revised definition of hypochondriasis for use with older patients would need to be broad enough to include not only those who have disproportionate concern over the state of their health, but also disproportionate disability. Secondly, the requirement that 'appropriate physical evaluation does not support the diagnosis of any physical disorder that can account for the physical signs or sensations' is particularly difficult when a clinical presentation may be partially explained by physical pathology and partially by psychosocial factors. Thirdly, the classification system as a whole, although multiaxial, does not adequately address the presence of multiple aetiological factors and, in many cases, the need for complex treatment interventions. Both classification systems, when applied to the elderly, implicitly require a judgement as to what are appropriate physical symptoms, whereas an ideal system would merely require one to list the various aetiological factors without any overt weighting of relative importance (see also Chapter 3).

Despite these methodological problems, several authors have used the DSM-IIIR classification in studies of elderly patients. For example, Barsky *et al.* (1991) compared a group of self-selected general medical out-patients over 65 years old fulfilling criteria for DSM-IIIR hypochondriasis with a group under 65 years. They found no significant differences between the two groups in measures of disease conviction, disease fear, bodily preoccupation, or somatic symptoms. The older subjects were more disabled but this was not associated with 'more hypochondriasis'. However, this study did not include many subjects over 75 years and the younger comparison group may have been more hypochondriacal than an unselected population (as the authors point out). Thus, the authors conclusion that 'hypochondriasis is found to some degree in all age groups' stands, but to say that hypochondriasis 'appears unrelated to age' may be misleading. Several authors have emphasized the role of psychosocial stressors in precipitating late-onset hypochondriasis (Busse 1976; Brink *et al.* 1981; Busse 1987), but unfortunately there is little empirical evidence concerning the development of hypochondriacal states in the elderly.

Social factors

Social support is an important factor which may change dramatically (for the worse) in old age. Common socio-economic changes occurring in old age are retirement from work, poorer housing, reduced income, restriction of social links, and changes in family relationships. One-quarter of those over 65 years in Britain have an income at or below supplementary benefit rates and a further 44 per cent live on the margins of poverty (Victor 1991). In addition, 36 per cent of people over 65 years live alone, though this does not necessarily imply separation from their families and society since nearly half the elderly people living alone see a relative or close friend on a daily basis (OPCS 1989).

Rozzini *et al.* (1988) found that the degree of support influenced somatic symptom scores regardless of disease and Busse (1976, 1987) has claimed that social stress and the loss of social opportunities are an important factor in precipitating a preoccupation with somatic symptoms in the elderly. Hence, complaints are more common in the widowed and separated elderly (Crook *et al.* 1984; von Korff *et al.* 1988) and Beitman *et al.* (1990) found those in his sample with panic disorder and atypical chest pain were all widows (compared to 40 per cent of those with atypical chest pain without panic disorder).

Health beliefs and attitude to old age

The self-perception of being in 'good health' falls with increasing age. This finding does not necessarily imply unnecessary handicaps or preoccupation with ill-health, however. With advancing age, people appear to take an increasingly practical view of good health as being active and free from acute illness, rather than absence of chronic symptoms (Abrams 1985; Copeland *et al.* 1986; Morgan *et al.* 1987; Victor 1991). Although older people in general appear remarkably resilient to physical disability and approaching death (Copeland *et al.* 1986), some individuals are not so phlegmatic. It is necessary to understand the individual's attitude to increasing age and disability in order to understand the significance of their somatic symptoms. For example, in a study of the characteristics of hypochondriacal patients (albeit largely a younger group than considered here) 'aversion to death and ageing' and a 'sense of body vunerability' were found to be highly correlated with hypochondriasis (Barsky and Wyshak 1989). Dysfunctional ideas about health are unusual in old people and primary care physicians and others should be aware that apparently unfounded complaints are a reason for further inquiry and possibly psychiatric referral.

A number of psychological theories have been proposed to explain why older people become preoccupied with somatic symptoms. These include

(1)   the impact of social isolation;

(2)   avoidance of emotional conflicts by shifting attention onto somatic processes;

(3)   the unconscious use of hypochondriacal symptoms to provide an excuse for social inadequacies and an escape from chronic criticism;

(4)   the focusing of older people on the inner self and their bodies, which is associated with psychological withdrawal from the outer world;

(5)   their inward turning of aggression (Busse 1976, 1987; Verwoedt 1981; Post 1982).

An illustrative case series

We have recently examined the characteristics of a small group of patients referred to local psychogeriatricians in whom unexplained physical symptoms were prominent. Patients were excluded if they suffered from severe cognitive impairment, if their physical symptoms were solely the 'biological' symptoms of depressive disorder (such as loss of appetite, weight loss, and constipation), or if reassessment demonstrated definite and untreated physical disease. The group comprised 18 patients, with a mean age of 77 years (range 68–84 years). All but one were referred from primary care. Physical investigation had been carried out before psychiatric referral in *only three patients*. In one case, investigation of prostatic symptoms preceded numerous physical symptoms and major depression. The other two patients had recently undergone investigation for deterioration of long-standing physical disease. In one of these cases the further physical assessment requested by the psychogeriatrician proved impossible to achieve because the patient would not leave the sofa and the physician would not leave the hospital!

Table 20.1 Examples of physical symptoms reported

Pain: abdominal, chest, pelvic, vaginal, and muscle headache
'Collapse', and 'legs are useless'
Nausea, dizziness, and shakiness
Belief of having cancer or eroding gums
Lump in throat

Table 20.2 Clinical characteristics of the patients ($n = 18$)

Group 1 (n = 11)	Group 2 (n = 7)
Short recent history (< 6 months)	Longer history (mean 4 years)
Presented with mood disturbance	Presented with functional loss and disability
Previous affective disorder	Marked restrictions in activities of daily living
Worrying beliefs about illness	Diagnostic uncertainty

The complaints of these 18 patients are shown in Table 20.1. Two main clinical groups were evident and their characteristic features are shown in Table 20.2. In the first group, depression was the commonest diagnosis. Many had overt mood symptoms as well as previous depressive episodes. These factors led to early recognition of mood disorder and early referral. There were few examples of overt symptom misinterpretation. However, three patients with major depression believed they had cancer and one with generalized anxiety believed that she had ME. We also found that the patients diagnosed as having generalized anxiety disorder, regardless of the length of history, had more concurrent physical illness.

Group 2 had longer histories and more restriction in activities of daily living. Referral was typically for help with the consequences of functional loss, for example 'getting stuck in the chair', 'legs are useless', and 'continuous stomach pain so I can't move'. It is possible that there seemed to be an acceptance of disability by carers and primary care workers in these people, so that referral only occurred after a prolonged period of treatment (without specialist geriatric or psychiatric intervention) when physical dependency had become difficult to manage.

Research on treatment

Just as there has been little research on the nature and epidemiology of persistent somatic symptoms in older people, there have been no adequate evaluations of treatment. It is not difficult to see why most published treatment studies excluded older people. In addition to the problems of recruitment and accurate diagnosis, the existence of multiple aetiological factors makes it unlikely that a single treatment could produce an easily demonstrated therapeutic benefit. Therefore, a comparison of standard treatment with standard treatment *plus* a single psychological intervention (such as cognitive therapy) may not be expected to yield much additional benefit. Furthermore, psychological treatments may need to be modified for use in the elderly if they are to be effective.

It has recently been suggested that hypochondriacal and other neurotic disorders of old age represent a changing 'chronic condition with a variety of symptoms resolving and recurring at various times' (Larkin *et al.* 1992). For example, an elderly person may lose her preoccupation with breathessness only to become housebound by agoraphobia. Uncertainty about the natural history and the possible change of symptoms over time means that any treatment study must include a long follow-up and a wide range of outcome measures. The authors believe that functional impairment is a more useful outcome measure than the severity of symptoms in elderly patients with functional somatic illness.

Practical guidelines for management

Assessment

The assessment of somatic symptoms in older people, whether due to actual physical disease or to an apparently functional somatic syndrome is similar. It involves identifying which physical, psychological, and social factors are relevant in the individual case. These factors are not hierarchical but dimensional and are likely to be *multiple*. Presentation is commonly non-specific and it is much more common than in younger age groups for functional symptoms to be intermingled with actual physical disease. It is probably inappropriate therefore to distinguish sharply between physical and functional somatic symptoms in the elderly patient. The assessment should include the following.

1. Set the stage for dual management, whereby both the physical and psychosocial aspects of the presenting somatic symptoms can be addressed constructively. It may be helpful to let the patient know at the outset that both physical symptoms and anxieties and worries are legitimate concerns and that both may need treatment in their own right.

2. Explore all the relevant factors, including those not initially presented by the patient to the doctor. For example, a patient may regard a

particular symptom simply as an inevitable part of ageing and may therefore feel that it does not need to be mentioned.

Assessment of physical state The aim is not simply to exclude the presence of physical disease (which will rarely be possible with elderly patients), but to determine whether the physical condition is a *sufficient explanation* for the severity of the somatic complaint or disability. This is a complex matter and the parallel psychosocial assessment is likely to be helpful. It is important to realize that lay informants' accounts of the elderly person's difficulties may be biased by negative expectations of health in old age. However, the opinions of the health visitor and district nursing staff may be useful because the assessment of activities of daily living may have been documented in their care plans.

Continuing physical review is important; it is more likely that an older person will develop further physical disease during the treatment of a chronic problem than a young person. The doctor should therefore establish a routine of care which includes physical examination of changing or new symptomatology and a thorough review of physical medication to ensure that this is not contributing to symptoms (for example, postural hypotension producing dizziness by over-treatment of hypertension).

Although investigation of symptoms is often necessary, laboratory tests in the elderly are often mildly abnormal and clinical judgement should inform both the instigation and interpretation of investigations.

Assessment of psychological state It is important to ascertain the *focus of the patient's concerns*. For example, old people are particularly at risk of loss of independence and there are often particular anxieties about the consequences of physical disability.

It is necessary here, as in all psychiatric assessments, to seek actively evidence of *depressive disorder* and *anxiety states*, because there may be simple and effective treatments for these. However, it is important also to be aware that the symptoms of physical illness frequently cause emotional distress (for example, the breathlessness of cardiorespiratory disease). The syndrome of 'fear of failing' (where after a transient ischaemic attack or other sudden episode the patient is afraid of walking unaided) (Lindesay 1991*a,b*) highlights the inter-relationship of physical and psychological factors.

Other major psychiatric illnesses should also be sought. Non-specific somatic symptoms can be the presenting features of almost any psychiatric illness in old people. Late-onset *paranoid states* are not uncommon and *dementias* may present with anxiety over many factors including physical health. *Depressive disorders* in the early stages of dementia may respond well to antidepressant treatment.

Social and family factors may be important, not only as precipitants, but also as maintaining influences. The way in which families respond to an episode of minor or major physical disease may perpetuate the elderly person's concern about somatic symptoms. Specific enquiry may be required because the involvement of others in care is often taken for granted. Indicators that such interpersonal factors are important include marked differences of opinion about the severity of the problems between carers and between the patient and their family. Similarly, the response of the caring agencies, such as home care or residential carers, should be assessed because these may, on occasion, also be inadvertently perpetuating the problem.

Treatment

Both presentation and management will commonly (although not exclusively) be within the primary care setting. We therefore offer guidelines on initial management applicable to general primary care, as well as an outline of specific treatments requiring more specialist resources.

Elderly patients may find it particularly difficult to accept an abrupt switch from a physical to a psychological treatment approach, not least because anxieties about the serious consequences of physical symptoms in later life may be exacerbated by an apparent change in the doctor's priorities. Addressing the patient's anxieties from the onset may help to prevent subsequent difficulties. It is also necessary to assess and respond to carers' worries because breakdown of care may occur if the complaints of fear or pain become too burdensome to tolerate.

General guidelines   The first step is to decide how many of the factors identified in the assessment can be addressed. The chosen interventions can often be simple, for example adjustment of medication for a chronic illness, an explanation of the bodily sensations of anxiety, and techniques to help the patient to manage anxiety themself.

Follow-up is important even when somatic complaints resolve after a single contact. This is especially true when there has been recurrent consultation or there is a mixed physical and functional presentation. The aim is to review not only the effectiveness of treatment and the absence of adverse effects, but also the effectiveness of advice given. For example, has the patient understood and remembered the explanations offered about bodily responses to fear associated with their chronic airways disease or been able to practice relaxation and distraction?

Referral to a physician (preferably a specialist geriatrician) may be indicated in the following circumstances.

1. In cases of diagnostic difficulty when further investigation needs to be considered or borderline results interpreted.

2. For advice on the possible need for further, more sensitive investigations or on which contributory physical factor should be treated.

The old age psychiatry team may be able to help with depression or anxiety, worry, or functional disability if these remain disproportionate to the severity of physical disorder and also in shared care of protracted functional illness.

Specific treatments

Treatment of psychiatric disorder Psychiatric illness (for example, depressive disorder) should be treated aggressively. If antidepressants are prescribed, particular attention should be paid to possible side-effects and their effect on patient compliance. The newer drugs such as the specific serotonin reuptake inhibitors may be useful in these patients because of their side-effect profile, but they are still relatively untried. Careful monitoring is just as important as choosing the right drug. Follow-up offers the opportunity to explain and follow side-effects and monitor progress in the light of developments in the treatment of concurrent physical illness and other changes (see also Chapter 4).

Anxiety management, which includes an explanation of physical symptoms of anxiety as well as practical techniques for managing this, may be required both in the presence and absence of actual physical disease. Techniques of relaxation, distraction, and control of hyperventilation or abnormal breathing patterns are used. When anxiety states make a major contribution to the somatic symptoms, we recommend techniques to improve problem-solving and coping stategies and also cognitive interventions which challenge negative thoughts and expectations (Garland 1992).

Medication may be required for anxiety when it is severely disabling.

Behavioural management Excessive help-seeking behaviour, whether it is directed at the family, other carers, or general practitioner, may need to be controlled. This approach is similar to that used with younger patients (see Chapter 7), although the social network may be different. It may also be more difficult to limit treatment, as a general practitioner may find it easier to take a firm stand about repeated claims of having had a heart attack by a 30-year-old, than by an 80-year-old with vascular disease.

When the likelihood of serious physical illness is high, explicit criteria may be needed to help the GP and carers decide how and when to respond. If family members are asked to alter their involvement, it is important to discuss any guilt feelings they may experience as a consequence of not always responding to the demands of their aged relatives.

Systemic approaches to treatment   A family systems approach may be useful in managing both functional and combined functional and physical symptoms. Sometimes, carers are drawn into a vicious circle of increasing disability of the patient and increasing care (Herr 1979). On other occasions, the old person's physical disability or somatic symptoms may actually stabilize the family by, for example, keeping the family in contact or by diverting attention away from the daughter's marital problems.

Family therapy is increasingly recognized as useful in treating the problems of elderly patients (Walsh 1989; Benbow *et al.* 1990; Ratna and David 1984) and even if formal family therapy is not possible there may be advantages to viewing the clinical problems in systemic terms (Jenkins and Asen 1992).

Specific individual therapies   Case studies support the usefulness of cognitive behavioural treatments for elderly people with hypochondriasis (Wattis and Church 1986). There is also evidence that cognitive therapy is effective in the treatment of depression in older people (Woods 1992), although some authors have suggested that older people have difficulty with the rather abstract techniques of cognitive therapy (such as monitoring automatic thoughts) (Little 1992). The therapies developed for younger patients with hypochondriacal problems should also be applicable in older people (see Chapter 9).

Brief psychotherapy may have an important place in the elderly, but with the specific aim of addressing age-related factors such as chronic illness and disability, death and dying, enjoyment in late life, and life review (Knight 1986).

Conclusion

In this chapter we have described the complexity of the problem of functional somatic symptoms in the elderly. We have emphasized the importance of specific age-related aetiological factors and of multifactorial aetiology. We consider it unfortunate that the role of psychiatric factors and treatments has been considerably underestimated in the elderly since many elderly patients with somatic symptoms may respond to simple interventions. As in younger patients, a minority with persistent and severe complaints will require more complex and specialized management. Much earlier recognition and more vigorous treatment of functional somatic symptoms would greatly improve the lives of many elderly people and their families.

References

Abrams, M. (1985). The health of the very elderly. In *Recent advances in geriatric medicine*, (ed. B. Isaacs), pp. 217–26. Churchill Livingstone, London.

Alarcon, R. (1964). Hypochondriasis in the elderly. *Gerontology Clinics*, **6**, 266–77.

Barsky, A.J. and Wyshak, G. (1989). Hypochondriasis and related health attitudes. *Psychosomatics*, **30**, 412–20.

Barsky, A.J., Frank, C.B., Cleary, P.D., Wyshak, G., and Klerman, G.L. (1991). The relation between hypochondrias and age. *American Journal of Psychiatry*, **148**, 923–8.

Beitman, B.D., Kushner, M., and Grossberg, G.T. (1900). Late onset panic disorder: evidence from a study of patients with chest pain and normal cardiac evaluations. *International Journal of Psychiatry in Medicine*, **21**, 29–35.

Benbow, S., Egan, D., Marriott, A., Tregay, K., Walsh, S., Wells, J., and Wood, J. (1990). Using the family lifecycle with later life families. *Journal of Family Therapy*, **12**, 321–40.

Bergman, K. (1971). The neuroses of old age. In *Recent developments in psychogeriatrics*, (ed. D.W.K. Kay and A. Walk), pp. 39–50. Headley, Kent.

Bergman, K. (1992). Functional psychiatric disorders. In *The Oxford textbook of geriatric medicine*, (ed. J.G. Evans and T.F. Williams), pp. 635–8, Oxford University Press, Oxford.

Bergmann, K. and Eastham, E.J. (1974). Psychogeriatric ascertainment and assessment for treatment in an acute medical ward setting. *Age and Ageing*, **3**, 174–88.

Blazer, D., Bachar, J.R., and Hughes, D.C. (1987). Major depression with melancholia: a comparison of middle-aged and elderly adults. *Journal of the American Geriatric Society*, **35**, 927–32.

Brink, T.L., Janakes, C., and Martinez, N. (1981). Geriatric hypochondriasis: situational factors. *Journal of the American Geriatric Society*, **1**, 37–9.

Busse, E.W. (1976). Hypochondriasis in the elderly: a reaction to social stress. *Journal of the American Geriatric Society*, **24**, 145–9.

Busse, E.W. (1987). Hypochondriasis in the elderly. *Comprehensive Therapy*, **13**, 37–42.

Campbell, A.J., Reinken, J., and McCosh, L. (1985). Incontinence in the elderly: prevalence and prognosis. *Age and Ageing*, **14**, 65–70.

Campbell, A.J., Borrie, M.J., and Speirs, G.F.S. (1989). Risk factors for falls in a community based prospective study of people 70 years and older. *Journal of Gerontology and Medical Science*, **44**, 112–17.

Copeland, J.R.M., Kelleher, M.J., Smith, A.M.R., and Devlin, P. (1986). The well, the mentally ill, the old and the old old: a community survey of elderly persons in London. *Ageing and Society*, **6**, 417–33.

Copeland, J.R.M., Dewey, M.E., Wood, N., Searle, R., Davidson, I.A., and McWilliam, C. (1987). Range of mental illness among the elderly in the community. *British Journal of Psychiatry*, **150**, 815–23.

Cox, B.D., Blaxter, M., Buckle, A.L.J., Fenner, N.P., Golding, J.F., Gore, M., *et al.* (1987). *The health and lifestyle survey*. The Health Promotion Trust, London.

Crook, J., Rideout, E., and Browne, G. (1984). The prevalence of pain complaints in a general population. *Pain*, **18**, 299–314.

Dewey, M.E., de la Camara, C., Copeland, J.R.M., Lobo, A., and Saz, P. (1993). Cross-cultural comparison of depression and depressive symptoms in older people. *Acta Psychiatrica Scandanivica*, **87**, 369–73.

Dover, S. and McWilliam, C. (1992). Physical illness associated with depression in the elderly in community based and hospital patients. *Psychiatric Bulletin of the Royal College of Psychiatrists*, **16**, 612–13.

Downes, J.J., Davies, A.D.M., and Copeland, J.R.M. (1988). Organization of depressive symptoms in the elderly population. *Psychology and Aging*, **3**, 367–74.

Evans, J.G. (1992). Hospital services for elderly people: the UK experience. In *The Oxford textbook of geriatric medicine*, (ed. J.G. Evans and T.F. Williams), pp. 703–6. Oxford University Press, Oxford.

Fairweather, D.S. and Campbell, A.J. (1991). Diagnostic accuracy: the effects of multiple aetiology and the degradation of information in old age. *Journal of the Royal College of Physicians of London*, **25**, 105–10.

Fogel, B.S. and Fretwell, M. (1985). Reclassification of depression in the medically ill elderly. *Journal of the American Geriatric Society*, **33**, 446–8.

Garland, J. (1992). Behaviour management. In *The Oxford textbook of geriatric medicine*, (ed. J.G. Evans and T.F. Williams), pp. 646–52, Oxford University Press, Oxford.

Gurland, B.J. (1976). The comparative frequency of depression in various age groups. *Journal of Gerontology*, **31**, 283–92.

Herr, J.J. (1979). *Counselling elders and their families*. Springer, New York.

Jenkins, H. and Asen, K. (1992). Family therapy without the family: a framework for systemic practice. *Journal of Family Therapy*, **14**, 1–14.

Knight, B. (1986). *Psychotherapy with older adults*. Sage Publications, London.

Kramer-Ginsberg, E., Greenwald, B.S., Aisen, P.S., and Brod-Miller, C. (1989). Hypochondriasis in the elderly depressed. *Journal of the American Geriatric Society*, **37**, 507–10.

Larkin, B.A., Copeland, J.R.M., Dewey, M.E., Davidson, I.A., Saunders, P.A., Sharma, V.K., McWilliam, C., and Sullivan, C. (1992). The natural history of neurotic disorder in an elderly urban population. *British Journal of Psychiatry*, **160**, 681–6.

Lewis, A. (1934). Melancholia. *Journal of Mental Science*, **80**, 277–92.

Lindesay, J. (1991a). Phobic disorders in the elderly. *British Journal of Psychiatry*, **159**, 531–41.

Lindesay, J. (1991b). Anxiety disorders in the elderly. In *Psychiatry in the elderly*, (ed. R. Jacoby and C. Oppenheimer), pp. 735–57. Oxford University Press, Oxford.

Lipsitz, L.A., Wei, J.Y., and Rowe, J.W. (1986). Syncope in institutionalised elderly: the impact of multiple pathological conditions and situational stress. *Journal of Chronic Disease*, **39**, 619–30.

Little, A. (1992). Psychological treatments. In *Psychiatry in the elderly*, (ed. R. Jacoby and C. Oppenheimer), pp. 400–15, Oxford University Press, Oxford.

McDonald, C. (1973). An age-specific analysis of the neuroses. *British Journal of Psychiatry*, **122**, 477–80.

Martin, J., Meltzer, H., and Elliot, D. (1988). *The prevalence of disability amongst adults: OPCS.* HMSO, London.

Morgan, K., Dallosso, H.M., Arie, T., Byrne, E.J., Jones, R., and Waite, J. (1987). Mental health and psychological well-being among the old and the very old living at home. *British Journal of Psychiatry*, **150**, 801–7.

Murphy, E. (1982). Social origins of depression in old age. *British Journal of Psychiatry*, **141**, 135–42.

Murphy, E., Smith, R., Lindesay, J., and Slattery, J. (1988). Increased mortality rates in late-life depression. *British Journal of Psychiatry*, **152**, 347–53.

Newmann, J.P., Engel, R.J., and Jensen, J.E. (1991). Changes in depressive-symptom experiences among older women. *Psychology and Aging*, **6**, 212–22.

OPCS (1982). *General household survey 1980.* HMSO, London.

OPCS (1988). *General household survey 1987.* OPCS, London.

O'Riordan, T.G., Hayes, J.P., Shelley, R., O'Neill, D., Walsh, B., and Coakley, D. (1989). The prevalence of depression in an acute geriatric medical assessment unit. *International Journal of Geriatric Psychiatry*, **4**, 17–21.

Oxman, T.E., Barrett, J.E., Barrett, J., and Gerber, P. (1990). Symptomatology of late-life minor depression among primary care patients. *Psychosomatics*, **31**, 174–80.

Post, F. (1982). Functional disorders. In *The psychiatry of late life,* (ed. R. Levy and F. Post), pp. 176–96. Blackwell Scientific Publications, Oxford.

Ramsay, R., Wright, P., Katz, A., Bielawska, C., and Katona, C. (1991). The detection of psychiatric morbidity and its effects on outcome in acute elderly medical admissions. *International Journal of Geriatric Psychiatry*, **6**, 881–6.

Ratna, L. and David, J. (1984). Family therapy with the elderly mentally ill: some strategies and techniques. *British Journal of Psychiatry*, **145**, 311–15.

Rozzini, R., Bianchetti, A., Carabellese, C., Inzoli, M., and Trabucchi, M. (1988). Depression, life events and somatic symptoms. *Gerontologist*, **28**, 229–32.

Sadavoy, J., Smith, I., Conn, D.K., and Richards, B. (1990). Depression in geriatric patients with chronic mental illness. *International Journal of Geriatric Psychiatry*, **5**, 187–92.

Schukit, M.A., Miller, P.L., and Hahlbohm, D. (1975). Unrecognised psychiatric illness in elderly medical-surgical patients. *Journal of Gerontology*, **30**, 655–60.

Shah, A., Phongsathorn, V., George, C., Bielawska, C., and Katona, C. (1992). Psychiatric morbidity among continuing care geriatric patients. *International Journal of Geriatric Psychiatry*, **7**, 517–25.

Swartz, M., Landerman, R., Blazer, D., and George, L. (1989). Somatization symptoms in the community: a rural/urban comparison. *Psychosomatics*, **30**, 44–53.

Turrina, C., Siciliani, O., Dewey, M.E., Fazzari, G.C., and Copeland, J.R.M. (1992). Psychiatric disorders among elderly patients attending a geriatric medical hospital. *International Journal of Geraitric Psychiatry*, **7**, 499–504.

Verwoerdt, A. (1981). Psychotherapy for the elderly. In *Health care of the elderly,* (ed. T. Arie), pp. 118–39, Croom Helm, London.

Vetter, N.J., Jones, D.A., Victor, C.R., and Phillip, A.E. (1986). The measurement of psychological problems in the elderly in general practice. *International Journal of Geriatric Psychiatry*, **1**, 127–34.

Victor, C.R. (1991). *Health and health care in later life*. Oxford University Press, Oxford.

Von Korff, M., Dworkin, S.F., Le Resche, L., and Kruger, A. (1988). An epidemiological comparison of pain complaints. *Pain*, **32**, 173–83.

Walsh, F. (1989). The family in later life. In *The challenging family life cycle: a framework for family therapy*, (ed. B. Carter and M. McGoldrick), pp. 311–32. Gardner Press, New York.

Wattis, J. and Church, M. (1986). *Practical psychiatry of old age*. Croom Helm, London.

Wells, K.B., Stewart, A., Hays, R.D., Burman, A., Rogers, W., Daniels, M. *et al.* (1989). The functioning and well-being of depressed patients. *Journal of the American Medical Association*, **262**, 914–19.

Woods, R. (1992). Psychological therapies and their efficacy. *Reviews in Clinical Gerontology*, **2**, 171.83.

PART 6 ORGANIZATION OF CARE

21 Management in primary care

Linda Gask

In this chapter Dr Gask describes the high prevalence of functional somatic symptoms in primary care settings and outlines those factors which predict poor outcome. She also describes a practical model for the detection, acknowledgement, and management of functional somatic symptoms which can be easily learned and used in primary care. Finally, the management of chronic somatization in primary care is described and the importance of shared care between the psychiatrist and primary health care team is emphasized.

Dr Gask uses the term somatization to describe patients with functional somatic symptoms. Whenever relevant, somatization is operationally defined, but in some instances the reader is advised to consult the cited reference.

Introduction

Functional somatic symptoms are common in primary care. In a well known British study Bridges and Goldberg (1985) surveyed 15 family practices in Manchester and found that approximately 19 per cent of patients fufilled the authors' research criteria for somatization, defined as follows:

(1) consulting for somatic symptoms;

(2) attributed these symptoms to a somatic disorder or took the view that the physical symptoms constituted the disorder;

(3) a DSM-III psychiatric disorder was present;

(4) in the view of the research psychiatrist, treatment of the affective disorder would reduce or eliminate the physical symptoms.

In a recent North American study (Kirmayer and Robbins 1991) similar rates were reported with 26.3 per cent of patients satisfying criteria for one or more forms of 'somatization'. Both of these studies are described in more detail in Chapter 3.

Relatively little is known however about the outcome of patients with functional somatic symptoms in primary care. For example, what proportion of patients with acute symptoms become chronic and why? In this chapter the detection and management of acute and subacute somatization in primary care is discussed and the management of patients with more chronic disorders outlined.

Outcome studies in primary care

There has been relatively little research on this topic. Acute and subacute somatization are very largely mood-related disorders in primary care and are common. (Bridges *et al.* 1991; Craig and Boardman, 1990; Goldberg and Bridges, 1988). But do these mood-related conditions eventually evolve into chronic disorders and, if so, what are the mechanisms involved in maintaining the process? Some clues may be found in recent studies carried out by Craig *et al.* 1993 in London, Bridges and Goldberg (1985) in Manchester, and Verhaak and Tijhuis (1992) in The Netherlands.

Craig *et al.* (1993) employed a two-stage screening procedure to identify patients with emotional disorder presenting with a recent onset of physical symptoms. The 44 patients defined as somatizers had an emotional disorder but physical symptoms that could not be attributed to organic disease at any time over the 2-year follow-up period. Decisions about the symptoms being 'organic' or 'functional' were made by a medically qualified researcher who was 'blind' to the ratings of emotional disorder. The authors developed this methodology to counteract the bias they felt was inherent in the definition provided by Bridges and Goldberg (1985), in which it is the psychiatric interviewer who decides not only whether physical symptoms can be explained by psychiatric disorder, but also whether these symptoms could be alleviated by suitable treatment.

The course and outcome of the somatizers was compared with three other groups:

(1)   patients with 'pure' emotional disorder;

(2)   'pure' physical disorder;

(3)   mixed conditions involving emotional disorder with concurrent physical disease.

The findings can be summarized as follows: the physical symptoms of somatizers were less likely to recover than those of the other groups and 16 (36 per cent) went on to develop chronic somatoform disorders. Among the somatizers, changes in the number of physical symptoms during the follow-up closely mirrored changes in emotional arousal, even when subjects whose symptoms could be regarded as psychophysiological in origin were removed from the analysis.

K. Bridges and D. Goldberg (personal communication) have followed up groups defined according to their original criteria as 'psychologizers', 'somatizers', and 'facultative somatizers' over a 6-month period. ('Facultative somatization' referred to patients who had somatized during the interview with the family doctor, but who were prepared to consider psychological factors as being relevant to their somatic symptoms when interviewed by a sympathetic psychiatrist.) They found that the outcome for psychologizers was worse than for somatizers, with the facultative somatizers in an intermediate position. It seems likely that the psychologizers were more ill than those identified as somatizers (in contrast to Craig *et al.*'s (1993) study where both groups developed chronic symptoms). It is possible that the somatizers were less depressed than the psychologizers in this study because somatization functioned as a defence against emotional distress.

These findings are similar to those of Verhaak and Tijhuis (1992), who recently reported a follow-up study of two groups of patients in general practice. During a 3-month period one group presented at least one articulated demand for psychosocial help, whereas the second presented at least one somatic complaint (considered by the general practitioner to be psychologically determined), without any psychosocial complaint. Objective needs for mental help in both cohorts were then assessed using the General Health Questionnaire and the two cohorts were followed up over 1 year. Recovery was found to be better in those patients presenting with somatic rather than psychological symptoms.

The different selection procedures used by the three research groups may go some way to explaining the apparent discrepancy between these findings, which leave many questions about the outcome of subacute somatization in primary care unanswered.

There is evidence that detection of psychiatric disorder in primary care can lead to improved outcome (Johnstone and Goldberg 1976; Tylee and Freeling 1989; Ormel *et al.* 1990), but in the only study to explore this (Bridges and Goldberg 1985) the process of detection appears to have been beneficial only to the 'facultative' group. We cannot yet identify clearly which interventions are likely to be most beneficial to which group of patients, but it seems likely that 'pure somatizers' and 'facultative somatizers' require different types of intervention.

Detection of psychiatric disorder alone may not be enough; 'acknowledgement' by the general practitioner of the patient's emotional distress may also be necessary. This means that the doctor must not only be able to acknowledge that the patient's emotional problems are worthy of discussion, but must also open up the topic to allow this to take place. This is clearly a very different matter from simply noting that the patient appears distressed without raising the issue explicitly in the interview. Indeed, Tylee and Freeling (1989) stress that *detection* and *acknowledgement* must be clearly distinguished and they believe that it is the latter which is the key to improvement when emotional problems are noted by the general practitioner. In the next section I focus on the development of a practical model for detection, acknowledgment, and management which can be easily learned and employed in primary care.

Improving the detection and management of subacute somatization

In their study of somatization primary care, Craig *et al.* (1993) found that 79 per cent of first presentations of mood disorder were couched in somatic terms alone. Like Bridges and Goldberg (1985) they found that this had a clear effect on the likelihood of detection. Only approximately 50 per cent of these emotional disorders were detected by the general practitioner compared with over 80 per cent of disorders which presented with emotional or psychosocial complaints. Detection also depended on the skills of the doctor. Goldberg has used the 'identification index' ('ii') as a measure of the doctor's ability to identify symptomatic cases (Goldberg and Huxley 1980). High ii and low ii general practitioners do not differ in their ability to identify cases presenting with emotional symptoms. However, the high ii general practitioners are significantly *less* likely to be misled by complaints of physical symptoms and more likely to diagnose the affective disorder correctly.

These findings suggest that there is an important *interaction* between the doctor and patient which has been further explored by Davenport *et al.* (1987). They rated videotapes of consultations of *high* and *low ii* doctors and found that *patients* who were high scorers on the General Health Questionnaire gave significantly more cues (they gave more verbal cues, had more distress in their voices, and tended to have more restless movements) when interviewed by a *high ii* doctor then by a *low ii* doctor. This was not the case for low scorers, for whom no significant difference between the groups was found. That is to say, *high ii* doctors seemed to encourage emotionally distressed patients to provide more cues.

General practitioners can be taught the skills required to detect and manage emotional problems and such training can have a significant impact on the accuracy with which general practitioners assess their patient's emotional distress (Gask *et al.* 1987, 1988). In training sessions we asked participants to make video recordings of surgery sessions in which the patient has completed the General Health Questionnaire and the doctor has made an independent rating of psychological disorder. In some cases a patient with a high General Health Questionnaire score is interviewed by a doctor who has not rated the presence of an emotional illness. These interviews can then be used in video feedback sessions which focus on the presence or absence of emotional cues and how these might have been responded to.

Screening questionnaires are probably only useful in the detection of somatization if the doctor has the requisite skills to raise, 'face to face' with the patient, those emotional problems reported on in the question-naire (Goldberg and Gask 1992). Both the General Health Questionnaire (Goldberg and Hillier, 1979) and the Hospital Anxiety and Depression rating scale (Zigmond and Snaith, 1983) are acceptable to patients in primary care and Wright (1992) has demonstrated how they can be adapted for the computerized administration in this setting.

In 1989 we proposed a simple model of consultation in order to improve the general practitioner's detection and management of patients presenting with subacute somatization (Goldberg *et al.* 1989). This has model has three main stages as well as a number of individual microskills and has been called the 'reattribution' model. The term 'reattribution' refers to the aim of helping the patient to move gradually from a physical to a psychological view of the aetiology of their symptoms. This model was never intended to provide a solution for those patients with chronic symp-toms, although some elements are appropriate whatever the duration of the complaints. We have demonstrated that the key elements of the model can be taught to general practitioner trainees (Gask *et al.* 1989; Kaaya *et al.* 1992), but it remains to be demonstrated whether general practitioners who have been taught the model can use the skills they have acquired to improve the outcome of patients under their care.

When general physicians interview patients with subacute rather than chronic symptoms they generally feel obliged to exclude organic patho-logy, even if they are fairly firmly convinced that none is present (see Chapter 10). This view is understandable, given that medical training instills the belief that organic pathology must not be missed at any cost. Two other approaches should also be considered however. First, that it is equally important not to miss *psychiatric* pathology. Although a valid point, this approach may result in further polarization between physical and psychological illness. A second approach, which derives directly from the findings of Bridges and Goldberg (1985) and others, is that physical and emotional problems often co-exist and as either or both may be responsible for the symptoms the consultation should address each accor-ding to the cues offered by the patient. In other words, to simply exchange the psychological explanation for the physical still does the patient no favours. A truly patient-centred approach will address both in accordance with the cues offered by the patient.

This model (see Table 21.1) has developed directly from our experience of viewing on videotape patients attending primary care and from our workshops with general practitioners in many different settings (Gask *et al.* 1991, 1992). It has been greatly influenced by the teaching of Lesser (1981, 1985), who spent many years teaching primary care physicians in North America. In order to address the issue of finding out exactly what the patient's problems are, the first stage of the three stage model is called *'feeling understood'*.

Table 21.1 The 'reattribution' model

Stage 1: feeling understood
1. Take a full history of the symptoms
2. Explore emotional cues
3. Explore social and family factors
4. Explore health beliefs
5. Brief focused physical examination

Stage 2: broadening the agenda
1. Feed back the results of the examination
2. Acknowledge the reality of the symptoms
3. Reframe the complaints: link physical, psychological, and life events

Stage 3: making the link
1. Simple explanation
    (i) Three-stage explanation for anxiety
    (ii) How depression lowers the pain threshold
2. Demonstration
    (i) Practical
    (ii) Link to life events
    (iii) 'Here and Now'
3. Projection or identification

See text for further explanation.

The doctor has a limited agenda of items to cover but must be led by the patient's cues. It is assumed that they will be aware of somatization, consider it particularly if the complaints are not obviously physical in origin, and remember that physical and psychological symptoms can and often do co-exist. Raising such awareness is a key matter for education. There are then five major task areas for this part of the consultation:

Stage 1

1. Taking a full history. Even though the doctor is unsure about physical cause, they should take a normal history. The aim is not only to explore the possibility of organic pathology, but also to reassure the patient that he or she is being taken seriously. It can be extremely useful to ask the patient to describe a typical 'symptom' day. Useful questions to ask are 'Do you notice anything else (when you get the symptoms)?' and 'What happens to the symptom during the day?'

2. Exploring emotional cues. The doctor should try to notice any verbal or non-verbal clues to emotional problems that the patient may offer and use empathic or supportive comments to promote discussion of

emotional issues, for example, 'You said the symptom is worrying you, how have you been feeling generally?' and 'You look quite tense, is that how you feel?' It is also important to inquire directly about the biological symptoms of depression and anxiety.

3. Exploring social and family factors. If possible these must be explored early in the assessment. Otherwise the patient may feel that the doctor is trying to dismiss the symptoms as emotional because they can't find anything else wrong.

4. Explore health beliefs. The patient should be asked what he/she believes is causing the symptoms. The aim is not only to explore possible aetiological factors (many patients in primary care worry about symptoms that resemble those experienced by relatives and friends), but also to provide a clear basis on which explanation and reassurance may be effective.

5. Carry out a brief focused physical examination. The doctor may want to do this to establish whether there is any relevant organic disease. Some will omit an examination if they believe the symptoms are somatized, but nevertheless it does serve an important purpose. A brief, focused examination may take only seconds and reassures the patient that his/her symptoms are being taken seriously.

Stage 2 The second stage of the model was originally called 'changing the agenda', but in retrospect is probably best called 'broadening the agenda' because the basic aim is to involve discussion of both emotional and physical topics during the consultation. (You may be particularly fortunate and manage to shift the agenda altogether but this isn't common.) Unless patients consciously present to the doctor with a somatic 'ticket' simply to test out whether more sensitive topics will be broached, most are worried by the somatic complaints themselves.

There are three key stages

1. Feedback the results of the examination. The findings should be described simply and if necessary clearly explained, for example some abdominal tenderness need not necessarily mean that serious pathology is present.

2. Acknowledge to the patient that his/her symptoms are real. This is a crucial stage and extremely important for the patient, who may have been told by an exasperated hospital doctor after negative investigations that there's nothing wrong with them.

3. Reframing the patient's symptoms and complaints. This means reminding the patients of all the complaints that have been mentioned, both physical and psychological, as well as the life events that he or she has talked about, for example 'You've told me about the stomach pains that you have had for the last month and how you have also had headaches and felt tense and worried and about the death of your father a month ago. I wonder if these are all linked in some way . . .' and 'I wonder if you've really been grieving for your father' . . .

At this stage it is important for the doctor not to be too emphatic and for the patient to be given a chance to discuss and to negotiate. The aim is to influence the patients' views in a significant way. This is best achieved if the patient feels that the doctor respects their point of view. Without first broadening the agenda it is difficult to obtain the patient's cooperation in treating underlying psychosocial problems.

Stage 3   The final stage in the model is called *'making the link'*. For some patients this may be superfluous if they have appreciated the importance of emotional factors and now want to move onto talking about them in more detail, but others may still want to know how the physical symptoms can be caused by psychosocial distress. There are a number of ways that the doctor can make this link.

1. Simple explanation. This is the most commonly used method. The doctor explains how anxiety can cause physical symptoms, for example 'When people are anxious they get tension in their neck muscles and this causes the headache'. In our revised teaching package (see below) we introduced the idea that such an explanation must clearly be in *three* stages, moving from emotional state, to physiological mechanism, to somatic symptoms. A related method is that of explaining how depression can make pain seem much worse because it lowers the pain threshold, for example 'If you are depressed or sad you feel pain or discomfort more and then start worrying that you may be sick'.

2. Demonstration. The technique of demonstrating in the surgery how symptoms are produced can be employed in three ways. First, by demonstrating to the patient how muscle tension can cause pain, for example pointing out how much arms and shoulders ache when carrying heavy objects. The patient can also be asked to hold a heavy weight with arm outstretched. This will demonstrate how tense muscles ache. Second, the patient's symptoms can often be linked in time to some stressful life event. Alternatively, it may be possible to ask a patient to note when symptoms are experienced during the day

and observe if there is any link with events or circumstances (using the information gained from inquiring about a typical day). Third, the somatic symptoms and feelings can be linked in the 'here and now' by getting the patient to say how the pain is at the moment and immediately also inquiring about feelings and emotions. For example, the patient may say that they have had abdominal pain quite badly since they have been talking to you and that they are worried about what you are going to tell them. The task here is to make this link between the worry and the intensity of the pain quite explicit.

3. Projection or identification. The final linking techniques involve asking if anyone else in the patient's family has ever suffered from similar symptoms. It may then be possible to help the patient to see that they have identified with the sick person (this may be a particularly important factor if a friend or family member has had similar symptoms associated with life-threatening illness). It may also be possible to help a patient to understand their own symptoms if other family members have also suffered similar symptoms at times of life stress. It is often much easier to appreciate psychological mechanisms in other people.

It may not be possible to move through all three of these stages in one consultation. Indeed, it might be necessary to organize investigations after the first stage, then continue when the results are available with a modified replay of stage two to feed back the results of investigations. Some investigations may be positive and others negative, indicating that a certain amount of disease pathology could explain some but not all of the symptoms. Such findings clearly complicate the picture, but the same principles of honesty about findings, acknowledgment, negotiation, and clear explanation apply.

We have never envisaged that more than one of the strategies in '*making the link*' would be employed at any one time; the doctor must choose what seems most appropriate in a particular consultation. Although our original report omitted any reference to involving the patient's family in the consultation, this can be very important in primary care settings where spouses, parents, and adult children may attend to provide 'support' for the patient and demand that 'something is done'. A joint session in which the agenda is broadened and links are make can be especially powerful and easily negotiated in primary care. It also has the potential to save considerable time later when inappropriate beliefs about health and illness may be further reinforced and further investigations demanded by other family members.

Evaluation of training in 'reattribution' skills

Following our original study in 1989 which demonstrated that the component skills of this model could be successfully taught to trainees attending a course in psychiatry for family doctors (Gask *et al.* 1989), we improved the teaching methods and then successfully replicated our findings (Kaaya *et al.* 1992). The teaching package (Gask *et al.* 1989) comprises a training videotape in which the model described above is demonstrated together with material for use in an interactive role-play session. An initial afternoon session, using the videotape both to demonstrate the model and to allow trainees working in pairs to practice the skills when prompted by cues from the tape, was followed by weekly small group video feedback sessions in which the trainees received teaching on both real and role-played consultations. Eighteen general practitioner trainees attending the annual 8 week course held at Manchester Royal Infirmary participated (Creed 1988). The teaching was evaluated by blind rating of skills demonstrated by the trainees during 10–15 min interviews with professional role-players. Ratings were made on pre-training and post-training videotaped interviews. The results demonstrated not only significant improvement in general interview skills but also in specific reattribution skills (see Table 21.2), with some improvement on the findings of our original study. It remains to be demonstrated whether such training will have an impact on patient outcome.

Further treatment

When the introductory stage has been successfully negotiated it should become possible to treat underlying psychiatric disorder using the usual combination of psychological, pharmacological, and social interventions. However, it may be necessary at times to repeat what has been discussed earlier. The concept of 'depression' or 'anxiety' may have to be 'sold' to the patient before treatment can begin and all suggestions for treatment plans must be negotiated. Depression may be viewed only in negative terms by a patient and it can be necessary to emphasize that depression is both common and treatable.

In primary care, patients often present with a range of symptoms, both somatic and psychological, which do not satisfy the criteria for a psychiatric diagnosis but nevertheless suggest emotional distress which is presenting as somatic complaints. For this group and also those for whom additional pharmacological intervention is indicated, a range of simple practical skills is required. Sell *et al.* (1990) have summarized treatment interventions in a training package produced in India and the following summary of 'where to go from here' is based on the interventions they suggest.

Table 21.2 Frequency of reattribution skills before and after training

	Number of trainees showing skill	
Takes full history of pain	Pre-training	Post-training
Asks about radiation site	8	15*
A typical pain day	6	13*
Elicits other symptoms	7	7 NS
Explores health beliefs	11	17*
		Mean score 4-point scale
Explores social and family factors	1.83	2.11**
		Consultations rated 'yes'
Acknowledge reality of symptoms	3	10*
Feedback results of physical examination	13	18*
Making the link: explanation	7	13*
		Mean score 4-point scale
Overall rating: making the link	0.89	1.78**

*$P < 0.05$ Binomial (one-tailed test).
**$P < 0.05$ Wilcoxon (two-tailed test).
***$P < 0.005$ Wilcoxon (one-tailed test).
From Kaaya *et al.* (1992).

Medication Patients with clear symptoms of depressive illness are likely to improve with a course of antidepressants. The rationale for prescribing must be clearly explained. Because of their heightened awareness of bodily sensations patients who present with somatic complaints are particularly prone to experience side-effects of medication, so it is crucial to provide clear information about side-effects before treatment begins (and about the delayed onset of action) in order to increase the likelihood of maintaining compliance. Each patient should then be seen again soon after starting treatment to reinforce these facts (for example 10–14 days). These points may be overlooked because patients who are complaining and demanding can be difficult to tolerate and there may be a temptation to see them less often!

Reassurance This is an effective intervention only after the doctor has successfully carried out the initial stages described above. It is frequently, as Balint (1964) so clearly described, offered prematurely. Doctors at all levels of experience make the mistake of saying 'There is nothing wrong with you'. Instead the aim should be to explain to the patient that serious disease does not account for the symptoms. Patients may also need reassurance that they are not 'going out of their mind'. Mental illness continues to carry a huge stigma and patients who present with somatic symptoms are frequently sensitive to and fearful of this.

Relaxation training   Simple relaxation techniques can be easily taught in primary care, using pre-recorded tapes or with the assistance of a community psychiatric nurse. Referral to a psychologist is rarely required, but may be useful if symptoms persist despite simple interventions. Traditional methods of meditation can also provide an effective means of relaxation training and where teachers of such skills are available, either directly or via adult education classes, their help can be usefully sought.

Problem solving   Problem-solving techniques can be used to enable patients to identify what changes they need to make in their lives. If the problem seems ultimately soluble then a session may be set aside to explore ways in which the problem can be tackled. It is crucial for goals to be broken down into simple and attainable steps. If the problem clearly cannot be solved, as may well be the case, some time will be needed to work with the patient in helping him or her to develop more realistic expectations and to focus on more positive aspects of life. Problem-solving sessions tend to take longer than the usual 10 min consultation, so practitioners may have to set aside a special long session at the end of a surgery for this purpose. In the long run this may be time-saving as problems can be addressed in more depth. There is preliminary evidence that problem-solving techniques are useful in patients with subacute somatization in primary care (Wilkinson and Mynors Wallis 1994).

Using other resources   A wide range of other resources/interventions can be employed in primary care for patients with emotional problems. General practitioners acquire information about self-help groups and frequently become involved in advocacy on behalf of their patients in liaison with housing departments, social services, and other agencies. Some practices have access to their own counsellor or to other members of the mental health care team. Sharing care between members of this team will be discussed in much more detail when we examine the management of chronic somatic complaints in primary care (below). The existence of a practice counsellor or easy access to a mental health team will not in itself improve the ability of the doctor to detect subacute somatization. Such patients will continue to present directly to the general practitioner because of their worries, fears, and convictions about somatic illness. Referral to mental health workers should therefore only be arranged *after* the stages described earlier have been successfully negotiated.

The management of chronic somatization in primary care

Specific treatments are discussed elsewhere, but these generally require referral to a specialist agency. The role of the general practitioner in managing chronic severe somatization is not an easy one. Few mental health professionals have an interest or even an adequate understanding of these patients and it is not uncommon to hear stories of how the patient was finally persuaded by their general practitioner to see a psychiatrist only to be told that 'there is no evidence of psychiatric illness'. In primary care many patients have received the label 'heartsink' (N. Mathers 1992). Few intervention studies have been carried out in this patient group and none in general practice in the UK. However, O'Dowd (1988) demonstrated that regular practice discussions, the aim of which was to formulate and discuss a management plan (described below), seemed to have some impact on both the practices' perception of the patients as 'heartsink' and on consultation rates. The general practitioner may have to work relatively unsupported in attempting to enable the patient to understand that emotional and/or social difficulties need to be tackled.

It can take a long time to engage a patient in exploring psychological aspects of their problems. The steps described in the 'reattribution' model are helpful but there may be difficulty in raising emotional issues (if few cues are given by the patient) and in exploring social and family difficulties in order to 'broaden the agenda'. Some authors are now beginning to emphasize the importance of management guidelines for the care of such patients. There is also now an increasing emphasis on education of the primary care doctor in a range of basic management skills. These can be summarized in the following recommendations, which are amalgamated from reviews by O'Dowd (1988), Bass and Murphy (1990), Goldberg *et al.* (1992), and Bass and Benjamin (1992).

1. *Reassurance that nothing is wrong does not help.* Clear information should be provided about clinical findings, which can then provide a basis for the provision of appropriate reassurance.

2. Contrary to what initially may appear to be the case, *the patient does not want simple straightforward symptom relief, but understanding.* Many patients can communicate distress only in the form of somatic symptoms and there is often a history of abuse or maltreatment in childhood. It may take a long time to change the agenda from the physical to the emotional pain, but this may ultimately be achieved by empathizing with the patient's past experiences of distress and

gradually helping them to feel understood. In this way a therapeutic relationship will be established and they will gradually appreciate that their pain, both emotional and physical, is being taken seriously.

3. What the patient wants is for the doctor to agree that he or she is sick. *Avoid challenging the patient but instead agree that there is a problem* and show a willingness to help to identify it.

4. *Little is gained by a premature explanation that the symptoms are emotional.* Such an explanation must be presented in such a way that the patient does not experience it as a rejection.

5. *A positive organic diagnosis will not cure the patient.* The emphasis should be on function not symptoms, with an assessment of how the patient copes and responds.

6. *Try and be direct and honest with the patient about areas that you agree on and those that you disagree on.* Be explicit about what you think he or she is capable of doing despite the symptoms and negotiate mutually agreed goals (for example, how far to walk, carrying out chores, helping family, etc.). Spurious organic diagnoses only lead to a subsequent breakdown in trust and less likelihood that the patient will accept an appropriate referral. Never give treatment for disorders that the patient has not got; this only confirms the patient's view that something is wrong.

7. *Regular scheduled appointments are required* so that the patient does not have to manifest symptoms in order to seek help. Paradoxically, this can be less time-consuming than frequent short visits which are taken up with fruitless reassurance.

8. *Clear agenda setting can be helpful in each consultation.* It can be very useful to work out a list of problems with the patient and agree to tackle one or two on each visit.

9. *Diagnostic tests should be limited.* Some focused examination can be helpful, with reliance more on signs than symptoms.

10. *Provide a clear model for the patient* which demonstrates that it is possible to have both organic pathology, which needs treatment, *and* emotional problems. It is important to challenge the dualistic model *which assumes* that illness is either physical or mental but never both, (that many patients (and doctors) believe).

11. *Involve the patient's family* so that spouse or children are aware of your treatment plan and can be involved in it if they wish to be.

12. *Involve colleagues in the primary care team* in discussion of the management plan so that the practice can present a consistent and agreed approach to management. Such practice meetings can provide essential support in managing a difficult patient. In O'Dowd's practice (1988) (mentioned above) the function of each lunchtime meeting was to share information, define apparent problems, formulate a plan of management, and provide support for the professional who was to be the primary carer for a particular patient. The management plan was then entered into the patient's case notes.

13. *Don't expect a cure.* Damage limitation is a more realistic ultimate goal but it may be difficult for the doctor to accept. Somatizers are difficult to treat because they are often angry with doctors and do not try to get better. Peer group discussion and support can help a doctor to understand their own reactions to such patients and learn how to deal with them.

It can be very difficult to know when to refer to a psychiatrist or other specialist. Some family doctors find it impossible to stop referring these patients to many different specialists because of their *own belief* that something will eventually be discovered. It is essential to be able to call a halt to further investigations at some point and to state that psychological and or social problems *must* be addressed. The patient and his or her family need to be clearly told the reasons for doing this.

Some patients can be effectively managed in primary care using the range of basic strategies described above. However, these patients can be very time-consuming and difficult to manage and at some point the general practitioner may feel the need to involve a psychiatrist or other psychological specialist. When this is arranged, it is crucial to be honest with the patient about who you are arranging for them to see. Suspicion and fear about being labelled 'mad' can be reduced by asking for the patient to be seen at the surgery or at home. Details about referral are also discussed further in Chapter 22.

Sharing the care of the somatizing patient in primary care

The concept of *shared care* between the primary and secondary care services is useful for such patients (see Chapters 10 and 22). This means not just professionals from both teams being involved in managing the patient, which often occurs anyway, but the existence of a *joint* treatment plan. Good channels of communication are needed to ensure that the patient receives the same message from all involved and to establish clear roles for all the professionals providing care. For example, the psychiatrist may be involved in overall planning of the management and may take a major responsibility for psychotherapeutic treatment, the general practitioner will review the patient's physical state regularly and is responsible for physical care and monitoring of medication, and the community psychiatric nurse will implement behavioural treatment of the patient such as planning and instituting an activity programme. All will arrange to meet regularly to discuss progress and to review the treatment plan.

Where it is difficult to engage psychiatric services in the management of such patients, it may be possible to operate a similar shared care approach within the primary care team by employing the approach described above by O'Dowd (1988). Peer supervision and discussion of a difficult case, preferably employing videotaped or audiotaped consultations, has been used by ourselves to help general practitioners learn new strategies in the management of such patients and to provide each other with the necessary supervision and support. It can be difficult and daunting to manage a patient with chronic somatic complaints who refuses to accept psychiatric referral but finally discloses, in the context of an empathic and trusting relationship with their general practitioner, that they were abused in childhood. The role of supervisor can be filled either by a psychiatrist with an interest in how emotional illness presents in primary care or by a similarly interested psychologist or suitably qualified practice counsellor familiar with the problems of somatization. It is preferable for these supervisors to regularly visit the practice for the specific purpose of discussing difficult patients.

Some practice counsellors have difficulty in coping with the problems presented by somatizing patients and may inadvertently reinforce their illness beliefs. Counsellors may lack appropriate training and qualifications and be referred patients who have problems which fall outside their previous experience (Sibbald *et al.* 1993). The difficulties caused by the principles of confidentiality may also make it problematic for doctors and counsellors to share information about the patient's emotional problems. In such a situation the doctor may not have access to the information necessary to help the patient make links between his or her emotional problems and physical symptoms because the counsellor feels unable to share such information without breaking confidentiality. Counsellors therefore need to learn the skills described above as necessary for general practitioners if they are to manage such patients effectively.

Conclusion

This chapter has reviewed the epidemiology and outcome of somatization in primary care. The management of subacute somatization has been discussed with specific reference to detection and early intervention. Chronic somatization poses a more difficult management problem, but a number of strategies are outlined and the importance of a clear management plan are emphasized.

In future, it is essential that more training in the management of somatization is included in the training of primary care doctors. This training should emphasize not only an awareness of the size and nature of the problem, but also confer the skills necessary to detect, assess, and manage these important clinical problems effectively (Goldberg *et al.* 1992).

Note

The teaching videotape referred to in this chapter is available from Mr N. Jordan, University Department of Psychiatry, Withington Hospital, Nell Lane, West Didsbury. Manchester M20 8LR, UK. Price £35 including postage and packing.

References

Balint, M. (1964). *The doctor, his patient and the illness*. Pitman, London.

Bass, C. and Benjamin, S. (1993). The management of chronic somatization. *British Journal of Psychiatry*, **162**, 472-80.

Bass, C. and Murphy, M.R. (1990). Somatization disorder: critique of the concept and suggestions for future research. In *Somatization: physical symptoms and psychological illness*, (ed. C. Bass). Blackwell, Oxford.

Bridges, K.W. and Goldberg, D.P. (1985). Somatic presentations of psychiatric illness in primary care settings. *Journal of Psychosomatic Research*, **32**, 137-44.

Bridges, K., Goldberg, D., Evan, G.B., and Sharpe, T. (1991). Determinants of somatization in primary care. *Psychological Medicine*, **21**, 473-83.

Craig, T.K.J. and Boardman, A.P. (1990). Somatization in primary care settings. In *Somatization: physical symptoms and psychological illness*, (ed. C. Bass). Blackwell, Oxford. pp. 73-103.

Craig, T.K.J., Boardman, A.P., Mills, K. *et al.* (1992). The South London Somatization Study: I Longitudinal course and influence of early life experiences. *British Journal of Psychiatry*, **163**, 579-88.

Creed, F. (1988). Course in psychiatry for family doctors. *Bulletin of the Royal College of Psychiatrists*, **11**, 193-4.

Davenport, S., Goldberg, D., and Millar, T. (1987). How psychiatric disorders are missed during medical consultations. *Lancet*, **i**, 439-40.

Gask, L., McGrath, G., Goldberg, D., and Millar, T. (1987). Improving the psychiatric skills of established general practitioners: evaluation of group teaching *Medical Education*, **21**, 362-8.

Gask, L., Goldberg, D., Lesser, A., and Millar, T. (1988). Improving the psychiatric skills of the general practice trainee. *Medical Education*, **22**, 132-8.

Gask, L., Goldberg, D., Porter, R., and Creed, F. (1989). Treatment of somatization: evaluation of a teaching package with general practice trainees *Journal of Psychosomatic Research*, **33**, 697-703.

Gask, L., Boardman, J., and Standart, S. (1991). Teaching communication skills: a problem-based approach. *Postgraduate Education for General Practice*, **2**, 7-15.

Gask, L., Usherwood, T., and Standart, S. (1992). Training teachers to teach communication skills. *Journal of Postgraduate General Practice*, **3**, 92-9.

Goldberg, D.P. and Bridges, K. (1988). Somatic presentation of psychiatric illness in primary care settings. *Journal of Psychosomatic Research*, **32**, 137-44.

Goldberg, D., and Gask, L. (1992). Primary health care and psychiatric epidemiology: a psychiatrist's perspective. In *Primary health care and psychiatric epidemiology*, (ed. B. Cooper and R. Eastwood). pp. 44-56, Routledge, London.

Goldberg, D.P. and Hillier, V.F. (1979). A scaled version of the general health questionnaire. *Psychological Medicine*, **9**, 139-45.

Goldberg, D. and Huxley, P. (1980). *Mental illness in the community*. Tavistock, London.

Goldberg, D., Gask, L., and O'Dowd, T. (1989). Treatment of somatization: teaching techniques of reattribution. *Journal of Psychosomatic Research*, **33**, 697-703.

Golberg, R.J., Novack, D.H., and Gask, L. (1992). The recognition and management of somatization: what is needed in primary care training. *Psychosomatics*, **33**, 55-61.

Johnstone, A. and Goldberg, D. (1976). Psychiatric screening in general practice: a controlled trial. *Lancet*, **20**, 605-9.

Kaaya, S., Goldberg, D., and Gask, L. (1992). Management of somatic presentation of psychiatric illness in general medical settings: evaluation of a new training course for general practitioners. *Medical Education*, **26**, 138-44.

Kirmayer, L.J. and Robbins, J.M. (1991). Three forms of somatization in primary care: prevalence, co-occurrence and socio-demographic characteristics. *Journal of Nervous and Mental Diseases*, **179**, 647-55.

Lesser, A. (1981). The psychiatric and family medicine: a different training approach. *Medical Education*, **15**, 398-406.

Lesser, A.L. (1985). Problem-based interviewing in general practice: a model. *Medical Education*, **19**, 299-304.

Mathers, N. (1992). An investigation of the heartsink patient. PhD thesis, University of Sheffield.

O'Dowd, T. (1988). Five years of heartsink patients in general practice. *British Medical Journal*, **297**, 528-30.

Ormel, J., Koeter, H., van den Brink, W., and van de Willinge, G. (1990). The extent of non-recognition of mental health problems in primary care and its effect on management and outcome. In *The public health impact of mental disorder*, (ed. D. Goldberg and D. Tantan). pp. 146-58. Hogrefe Huber, Basel.

Sell, H.L., Srinivasa Murthy, R., Seshadri, A. *et al.* (1990). Recognition and management of patients with functional complaints (psychosocial problems, ill-defined somatic complaints). A training package for the primary-care physician. In *Psychological disorders in general medical settings*, (ed. N. Sartorius, D. Goldberg, G. de Girolamo *et al.*), pp. 189-200. WHO/Hogrefe and Huber, Toronto.

Sibbald, B., Addington-Hall, J., Brenneman, B., and Freeling, P. (1993). Counsellors in English and Welsh general practices: their nature and distribution. *British Medical Journal*, **306**, 29-33.

Tylee, A., and Freeling, P. (1989). The recognition, diagnosis and acknowledgment of depressive disorders by general practitioners. In *Depression: an integrative approach*, (ed. E. Paykel and K. Herbst). pp. 216-31. Heinemann, London.

Verhaak, P.F. and Tijhuis, M.A.R. (1992). Psychosocial problems in primary care: some results from the Dutch National Study of Morbidity and Interventions in General Practice. *Social Science and Medicine*, **35**, 105-10.

Wilkinson, P.B. and Mynors-Wallis, L. (1994). Problem solving in the treatment of unexplained physical symptoms in primary care: a preliminary study. *Journal of Psychosomatic Research*, **38**, 591-8.

Wright, A. (1992). The computer will see you now: meeting the challenge of hidden psychiatric morbidity in general practice. In *The prevention of depression and anxiety: the role of the primary care team*, (ed. R. Jenkins, J. Newton, and R. Young). HMSO, London.

Zigmond, A.S. and Snaith, R.P. (1983). The hospital anxiety and depression rating scale. *Acta Psychiatrica Scandinavica*, **67**, 361-70.

22 The management of patients with functional somatic symptoms in the general hospital

Christopher Bass, Michael Sharpe, and Richard Mayou

In this chapter we propose that patients with functional somatic symptoms are best managed by a combination of improvements in routine care by medical and surgical teams and greater provision of specialist care by psychiatrists and clinical psychologists. These improvements would, however, require better training for all those involved. Although some initial increase in resources would be required, significant savings from the reduction of the inappropriate and ineffective use of existing hospital and primary care resources could be expected. Both clinical experience and evaluative research suggest opportunities for improved outcomes for many patients.

Introduction

Whilst the majority of patients with functional symptoms and syndromes are seen and managed in primary care, those referred to general hospitals pose a particularly important clinical problem. This is because of the following.

1. Patients with functional somatic symptoms form a large proportion of general hospital attenders. As many as half the patients seen in hospital out-patient clinics have functional problems (Kroenke *et al.* 1990), the most common symptoms being pain and fatigue. Patients with functional problems also constitute a significant proportion of hospital in-patients in some specialties (Creed *et al.* 1990).

2. As well as having troublesome symptoms the disability and distress suffered by such patients are often severe (for example, Sharpe *et al.* 1992).

3. Standard medical and surgical management is relatively ineffective, often leaving the patient dissatisfied (Kroenke *et al.* 1990) and the doctor frustrated (Lin *et al.* 1991).

4. The management of these patients as currently practised is both expensive in time and wasteful in resources (Shaw and Creed 1991). As a result, the management of patients with multiple functional complaints may consume a significant proportion of the budget of the entire hospital service (Fink 1992).

Despite the importance of functional somatic symptoms as a clinical problem few hospitals have specialist expertise in the management of this patient group or devote resources specifically to them. Many medical and surgical clinics are already extremely busy and have little opportunity for greater discussion of findings with patients and their relatives. Even in those hospitals with specific services, the provision of care may be patchy and limited by the availability and expertise of staff. Whilst responsibility for the care of the majority of patients with functional somatic symptoms must remain with the physicians and surgeons to whom they present we also believe that psychiatrists and psychologists should make greater efforts to acquire the special skills necessary to contribute effectively to their care (Bass and Benjamin 1993). Other disciplines also make an important contribution and treatment should ideally be multidisciplinary, with each discipline making its own distinctive contribution (Table 22.1).

Table 22.1 Disciplines involved in the management of patients with functional somatic symptoms

Consultation–liaison psychiatrists	Occupational therapists
Clinical psychologists	Physiotherapists
Specialist psychiatric nurses	Social workers

Care by general hospital teams

The ways in which we suggest the hospital care of patients with functional somatic symptoms might be improved are listed in Table 22.2. We believe that the necessary modifications in routine medical and surgical practice would require little extra medical time and only a small amount of additional resources. Such improvements would, however, require improvements in training and some changes in the organization of services. The selective use of additional clinical resources to fund specialist services could result in substantial benefits to the important minority of patients with persistent and severe disabling functional symptoms.

Table 22.2 Improved hospital management

Changes in referral
Improved routine care
   Information: leaflets, audiotapes, videotapes, etc.
   More advice and treatment by medical staff
   More advice and treatment by nursing and other staff
   Self-help groups
Extra resources for medical and surgical teams
   Specialist nurses
   Clinical psychologists
Specialist services
   Consultation–liaison psychiatry
   Behavioural medicine

The referral of patients with functional somatic symptoms to hospital

Clearly one way of reducing the size of the problem in hospitals would be to improve the diagnosis and management of patients with functional somatic symptoms in primary care (see Chapter 21). General practitioners will however continue to refer such patients to hospital for a number of reasons:

(1)   concern that the patient may have serious organic disease;

(2)   the co-existence of functional somatic symptoms with proven organic disease;

(3)   the general practitioner's inability to effectively manage the patient in primary care;

(4)   the patient's demand for hospital treatment.

Although it would be inappropriate to block such referrals, it is desirable that the referring doctor make the reason for referral more explicit to both the hospital doctor and to the patient. In this way hospital referral could be made a constructive part of a coordinated management plan which would be continued in primary care after discharge from hospital.

Improvements in routine care

The task of managing patients with functional somatic symptoms falls almost entirely to specialist medical and surgical services designed for the rapid assessment and treatment of large numbers of patients with specific

Table 22.3 Simple psychological and educational interventions

Initial assessment
  Include psychosocial assessment
  Explanation and advice to patient
  Information to general practitioner (and other doctors)
  Arrange follow-up review
  Identify problem patients; consider referral

Follow-up
  Extra explanation and advice
  Identify problem patients; consider referral

Persistent problem
  Treatment by specialist nurse or clinical psychologist
  Refer to liaison psychiatrist or clinical psychologist

Table 22.4 Essential tasks for the non-psychiatrist

1. Be *aware* of psychosocial problems
2. Ask some basic *screening questions*, for example how do you feel in your mood? and what do you think is causing the pain?
3. Perform the *minimum* number of investigations
4. Provide *unambiguous reassurance* when there is no evidence of *relevant* organic disease
5. Provide a *satisfactory alternative explanation* for the pain/symptoms
6. Withdraw *unnecessary* medication
7. Know *when* to refer for psychiatric/psychological opinion
8. Know *how* to expedite such a referral

diseases. Such services are ill equipped to manage patients with functional somatic symptoms. Staff are likely to lack specialist knowledge of the problem, to possess only limited skills in psychological management, and to have limited access to specialist psychosocial care. It is therefore necessary to establish simple procedures for improving assessment, clarifying the role of follow-up, and offering extra treatment to those patients who pose particular problems (Table 22.3).

We believe that physicians and surgeons could do more to provide convincing explanations of symptoms, to answer patients' questions, and to indicate the value of simple psychological and social interventions (Tables 22.3 and 22.4). National and local guidelines can be helpful in achieving such changes in practice (Delamothe 1993).

The task of informing patients about their illnesses and advising them about how they may help themselves can be supplemented by a greater use of educational materials (leaflets, audio, and videotapes). In particular the new interactive programmes can go a long way to meeting individual patients' needs for advice about their own particular functional symptoms (Troop *et al.* 1993).

Extra resources for the general hospital team

Even those consultants who are aware of the problem of functional somatic symptoms and who want to manage the patients in the most constructive way possible, often find that the constraints of current working practice and the absence of appropriate support services leaves them feeling unable to take effective action (Sharpe *et al.* 1994). It is unrealistic to expect the orthopaedic surgeon or gastroenterologist seeing perhaps 30 patients in a clinic to administer complex psychological treatment. There is, however, no reason why an experienced and suitably trained and supervised nurse should not be able to adequately undertake the management of a patient with, for example non-cardiac chest pain or non-ulcer dyspepsia. The efficacy of such interventions is not known, but a controlled study evaluating an educational and treatment 'package' for patients with noncardiac chest pain, administered by a trained cardiac nurse, began in Oxford in 1993. The nurse therapist is taking an increasingly important role in such services. Nurses have the advantages of being familiar with the culture and working of general hospitals and being non-threatening to patients. Furthermore, they are proving themselves to be effective therapists. Patients with complex somatoform disorders can respond to psychological treatments administered by trained nurses (Butler *et al.* 1991).

Access to specialist care

Physicians and surgeons need easy access to specialist psychiatric and psychological services. Simple availability is not enough, however. It is also necessary that referral to them is seen to be worthwhile by both referrer and patient. We suggest that the all too common lack of interest in and therapeutic pessimism concerning patients with functional somatic symptoms amongst psychiatrists has been one of the most important reasons for the lack of progress in improving their management.

More recently the growth of liaison psychiatry and behavioural medicine services have offered an important opportunity to change this situation. Unfortunately, rivalries between the psychiatrists and psychologists are all too common and threaten the development of services in which the coordination of care is of fundamental importance.

Specialist services

Consultation liaison psychiatry

The clinical work of the psychiatrist in the general hospital is traditionally divided into the overlapping tasks of liaison and consultation.

Liaison with hospital staff Meetings with hospital staff in order to discuss the management of patients with psychosocial problems has been referred to as liaison. Such meetings can be used to improve the non-psychiatric staff's knowledge of the presentation and management of patients with functional somatic symptoms in medical and surgical clinics and to ensure that referrals to specialist psychiatry and psychology services are appropriately chosen and effectively made.

A useful opportunity to educate colleagues is also provided by regular joint clinical or research meetings. It is sensible to target both those hospital departments which see a large number of patients with functional somatic symptoms and those which may be especially lacking in the requisite knowledge and expertise. Departments which see a particularly large number of patients with functional somatic symptoms include gastroenterology, cardiology, neurology, and obstetrics and gynaecology. Departments in particular need of education may include the accident and emergency department, especially if it is staffed by trauma surgeons who may not have well developed skills in psychological assessment and who may need formal tuition about the management of patients presenting with functional somatic symptoms.

Collaborative research and audit provide an important opportunity to develop closer personal and intellectual links between psychiatry and medicine. Psychiatrists should always be alert to the possibility of presenting the results of their research at departmental meetings in the general hospital. Creed (1992) has suggested that one product of such collaboration could be agreed local guidelines or algorthims for the management of special clinical problems including functional somatic symptoms. For example, the initial assessment of a patient with functional abdominal pain requires equal emphasis on physical and psychological aspects of the presentation. Such an approach readily lends itself to audit, which could become a routine exercise and lead to continual updating and improvement of the guidelines.

Consultation Consultation involves the assessment of individual patients and the provision of recommendations to the referrer. Most of the specialist management of patients with functional somatic symptoms is currently done in this way. Thomas (1983) estimated that patients with

Table 22.5 DSM-III diagnoses (per cent) in patients referred for psychiatric evaluation of unexplained somatic symptoms

	Katon *et al.* (1984) (*n* = 100)	Slavney and Teitelbaum (1985) (*n* = 100)	Lloyd (1985) (*n* = 85)
Affective disorders	48	9	33
Somatoform disorders	29	34	11
Psychological factors affecting physical disorder	9	14	–
Substance use/alcoholism	8	1	–
Adjustment disorder	7	8	–
Factitious disorder	4	1	–
Eating disorder	–	1	4
Generalized anxiety	–	–	14
Panic disorder	4	–	4
Anxiety disorder, unspecified	–	7	–
Schizophrenia	–	–	2
Other diagnosis	4	10	12
No psychiatric diagnosis	–	15	18

Reproduced with permission from Lloyd (1986).

functional somatic symptoms were responsible for 30 per cent of referrals to a UK liaison service, while Katon *et al.* (1984) reported that they formed 38 per cent of referrals to a liaison service in the USA. There is a paucity of studies on out-patient samples in general hospital clinics, but in those studies of referrals to liaison psychiatry services with somatic symptoms, the majority of patients are found to have somatoform and affective disorders (Lloyd 1986; Table 22.5).

There are important limitations to this way of working and the proportion of patients offered specialist treatment by liaison psychiatrists is very small. The majority of referrals are of difficult in-patients and of those who present as emergencies. These are usually briefly assessed and the management limited to the provision of simple recommendations to the referrer which are frequently ignored (Goldberg 1992).

Specialist out-patient clinics for patients with functional somatic symptoms In recent years some consultation liaison units have begun to establish more sophisticated specialist treatment programmes (Fava *et al.* 1987; Dolinar 1993). It is the opinion of the authors that the specialist 'somatization' or 'psychosomatic' out-patient clinic in the general hospital is the most appropriate place to assess and manage patients who present with particularly severe or chronic functional illnesses. A multidisciplinary pain clinic can also provide an ideal setting for the assessment of patients with these disorders (Sullivan, 1993) and may comprise both individual and group programmes.

Individual treatment programmes   Individual treatment programmes for specific functional syndromes are outlined in other chapters. These consist principally of psychological therapies, antidepressant drugs, or a combination of these. Psychological treatments can be effective but require considerable amounts of staff time and skill.

Group programmes   Group programmes potentially offer a saving of skilled therapist time. There is some evaluation of out-patient group programmes for the treatment of patients with functional somatic symptoms (Melson and Rynearson 1986). Groups have been successfully used to treat hypochondriasis (Stern and Fernandez 1991), chronic somatization (Ford and Long 1977; Roskin *et al.* 1980), and chronic pain (Skinner *et al.* 1990; Pither and Nicholas 1991).

Specialist multidisciplinary in-patient units   As well as out-patient services there is almost certainly a place for the limited provision of specialist in-patient units employing multidisciplinary treatment programmes. Several of these already exist for the management of patients with chronic pain complaints (Benjamin 1989; Williams 1993).

In-patient treatment programmes for patients with mixed somatic complaints have also been described (Lipowski 1988). In this unit comprehensive assessment by social workers, occupational therapists, psychologists, and psychiatrists is supplemented by a work history and by assessment of the patient's level of functioning in daily activities. During a 6–12 week admission each patient receives an individually tailored set of treatments that includes individual and group psychotherapy, family therapy, occupational therapy, physiotherapy, relaxation training, psychotropic drugs, and vocational counselling. In frequent group meetings patients are encouraged to become self-assertive and to set their own goals for the future after leaving hospital.

The success of such treatment in reducing subsequent health costs and functional disability in patients with chronic functional somatic symptoms remains uncertain, however. Abbey *et al.* (1992) have suggested that those patients with symptoms of relatively short duration, concomitant depressed mood and a history of stable interpersonal relationships were more likely to benefit.

Behavioural medicine

Clinical psychologists have increasingly become involved in developing services for the general hospital. These are usually referred to as behavioural medicine or medical psychology units. Such ventures have sometimes been developed in collaboration with consultation liaison psychiatry, but sometimes as rival services (Agras 1992). Clinical psychologists have made very important contributions to the management of patients with functional somatic symptoms; perhaps the most prominent example has been in their work in multidisciplinary pain clinics (Pearce and Erskine 1993; Williams 1993). It is clear that effective collaboration between psychiatry and psychology is desirable for optimum patient care.

Implications for training

Most of our proposals for improved care depend on greater recognition of functional somatic symptoms as a problem and on the acquisition of the necessary clinical skills by both those working in general hospital clinical teams and those providing specialist psychiatric and psychological services. How is this going to be achieved? Clearly education and training are an important part of any attempt to improve the management of patients with functional somatic symptoms.

What needs to be taught?

1. Knowledge: all clinical staff need to be aware of the prevalence of functional somatic symptoms, their importance in terms of distress, disability, and health care expenditure, their frequent association with emotional disorders, and how they may be treated.

2. Skills: it is desirable that all clinicians be able to effectively perform a number of basic clinical tasks. These are listed in Table 22.4. Many physicians and surgeons already possess these skills. Specific training programmes in psychological management for interested medical staff have been shown to be effective in training those who do not (Maguire and Faulkner 1988).

3. Beliefs and attitudes: although attitudes are not simply taught they are an important factor in determining how patients with functional somatic symptoms are managed in practice and need to be addressed in educational programmes. In our opinion two beliefs are especially unhelpful:

(1) symptoms are only 'real' if the doctor can find disease;

(2) symptoms can only be diagnosed as functional after exhaustive investigation.

These issues are discussed further in a series of articles by Todd (1984*a,b,c*).

Who needs to be taught?

Medical students Medical student training pays little attention to functional somatic symptoms. This is because little attention is given to patients with functional somatic symptoms in medical and surgical training and most psychiatric training is carried out on general psychiatry in patient units. One way to improve this situation is for more students to have the opportunity of an attachment to a liaison psychiatry unit. Where this has been tried it has been found to be both popular and of educational value (Weddington *et al.* 1978). However, both specialist services and the number of psychiatrists with the requisite expertise are too few to effectively remedy this deficiency in doctor training.

Post-graduate medical training Specialist medical and surgical training offers a further opportunity to educate doctors about functional somatic symptoms. Recent collaborative working groups between the Royal College of Psychiatrists and Royal College of Physicians (Creed *et al.* 1992) with joint conferences and publications are an important step in this direction, but much remains to be done. The training of psychiatrists also needs improving in this respect. To date few psychiatrists have shown an interest in the management of functional somatic symptoms and many will assess referrals with functional somatic symptoms as either not suffering from psychiatric disorder or as not suitable for psychological treatment. Whilst liaison psychiatry is increasingly recognized as a substantial component of psychiatric training, this development has so far had little impact on general clinical practice.

The recent moves in many countries to ensure competence and require the reaccreditation of fully trained hospital doctors have resulted in continuing medical education becoming increasingly important. This new emphasis provides an important opportunity to offer education in the management of functional somatic symptoms to doctors who did not receive relevant training earlier in their career and who are now aware of their lack of expertise in managing such problems.

Training for non-medical staff It is also important to improve the training of nursing and other non-medical staff. In a period where nurse training is undergoing change in many countries it would be desirable to achieve a greater priority for systematic methods of psychological assessment and treatment. Once trained, nurses will also require continuing opportunities for supervision and for the development of skills. Senior nurses or medical in-patient wards in particular should know about the management of functional somatic symtoms. Indeed, observant nurses may be the first to detect patients with functional complaints and to inform the medical staff. Senior nurses in the accident and emergency department may benefit specifically from education about panic attacks and factitious illness.

Other non-medical professions also have important roles. For example, physiotherapists often have to manage patients with physical disabilities associated with functional syndromes. They need to know how to identify these patients and to be aware of abnormal or exaggerated illness behaviour (Mechanic 1962). A physiotherapist could notify the referring doctor of this observation and arrange for a psychiatric referral. Trained physiotherapists can identify and refer patients with disproportionate breathlessness (hyperventilation) and gross disability secondary to a hysterical conversion.

Who should do the teaching?

Few doctors have the expertise necessary to teach the management of functional somatic symptoms. In practice teaching about functional somatic symptoms is likely to fall to psychiatrists in general and liaison psychiatrists in particular. This is not ideal because it is likely to perpetuate the attitude that the management of functional somatic symptoms is a 'psychiatric' problem, rather than an integral part of general medical practice. It is therefore better for senior physicians to teach the topic (Engel 1982).

Practical issues for specialist services

A specialist service for patients with functional somatic symptoms depends on:

(1) identification of patients with functional somatic symptoms who might benefit from specialist treatment;

(2) ensuring that patients referred for a specialist opinion attend an assessment interview (see Chapters 5 and 11) and;

(3) the provision of effective treatment (see Chapter 7);

Table 22.6 Identification of patients for extra treatment

1. Clinical assessment
2. Screening instruments
3. Specialist nurse
4. Psychiatrist or psychologist liaison
    (i) Joint clinics
    (ii) Medical review meetings
    (iii) Joint ward rounds

(4) effective communication with the patient's consultant, general practitioner, and others health professionals involved in their care.

Identification of patients with functional somatic symptoms

The aim is to identify all the cases who require treatment, a process that requires systematic screening (Table 22.6). This can be achieved in a number of ways:

1. Clinical assessment. General awareness of the nature of functional symptoms and the need to ask general questions about patients' beliefs, behaviour, and mood can be incorporated in the briefest of medical interviews.

2. Screening instruments. These can be a useful adjunct to clinical assessment. There are simple interviewer rated measures available for rating how 'difficult to help' the patient is (Sharpe *et al.* 1994) or the degree to which the patient's complaints are functional (Creed *et al.* 1990). Patient completed questionnaires may also be used. Popular scales include the General Health Questionnaire (Goldberg and Hillier 1979), the Hospital Anxiety and Depression Scale (Zigmond and Snaith 1983), and the Whiteley Index (Pilowsky 1967). Rating scales are discussed in more detail by Gask (see Chapter 21). One of us routinely sends patients a 'problem list' to be mailed back before the out-patient visit (Table 22.7).

3. Joint clinics. A much more elaborate method of detection is for the psychiatrist to be present in the medical/surgical clinic. However, resources rarely allow such a luxury except in research settings (for example, Guthrie *et al.* 1991).

4. Joint meetings. Physicians and surgeons may on occasion ask the psychiatrist or psychologist to join them in the assessment of an individual patient. This 'one-stop' approach can be both efficient and therapeutic. It does however require planning and the patient's permission. Psychiatrists,

Table 22.7 Problem list mailed back by patients *before* out-patient visit

It would be very helpful if you could complete the following problem list before the doctor sees you at clinic. Do not worry if you are unable to answer any of the questions.

What are the main *problems* at present?

1. Pain   Yes/No

   If Yes, state site(s) of pain(s)

2. Other physical complaints   Yes/No

   If Yes, state complaints

3. Problems at work   Yes/No

4. Family problems   Yes/No

5. Problem with others, for example with colleagues, friends   Yes/No

6. Financial problems   Yes/No

7. Physical disabilities   Yes/No

   List one or two activities you can no longer carry out since the symptoms began

8. Other problems not included from 1–7   Yes/No

   If Yes, please list here

---

psychologists, and anaesthetists do already collaborate in joint assessment clinics for patients with chronic pain. These clinics provide important opportunities for the training of non-psychiatrists.

5. Joint ward rounds are regrettably rarely worthwhile. A regular 'psychosocial' meeting with the members of the general hospital team to discuss difficult in-patients or current out-patients may be a more efficient arrangement.

Coordination of hospital and primary medical care

The coordination of hospital and primary care in the management of patients with functional somatic symptoms is generally desirable and in many cases essential. For some patients we advocate a 'shared care' approach, with an agreed care plan which involves the patient alternating visits between the family doctor and the hospital. In these cases it is often

Table 22.8 Ground rules for chronic, persistent somatizers

1. Do not allow out-patient visits to become symptom-contingent
2. Do not see out of hours
3. No more than one phone call per week
4. Discuss plan with receptionists and secretaries
5. Inform GP and family
6. Keep your own set of notes (if psychiatric and medical notes are in single case folder)
7. Arrange support with other members of clinical team

helpful to review the family doctor's file, which may reveal a pattern of persistent and repetitive complaint behaviour that may have a bearing on the management plan.

For patients who have become excessively dependent or demanding, written ground rules (Table 22.8) may be explicitly agreed by all the hospital staff involved and similar guidelines sent to the general practitioner to ensure a consistency of approach (Bass 1990) (see Table 22.9, overleaf).

Funding

If the service developments outlined above are to be implemented adequate funding will be required. How much money should be devoted to patients with functional somatic symptoms and where it should come from are controversial issues: should services be funded by general medical or mental health services? Will purchasers regard the treatment of patients with functional somatic symptoms as a priority? We believe that there is a good case for the allocation of funds specifically this purpose. Whilst it is probably unrealistic to expect large sums of money to be spent on a comprehensive specialist services, even small amounts of money spent on improved education could have a significant impact on the management of functional somatic symptoms by non-specialist staff.

Conclusions

1. This chapter describes the *organization* of general hospital services for patients with functional somatic symptoms. General and specific management strategies are dealt with in other chapters.

2. Non-psychiatrists need to learn a minimum number of basic skills. These include providing unambiguous reassurance, giving the patient new information about the possible causes of the somatic symptoms and knowing how to refer a patient to a psychiatrist.

Table 22.9 Managing the heartsink patient/frequent attender/chronic somatizer: guidelines for general practitioners

1. Try to be *proactive* rather than *reactive*. That is to say, arrange to see the patient at *regular, fixed* intervals rather than allow him/her to dictate the timing and frequency of visits. Appointments should take place at approximately the frequency with which the patient has been visiting the doctor, that is every 2, 4, or 6 weeks. Once this pattern of visits is established, the time between visits can be gradually extended

2. During these visits aim to *broaden the agenda* with the patient. This involves establishing a *problem list*, eliciting current and relevant *psychosocial problems*, and allowing the patient to discuss his/her emotional problems. Try to avoid an 'organ recital', that is, a long discourse about the many and varied somatic-symptoms. Asking the patient to draw up a *problem list* can be useful. Individual problems can then be addressed in turn

3. Reduce unnecessary drugs. Often more than one analgesic or psychotropic drug is being prescribed. Try to negotiate a *gradual* withdrawn of *one drug a time*, for example DF118, followed by Valium. Psychotropic drugs should always be *tapered* over the course of 6–10 weeks

4. Treat any co-existing psychiatric disorder, for example panic attacks or depression with psychotropic drugs if necessary. Some chronic attenders have these concurrent disorders, which should be treated in the normal way

5. Whenever possible try to *minimize* the contact these patients have with other specialists or practitioners (including alternative practitioners). The reasons for this are:
    (i) the potential for *iatrogenic harm* is greater if patients are visiting many doctors (and being told different things by each one);
    (ii) *containment* is easier if only one (or at most two) practitioners are involved

6. Always interview the patients nearest relative and inform him/her of the management plan. Your best efforts can be sabotaged by spouses or partners and so try to co-opt a relative as a *therapeutic ally*

7. Try to reduce your *expectation of cure* with these patients. The multiple psycho-social and/or medical problems are often chronic and intractable and may be insoluble. Try to aim for *containment* and *damage limitation*, that is, limit the iatrogenic damage that may result from doctor-shopping, as well as the damage to your own self-esteem as a doctor. If you encourage the patient (and yourself) to think in terms of *coping* and not curing, you will feel less frustrated and demoralized

8. Don't expect rapid changes. Patients will become less demanding over a matter of months, especially if they feel that their complaints and symptoms are being taken seriously

9. If you are in a group practice then *inform your partners* of your management plan. Share it with them and develop contingency plans for when you are off duty, on leave, etc.

10. Finally, arrange some support for yourself, either from your colleagues or from someone with experience of managing these patients

3. Education of medical students and non-psychiatric colleagues (both medical and non-medical) is a crucial activity and methods of implementing this in a general hospitals are discussed.

4. Collaborative research activity often leads to the development of service links and, in some cases, important service developments. These in turn have implications for staffing and the organization of the liaison psychiatry service.

5. Future studies should concentrate on educating non-psychiatric staff to carry out simple interventions in relatively homogeneous patient groups with functional somatic symptoms, as well as on the evaluation of specialist services for 'difficult cases'. Studies of this nature should always include economic analyses and potential cost savings to the health service.

6. The funding of specialist services for the management of patients with functional somatic symptoms is problematic, falling as it does between psychiatry and medicine. Funds are increasingly, albeit reluctantly, being found from general medical rather than from psychiatric budgets. It remains uncertain how these services will be funded in the future.

References

Abbey, S.E., Gillies, L.A., Singh, M., and Lipowski, Z.J. (1992). Inpatient treatment of persistent somatization. *Psychosomatics*, **33**, 295–301.

Agras, W.S. (1992). Some structural changes that might facilitate the development of behavioral medicine. *Journal of Consulting and Clinical Psychology*, **60**, 499–504.

Bass, C. (1990). The frequent attender in general practice. *Hospital Update* March, 494–501.

Bass, C. and Benjamin, S. (1993). The management of chronic somatization. *British Journal of Psychiatry*, **162**, 472–80.

Bass, C. and Murphy, M. (1993). Somatization, somatoform disorders and factitious illness. In *College seminars in psychiatry. Textbook of liaison psychiatry*, (ed. F. Creed and E. Guthrie). Royal College of Psychiatrists. (in press) London.

Benjamin, S. (1989). Psychological treatment of chronic pain: a selective review. *Journal of Psychosomatic Research*, **33**, 121–31.

Butler, S., Chalder, T., Ron, M., and Wessely, S. (1991). Cognitive behaviour therapy in chronic fatigue syndrome. *Journal of Neurology, Neurosurgery, and Psychiatry*, **54**, 153–8.

Creed, F. (1992). The future of liaison psychiatry in the UK. *International Review of Psychiatry*, **4**, 99–107.

Creed, F., Firth, D., Timol, M., Metcalfe, R., and Pollock, S. (1990). Somatization and illness behaviour in a neurology ward. *Journal of Psychosomatic Research*, **34**, 427–37.

Creed, F., Mayou, R.A., and Hopkins, A. (1992). *Medical symptoms not explained by organic disease*. The Royal College of Psychiatrists and the Royal College of Physicians of London, London.

Delamothe, T. (1993). Wanted: guidelines that doctors will follow. *British Medical Journal*, **307**, 218.

Dolinar, L.J. (1993). A historical review of out-patient Consultation–Liaison psychiatry. *General Hospital Psychiatry*, **15**, 363–8.

Editorial (1992). Negative investigations. *Lancet*, **340**, 213.

Engel, G. (1982). The biopsychosocial model and medical education. Who are to be the teachers? *New England Journal of Medicine*, **306**, 802–5.

Fava, G.A., Trombini, G., Grandi, S., Bernardi, M., and Canestrari, R. (1987). A psychosomatic outpatient clinic. *International Journal of Psychiatry in Medicine*, **17**, 261–7.

Fink, P. (1992). The use of hospitalizations by persistent somatizing patients. *Psychological Medicine*, **22**, 173–80.

Ford, C.V. and Long, K.D. (1977). Group psychotherapy of somatizing patients. *Psychotherapy and Psychosomatics*, **28**, 294–304.

Goldberg, D. (1992). The treatment of mental disorders in general medical settings. *General Hospital Psychiatry*, **14**, 83–5.

Goldberg, D., Gask, L., and O'Dowd, T. (1989). The treatment of somatization: teaching techniques of reattribution. *Journal of Psychosomatic Research*, **33**, 689–95.

Goldberg, D. and Hiller, V.F. (1979). A scaled version of the general health questionnaire. *Psychological Medicine*, **9**, 139–45.

Guthrie, E. Creed, F.H., Dawson, D., and Tomenson, B. (1991). A controlled trial of psychological treatment for the irritable bowel syndrome. *Gastroenterology*, **100**, 450–7.

Katon, W., Ries, R.K., and Kleinmann, A. (1984). A prospective study of 100 consecutive somatization patients. *Comprehensive Psychiatry*, **25**, 305–14.

Kroenke, K., Arrington, M.E., and Manglesdorff, D. (1990). The prevalence of symptoms in medical outpatients and the adequacy of therapy. *Archives of Internal Medicine*, **150**, 1685–9.

Lin, E.H.B., Katon, W.J., Von Korff, M. *et al.* (1991). Frustrating patients: physician and patient perspectives among distressed high utilizers of medical services. *Journal of General Internal Medicine*, **6**, 241–6.

Lipowski, Z.J. (1988). An inpatient programme for persistent somatizers. *Canadian Journal of Psychiatry*, **33**, 275–7.

Lloyd, G.G. (1986). Psychiatric syndromes with a somatic presentation. *Journal of Psychosomatic Research*, **30**, 113–20.

Maguire, P. and Faulkner, A. (1988). How to improve the counselling skills of doctors and nurses in cancer care. *British Medical Journal*, **297**, 847–9.

Mechanic, D. (1962). The concept of illness behaviour. *Journal of Chronic Diseases*, **15**, 189–94.

Melson, S.J. and Rynearson, E.K. (1986). Intensive group therapy for functional illness. *Psychiatric Annals*, **16**, 687–92.

Pearce, S. and Erskine, A. (1993). Evaluation of the long-term benefits of a cognitive-behavioural out-patient programme for chronic pain. In *Psychological treatment in disease and illness*, (ed. M. Hodes and S. Moorey), pp. 114–39. Gaskell and the Society for Psychosomatic Research. London.

Pither, C.E. and Nicholas, M.K. (1991). Psychological approaches in chronic pain management. *British Medical Bulletin*, **47**, 743–61.

Roskin, G., Mehr, A., Rabiner, C.J., and Rosenberg, C. (1980). Psychiatric treatment of chronic somatizing patients: a pilot study. *International Journal of Psychiatry in Medicine*, **19**, 181–8.

Sharpe, M., Mayou, R., Seagroatt, V., Surawy, C., Warwick, H., Bulstrode, C., Dawber, D., and Lane, D. (1994). Why are some patients difficult to help? A study of three outpatient clinics. *Quarterly Journal of Medicine*. **87**, 187–93.

Sharpe, M., Peveler, R., and Mayou, R. (1992). The psychological treatment of patients with functional somatic symptoms: a practical guide. *Journal of Psychosomatic Research*, **36**, 515–31.

Shaw, J. and Creed, F. (1991). The cost of somatization. *Journal of Psychosomatic Research*, **35**, 307–12.

Skinner, J.B., Erskine, A., Pearce, S., Rubenstein, I., Taylor, M., and Foster, C. (1990). The evaluation of a cognitive behavioural treatment programme in outpatients with chronic pain. *Journal of Psychosomatic Research*, **34**, 13–19.

Slavney, P.R. and Teitelbaum, M.L. (1985). Patients with medically unexplained symptoms: DSM-III diagnoses and demographic characteristics. *General Hospital Psychiatry*, **7**, 25–35.

Stern, R. and Fernandez, M. (1991). Group cognitive and behavioural treatment for hypochondriasis. *British Medical Journal*, **303**, 1229–31.

Sullivan, M.D. (1993). Psychosomatic clinic or pain clinic, which is more viable? *General Hospital Psychiatry*, **15**, 375–80.

Thomas, C. (1983). Referrals to a British liaison psychiatry service. *Health Trends*, **15**, 61–6.

Todd, J. (1984*a*). Wasted resources: referrals to hospital. *Lancet*, **ii**, 1089.

Todd, J. (1984*b*). Wasted resources: Investigations. *Lancet*, **ii**, 1146–7.

Todd, J. (1984*c*). Wasted resources: hospital treatment. *Lancet*, **ii**, 1266.

Troop, N., Treasure, J., and Schmidt, U. (1993). From specialist care to self-directed treatment. *British Medical Journal*, **307**, 577–8.

Weddington, W.W., Hine, F.R., Houpt, J.L. and Orleans, C.S. (1978). Consultation–liaison versus other psychiatry clerkships: a comparison of learning outcomes and student reactions. *American Journal of Psychiatry*, **135**, 1509–12.

Williams, A. (1993). In-patient management of chronic pain. In *Psychological treatment in disease and illness*, (ed. M. Hodes, and S. Moorey), pp. 114–39. Gaskell and the Society for Psychosomatic Research. London.

Zigmond, A.S. and Snaith, R.P. (1983). The hospital anxiety and depression rating scale. *Acta Psychiatrica Scandinavica*, **67**, 361–70.

23 Alternative and complementary treatments

Christopher Bass and Richard Mayou

The two forms of non-conventional medicine, complementary, and alternative treatment are described and the reasons patients consult non-orthodox practitioners are outlined. It is suggested that the increased interest in non-conventional therapies is in part a consequence of dissatisfaction with orthodox medicine and, by implication, the training of doctors.

The efficacy of alternative treatments is reviewed and the evidence for most but not all therapies is found to be unconvincing. For example, some of the manipulative therapies may be effective but others such as iridology and reflexology appear to be useless.

The importance of popular beliefs and media campaigns in shaping public views of illness is emphasized, and the example of 'environmental illness' is used to illustrate this.

Finally, the authors acknowledge the role of some non-conventional procedures, but express concern that their use is often indiscriminate and uncritical and frequently associated with the rejection of orthodox medical treatment.

Underlying the continuing controversy about alternative medicine are deeper issues about public perceptions of psychological problems and treatments. There is scope for more public education about functional somatic symptoms and the treatments that are most effective in relieving them.

Introduction

Approximately 75 per cent of 'abnormal' symptoms reported in general population surveys do not result in consultation with the professionals (Wadsworth *et al*. 1977). Many people medicate themselves or seek help from those not practising traditional medicine (Kleinman 1985), their choice being influenced by the patient's explanation of the symptoms and by the types of help available (Furnham 1988).

Self-care

Many people regularly take non-prescription drugs such as analgesics or popular folk remedies, such as herbal teas. The results are usually good, although it is not clear whether the explanation is the effectiveness of the medication, placebo effects, or the self-limiting nature of the condition. However, prolonged and unsuccessful self-medication may lead to unwanted side-effects and to delay in obtaining proper investigation and treatment for a possibly serious condition.

It would be inappropriate to discourage patients from self-care of what are accepted as minor complaints as long as we also promote professional assessment of persistent complaints. Indeed in the UK and elsewhere there is increasing official encouragement for pharmacists and others to give simple advice and guidance about self-care as well about when to consult doctors.

Table 23.1 Types of non-conventional therapy

Acupuncture	
Alexander Technique	Postural education
Aromatherapy	Massage with plants oils
Bach Flower Remedies	Infusions from wild plants
Chiropractice	Joint adjustment, manipulation, and massage
Crystal Therapy	Use of crystals, gems, and elixirs
Healing	Non-physical procedures, often 'laying on of hands'
Herbalism	
Homeopathy	Diluted forms of natural substance which would bring on symptoms similar to the patient's complaints
Hypnotherapy	
Iridology	Diagnosis by observation of the iris
Kinesiology	Testing muscles use of pressure, diet, to restore 'balance'
Massage	
Osteopathy	Manipulation
Radionics	Measures to provide 'correctional energies' by contact medication and broadcasting
Reflexology	Compression or massage of 'reflex parts' in the hands and feet
Shiatsu	Massage on 'surface points'

Complementary and alternative therapies

Various terms have been used for non-orthodox treatments which have different connotations. *Complementary medicine* implies working along-side orthodox medicine whilst *alternative therapies* are rival treatments. A British Medical Association working party (1993) has preferred the term *non-conventional therapies* which it defines as 'those forms of treatment which are not widely used by orthodox health care professionals, and skills of which are not taught as part of the undergraduate curriculum of ortho-dox medicine and medical health care courses'. These non-conventional therapies are very diverse (see Table 23.1) ranging from those that are widely accepted by orthodox practitioners (such as chiropraxy and osteopathy) to alternative procedures (such as radionics) which are rejected by virtually all doctors.

Although the variety of therapies makes it impossible to generalize, it is apparent that there has been a considerable growth in their availability and variety in the last 30 years. It was estimated that one-third of American adults used some form of non-conventional therapy in 1990 (Eisenberg *et al.* 1993) and an increasing number of doctors are recommending, even using, some therapies, especially those involving manipulation for musculoskeletal complaints.

Whilst folk medicine and self-medication are widely accepted, there is a long history of official condemnation of non-conventional therapies. Fuller (1989) has shown the parallels between current controversies about New Age beliefs and nineteenth-century debates about a bewildering variety of therapeutic and religious movements in the USA. Recent arguments have centred on regulation and the extent to which non-conventional methods should be made available as part of publically funded health care (British Medical Association, 1993).

Why do patients consult alternative practitioners?

It is common for patients to consult orthodox practitioners at the same time as seeking alternative care (Fulder and Munro 1985; Thomas *et al.* 1991). Others avoid orthodox care and seek out alternative medicine.

There are a number of reasons why people choose non-conventional care:

(1) they may hold different theories as to the cause and cure of illness from those advocated in orthodox medicine (Helman 1984);

(2) they may be more aware of and ascribe greater importance to the relevance of life-style to health or express a preference for 'natural' as opposed to a pharmacological solution to their problem;

(3) they may be dissatisfied with the medical care they are getting; sadly, all to often this dissatisfaction is the result of misdiagnosis, mismanagement, or poor communication by their orthodox doctors (Pearson 1986);

(4) there are a number of areas of complementary practice, such as forms of manipulation and treatment of muscular aches and pains, that are widely accepted within the medical profession and whose uses often are actually encouraged.

There are differences in beliefs and behaviour between those who normally consult orthodox medicine and those who first choice is alternative medicine. In a study comparing and contrasting the beliefs and expectations of two groups — the one choosing to visit an orthodox medical practitioner, the other an alternative medicine homeopath — Furnham and Bhagrath (1993) found that homeopathic subjects differed from the general practitioner sample in a number of different ways. First, they were more dissatisfied with orthodox medicine, although some continued to consult orthodox practitioners. Second, they scored higher on a rating of psychiatric morbidity, suggesting a greater vulnerability to react to stressful life events with undifferentiated symptoms, a process described by Barsky (1988). Third, they had more faith in the healing power of their own bodies, which they promoted with homeopathic treatment. Interestingly, they also believed that they were *more* susceptible to certain illnesses, for example asthma. Fourth, they had a greater knowledge of personal health care and general health awareness than general practitioner patients. Murray and Shepherd (1993) have also described a study of general practice population. They found that 34 per cent of men and 46 per cent of women had had alternative treatment over a year period with limited satisfaction with the outcome. Such treatment was associated with a high consulting rate in general practice and notes commenting on psychosocial problems. The subjects did not seem to expect a rapid cure but were seeking an alternative explanation of chronic symptoms and greater feeling of autonomy in dealing with them. Most continued to consult orthodox practitioners for new acute medical complaints.

Why orthodox medicine fails patients with functional complaints

Non-conventional medical therapy — especially osteopathy, acupuncture, and homeopathy — attract increasingly large numbers of patients with functional somatic symptoms. The principal reason for this is that patients have become dissatisfied with orthodox medicine because it has failed them in their search of a cause or 'label' for their symptoms. This is understandable — many patients are told, after a series of negative investigations, what diseases they do not have and are not always provided with a credible or comprehensible explanation for their somatic complaints. Unfortunately medical education does not equip doctors with the skills to recognize or manage the myriad non-specific illnesses and chronic diseases that occur in general practice and other medical settings. Medical training programmes remain biologically orientated and insufficient time is assigned to the psychological and social factors that influence the presentation and outcome of illnesses.

In contrast, alternative therapists often provide an explanation and, furthermore, they are often effective communicators: a plausible explanation is often accompanied by careful listening. When there is acknowledgement of the patient's experience, and clear explanation of the diagnostic and treatment plan, then patient compliance is likely to be very high (Buckman and Sabbagh 1993). These explanations also have an appeal to many patients, who may equate conventional medicine (and medication) as unnatural, 'toxic' even, or tampering in some way with the natural bodily processes. Furthermore, alternative approaches assume an intuitive belief in some form of life force. The therapies and disease models that are applied within the field of alternative medicine are designed to specify subtle imbalances within the body and 'rebalance' the individual, thereby returning them to a state of health (Lewith 1988). The popularity of alternative and complementary treatment attests to the popularity of these explanatory illness (and treatment) models. Alternative practitioners will continue to flourish for as long as the education of future doctors remains out of step with the needs of their patients (Bass and Wessely 1989).

Alternative and complementary medicine — does it work?

There have been far too few adequate evaluations for alternative and complementary treatments, partly because many alternative practitioners reject the concept of a randomized controlled trial (British Medical Association 1993). However, it is important to avoid general statements about non-conventional treatments, since they are diverse and vary from the bizarre to rationally formulated procedures.

Although there have been few convincing evaluations of non-conventional therapies, there have, however, been two major randomized trials of chiropractic manipulation for low back pain. Both have shown that chiropractic manipulation produces better relief of the back pain than treatment in a hospital orthopaedic department or by the family doctor (Meade *et al.* 1990).

There have been very few systematic studies of alternative therapy in other discrete functional syndromes excepting hypnotherapy in irritable bowel syndrome (Whorwell *et al.* 1992) and electroacupuncture in fibromyalgia (Deluze *et al.* 1992)]. However, acupuncture has been evaluated in chronic pain and a recently published meta-analysis concluded that 'the efficacy of acupuncture in the treatment of chronic pain remains doubtful' (Ter Riet *et al.* 1990).

Knipschild (1993) has recently carried out exhaustive literature searches on the effectiveness of some alternative treatments (in particular homeopathy and iridology). A meta-analysis of more than 100 controlled studies of homeopathy (Kleijnen *et al.* 1991) noted the problems of low methodological quality and publication bias. However, to the astonishment of the authors, beneficial effects for homeopathy were reported in many (but not all) well-performed trials. By contrast, iridology was completely useless for discriminating between patients with gall-bladder disease and controls (Knipschild 1988). Knipschild 1993 urges alternative practitioners to carry out further randomized control trials, emphasizing that the burden of proof lies mainly with its exponents.

Advantages and disadvantages

As with self-care, non-conventional therapy may offer the patient an acceptable answer to symptoms which are of short duration and not of serious medical significance. This is because

(1)   some, such as the manipulation therapies, appear to be effective;

(2)   placebo benefits can be considerable, especially with functional symptoms;

(3)   a number involve relaxation and distraction which may provide useful anxiety management.

The dangers are that more appropriate and effective orthodox treatments will be delayed or missed, that the patients may pay large sums of money that can be ill afforded for unsuccessful therapies, and that the alternative medicines may themselves have side-effects (Chan *et al.* 1993).

It is unfortunate that some alternative practitioners neither confine their treatments to clearly defined conditions nor encourage the complementary use of orthodox medicine. Instead, some make grandiose claims and seek to prevent their clients from consulting doctors. Recent moves towards the official registration and regulation of certain forms of complementary therapy in the UK and the European Community have rightly emphasized the importance of defining areas of expertise and relationships with other professions (British Medical Association 1993).

The example of patients with environmental sensitivity

Elsewhere in this book Wessely and Sharpe (Chapter 16) illustrate the importance of popular beliefs and media campaigns in the shaping of public views about chronic fatigue. Another conspicuous recent example of the development of popular beliefs and of alternative therapies are alleged syndromes of multiple food and environmental allergies; these have been widely attributed to physical processes but after scientific investigation appear to be of predominantly psychological origin (Howard and Wessely 1993).

A central influence has been the *clinical ecology* movement, founded in the 1950s by the American allergist, Dr Theron Randolf, which is based on the belief that certain people are unusually susceptible to the adverse affects of their environment. These are said to suffer from disease which clinical ecologists call 'environmental illness' but which has several names, including 'total allergy syndrome', '20th century disease', and 'food and chemical sensitivity (Kay 1993). Environmental chemicals and foods are said to be responsible for an unlimited variety of symptoms which occur in the absence of physical findings or abnormal laboratory results. Nevertheless, many patients continue to believe that their somatic symptoms are attributable to modern chemicals. Some believe they are so sensitive that they will die unless they live in isolated bubbles or sleep outside the house.

The idea that the environment is responsible for a multitude of human health problems is appealing and the media have made an important contribution to this belief by reporting alarming statements, without analysis or criticism, as if they were an accepted fact. The concept of 'environmental illness' is, in fact, unfounded and the claims of clinical ecologists are invalid because they do not properly control their studies or define objective parameters of illness. Indeed, a report by the Royal College of Physicians Committee on Clinical Immunology and Allergy stated 'the public should be warned against (all) methods of diagnosis and treatment which have not been validated' (Royal College of Physicians 1992). Significantly, when patients with these disorders were made the subject of a television programme no mention was made about their high rates of psychiatric morbidity (Richmond 1992).

Systematic psychiatric studies using standard rating scales confirm that most patients with 'environmental illness' and 'food allergy' suffer from psychiatric illness. For example, in a study of 23 patients who attributed a wide variety of symptoms to food allergy, hypersensitivity to injected substances was confirmed in four, each of whom presented with typical atopic symptoms. By contrast, all but one of the remaining 19 polysymptomatic patients had evidence of psychiatric disorder (Pearson *et al.* 1983). Significantly, all of these patients were hostile to the idea that any of their symptoms were 'psychological'; they considered that this idea could suggest that their symptoms were imaginary or that the diagnosis of psychological illness implied moral censure (Rix *et al.* 1984).

In a North American study of 18 patients with a disorder, described as '20th century disease' or 'total allergy syndrome', Stewart and Raskin (1985) found that only two patients had a documented history of allergies or atopy, but 12 had consulted psychiatrists. All of the patients were found to be suffering from psychiatric disorder: seven had somatoform disorders, ten suffered from a psychosis or from an affective disorder, and one had a personality disorder. In a subsequent study of 50 such patients Stewart (1990) found very high rates of invalidism (none of the patients were employed at the time of assessment). They believed themselves to be seriously disabled with only 34 per cent expecting to return to other employment in the future. Although only 30 per cent had somatization disorder, symptoms of somatization were universal in this group.

Sadly, providing a false diagnosis adds to the patient's disability, reinforces maladaptive behaviour, and ensures that what might have been a brief illness becomes refractory to treatment. Furthermore, some of the techniques used by clinical ecologists, which centre on avoiding environmental stimuli, can worsen psychological distress and physical disability.

Should patients with functional somatic symptoms be advised to consult complementary and alternative practitioners?

In increasingly consumer-led health services, should we tolerate or even welcome this expansion in the availability of non-conventional treatments for patients with functional somatic symptoms? Our answer is an emphatic no to alternative therapies and guarded acceptance of some well-regulated complementary medicine and care. We recognize the effectiveness of some non-conventional procedures and the placebo benefits of a wider variety of treatments which appeal to individual patients, but we are concerned that their use is indiscriminate and uncritical and is frequently associated with the active rejection of orthodox medical investigation and treatment. Furthermore, some alternative treatments are not without danger; the toxic effects of some herbal medicines have been documented (MacGregor *et al.* 1989). The danger is that the patient's illness beliefs may become entrenched, the illness will develop a more chronic course, and the underlying psychosocial problems, because the are being neglected, will eventually become more refractory to psychological treatment.

We usually advise patients to avoid alternative medicine unless

(1) It is likely to lead to non-specific improvement, for example massage in an anxious patient or processes leading to relaxation;

(2) the patient has a musculoskeletal condition in which osteopathy and chiropractic manipulation may be effective;

(3) there is an opportunity to communicate and work with the complementary therapist.

Conclusions

The many forms of non-conventional therapies are attractive to patients with functional somatic symptoms. However, clinical trials have demonstrated that few of these treatments are effective and many of the therapeutic approaches can add to the patients' disability, reinforce maladaptive behaviour, and ensure that what might have been a brief illness becomes refractory to treatment. The fragmentation of care exacerbates the problems which can result from the involvement of several orthodox therapists. Complementary medicine needs to be subjected to proper regulations with clear codes of practice. The opportunity to be truly complementary is analogous to the manner in which the orthodox mental health services are developing in underdeveloped countries alongside traditional native healers, who are being trained to recognize the problems for which they have no answer and which require consultation with doctors.

Underlying the continuing controversy about alternative medicine are deeper issues about public perceptions of psychological problems and treatments. First, there is a prevalent view (even within the medical profession) that physical and psychological disorders are mutually exclusive and, second, that psychological care is only given to individuals without 'real' illnesses. Both views are wrong. Indeed, there are currently at least five clinical trials progress in the treatment of chronic fatigue syndrome, all led by psychiatrists. As Wessely (1993) has pointed out, this would hardly be the case if doctors felt the illness was 'imaginary' or 'unreal'.

In our view there is an important lack of public education about how patients with functional somatic symptoms should be encouraged to receive treatment that is appropriate to their needs. Improving understanding within the medial profession with better medical recognition of anxiety and depressive disorders, especially when they present with somatic symptoms, is equally important.

References

Barsky, A.J. (1988). *Worried sick. Our troubled quest for wellness*. Little Brown, Boston.

Bass, C. and Wessely, S. (1989). Alternative medicine. *The Times*, 30 November. p. 15.

British Medial Association (1993). *Complementary medicine. New approaches to good practice*. Oxford University Press, Oxford.

Buckman, R. and Sabbagh, K. (1993). *Magic or medicine? An investigation into healing*. Macmillan, London.

Chan, T.Y.K., Chan, J.C.N., Thomlinson, B., and Critchley, J.A.J.H. (1993). Chinese Herbal Medicines revisited: a Hong Kong perspective. *The Lancet*, 342, 1532–4.

Deluze, C., Bosia, L., Zirbs, A., Chantraine, A., and Vischer, T.L. (1992). Electroacupuncture in fibromyalgia: results of a controlled trial. *British Medical Journal*, 305, 1249–51.

Eisenberg, D.M., Kessler, R.C., Foster, C. Norlock, F.E., Calkins, D.R., and

Delbanco, T.L. (1993). Unconventional medicine in the United States, prevalence costs and patterns of use. *New England Journal of Medicine*, 328,

Fulder S.J. and Munro, R.C. (1985). Complementary medicine in the UK: patients, practice and consultations. *Lancet*, 2, 542-5.

Fuller, R.C. (1989). *Alternative medicine and American religious life*. Oxford University Press, New York.

Furnham, A. (1988). *Lay theories*. Pergamon Press, Oxford.

Furnham, A. and Bhagrath, R. (1993). A comparison of health beliefs and behaviours of clients of orthodox and complementary medicine. *British Journal of Clinical Psychology*, 32, 237-46.

Helman, C. (1984). *Culture, health and illness*. Wright, Bristol.

Howard, L.M. and Wessely, S. (1993). The psychology of multiple allergy. *British Medical Journal*, 307, 747-8.

Kay, A.B. (1993). Alternative allergy and the General Medical Council. *British Medical Journal*, 306, 122-4.

Kleijnen, J., Knipschild, P., and Ter Riet, G. (1991). Clinical trials of homeopathy. *British Medical Journal*, 30, 316-23.

Kleinman, A. (1985). *Patiets and healers in the context of culture*. University of California Press, Berkeley, CA.

Knipschild, P. (1988). Looking for gall bladder disease in the patient's iris. *British Medical Journal*, 297, 1578-81.

Knipschild, P. (1993). Searching for alternatives: loser pays. *Lancet*, 341, 1135-6.

Lewith, G.T. (1988). Undifferentiated illness: Some suggestions for approaching the polysymptomatic patient. *Journal of the Royal Society of Medicine*, 81, 563-5.

MacGregor, F., Abernethy, V.E., Dahabra, S., Cobden, I. and Hayes, P.C. (1989). Hepatotoxicity of herbal remedies. *British Medical Journal*, 299, 1156-7.

Meade, T.W., Dyer, S., Browne, W., Townsend, J., and Frank, A.O. (1990). Low back pain of mechanical origin: randomised comparison of chiropractic and hospital out-patient treatment. *British Medical Journal*, 300, 1431-7.

Murray, J. and Shepherd, S. (1993). Attitudes on alternative medicine. An exploratory study in general practice. *Social Science and Medicine*, 37, 983-8.

Pearson, D.J. (1986). Pseudo food allergy. *British Medical Journal*, 292, 221-2.

Pearson, D.J., Rix, K.J.B. and Bentley, S.J. (1983). Food allergy: how much in the mind? A clinical and psychiatric study of suspected food hypersensitivity. *Lancet*, i. 1259-61.

Richmond, C. (1992). They call themselves human canaries. *The Independent*, 14 January, 13.

Rix, K.J.B., Pearson, D.P., and Bentley, S.J. (1984). A psychiatric study of patients with supposed food allergy. *British Journal of Psychiatry*, 145, 121-6.

Royal College of Physicians Committee on Clinical Immunology and Allergy (1992). *Allergy, conventional and alternative concepts*. Royal College of Physicians London.

Stewart, D. (1990). Emotional disorders misdiagnosed as physical illness. environmental sensitivity, candidiasis syndrome. *International Journal of Mental Health*, 19, 56-8.

t, D.E., and Raskin, J. (1985). Psychiatric assessment of patients with '20th
tury disease' ('Total allergy syndrome'). *Canadian Medical Association Jour-
al*, **133**, 1001-6.

r Riet, G., Kleijnen, J., and Knipscild, P. (1990). Acupuncture and chronic
pain: a criteria-based meta-analysis. *Journal of Clinical Epidemiology*, **43**,
1191-9.

Thomas, K.J., Carr, J., Westlake, L., and Williams, B.T. (1991). Use of non-
orthodox and conventional health care in Great Britain. *British Medical Journal*, **302**, 207-10.

Wadsworth, M., Butterfield, W., and Blaney, R. (1977). *Health and sickness: the
choice of treatment*. London, Tavistock.

Wessely, S. (1993). Alternative allergy and the GMC. *British Medical Journal*,
306, 330.

Wessely, S. (1993). Why ME is not all in the mind. *The Times*, 27 July, p. 13.

Whorwell, P.J., Houghton, L.A., Taylor, E., and Maxton, D.G. (1992).
Physiological effects of emotion: assessment via hypnosis. *Lancet*, **340**, 69-72.

Index